An Introduction to

Clinical

Laboratory

Science

An Introduction to

Clinical Laboratory Science

Connie Mahon, MS, MT(ASCP) CLS
Associate Professor
Department of Clinical Laboratory Sciences
School of Allied Health Sciences
The University of Texas Health Science Center at San Antonio
San Antonio, Texas

Linda A. Smith, PhD, MT(ASCP) CLS
Associate Professor
Department of Clinical Laboratory Sciences
School of Allied Health Sciences
The University of Texas Health Science Center at San Antonio
San Antonio, Texas

Cheryl Burns, MS, MT(ASCP) CLS
Associate Professor
Department of Clinical Laboratory Sciences
School of Allied Health Sciences
The University of Texas Health Science Center at San Antonio
San Antonio, Texas

W.B. SAUNDERS COMPANY
A Division of Harcourt Brace & Company
Philadelphia   London   Toronto   Montreal   Sydney   Tokyo

W.B. SAUNDERS COMPANY
A Division of Harcourt Brace & Company

The Curtis Center
Independence Square West
Philadelphia, Pennsylvania 19106

Library of Congress Cataloging-in-Publication Data
Mahon, Connie
    An introduction to clinical laboratory science / Connie Mahon,
Linda Smith, Cheryl Burns.
        p.   cm.
  ISBN 0-7216-4990-4
  1. Medical laboratory technology.   I. Smith, Linda, Ph. D.
II. Burns, Cheryl.   III. Title.
  [DNLM: 1. Anatomy—laboratory manuals. 2. Physiology—laboratory
manuals. 3. Diagnosis, Laboratory—methods—laboratory manuals.
QS 25 M216i 1998]
RB37.M237 1998
616.07'56—dc21
DNLM/DLC
                                      97-36630
                                         CIP

AN INTRODUCTION TO CLINICAL LABORATORY SCIENCE   ISBN 0-7216-4990-4

Printed in the United States of America.

Last digit is the print number: 9   8   7   6   5   4   3   2   1

Contributors

Barbara G. Border, PhD
Assistant Professor, Clinical Chemistry, Texas Tech University Health Sciences Center, Lubbock, Texas
Laboratory Mathematics

Lisa Denny, MT(ASCP)
Instructor and Education Coordinator, Kilgore College, Kilgore, Texas
The Cardiopulmonary System

Janice F. Gaska, MT(ASCP)
Clinical Assistant Professor, Department of Clinical Laboratory Sciences, University of Texas Health Science Center at San Antonio, San Antonio, Texas
The Urinary System

George B. Kudolo, PhD, FAIC, CPC
Assistant Professor, Department of Clinical Laboratory Sciences, University of Texas Health Science Center, San Antonio, Texas
The Musculoskeletal System; The Reproductive System

Cynthia A. Martine, MEd, MT(ASCP)
Assistant Professor of Medical Technology, University of Texas Medical Branch at Galveston, School of Allied Health Sciences, Galveston, Texas
The Central Nervous System

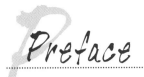

Preface

Students who would like to pursue a profession in laboratory medicine need to understand the critical role they will play in the health care arena as clinical laboratory practitioners. They must recognize that they will be required to perform their tasks in the clinical laboratory as well as to interact with other health care professionals. Therefore, we felt that clinical laboratory science (CLS) and clinical laboratory technician (CLT) students must be introduced to the technical and clinical functions of the profession as well as to the professional aspects of clinical laboratory science. With this intent, we wrote *An Introduction to Clinical Laboratory Science* as an introductory textbook that provides general information for students entering the CLS profession. The textbook has been written at a basic level and is primarily intended for CLS/CLT or medical technology/medical laboratory technology (MT/MLT) students taking an introductory course to clinical laboratory science or medical technology. An introduction to medical terminology, basic physiology, and bodily functions are highlights of this text. The book is divided into two major parts: Part I provides general information and laboratory mathematics; Part II describes the anatomy and physiology of major organ systems.

The text begins with an introduction to the profession, which provides a brief history of the education of clinical laboratory practitioners. This chapter also describes places of employment, the clinical disciplines in the hospital laboratory, and the skills required to function as a clinical laboratory practitioner. In addition, the book includes a chapter that provides information regarding certification, licensure, and professional organizations. In Part I, the student is also introduced to medical terminology by learning how medical terms are derived or formed. This chapter includes exercises for students to practice and enhance their skills in recognizing medical terms. Part I also contains a chapter on applications of mathematics in the laboratory. There are math problems at the end of the chapter for students to practice their skills.

Part II provides discussions of the body systems. Each chapter contains illustrations of the organ system and describes the anatomy and functions as well as the disease states encountered or associated with that particular organ system. In addition, the discussion includes the more common laboratory tests associated with the diseases of that organ system and how the results are utilized in diagnosis. Part II includes a chapter of case studies that will allow students to "tie everything together." Study questions at the end of each chapter also give students a chance to review and meet the objectives of the chapter.

We believe that students entering the clinical laboratory science profession are not aware of the clinical and technical as well as the professional aspects of clinical laboratory science. We hope this textbook will provide students with a better understanding of the critical role they will play as health care providers and how they will interact with other health care professionals.

Acknowledgments

We would like to thank our contributing authors, George Kudolo, Lisa Denny, Jan Gaska, Cindy Martine, and Barbara Border and the many other individuals who have provided encouragement and support to complete this project. Our appreciation also goes to Shirlyn B. McKenzie for her invaluable comments and suggestions and to Selma Kaszczuk for her assistance and motivation. Our thanks to Rachael Kelly for making sure we got the manuscript in on schedule.

Contents

Part I   General Information

CHAPTER 1   Introduction to the Profession   2

CHAPTER 2   Introduction to Medical Terminology   18

CHAPTER 3   Disciplines in Laboratory Medicine and Applications to Functions of the Body Systems   34

CHAPTER 4   Laboratory Mathematics   48

Part II   Clinical Disciplines and Applications to Functions of the Body System

CHAPTER 5   The Musculoskeletal System   72

CHAPTER 6   The Cardiopulmonary System   88

CHAPTER 7   The Urinary System   110

CHAPTER 8   The Digestive System   144

CHAPTER 9   The Hepatic System   164

CHAPTER 10   The Central Nervous System   186

CHAPTER 11   The Hematopoietic and Lymphatic Systems   208

CHAPTER 12   The Endocrine System   236

CHAPTER 13   The Reproductive System   268

CHAPTER 14   Case Studies   293

APPENDIX A   Answers to Review Questions   305

APPENDIX B   Answers to Case Studies   315

INDEX   323

Color Plates follow

An Introduction to

Clinical

Laboratory

Science

Color Plates

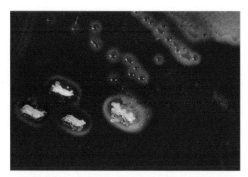

Color Figure 1 Blood agar plate (BAP) showing beta-hemolytic colonies (clear zone around colony) of Group A streptococci, the organism that causes bacterial pharyngitis.

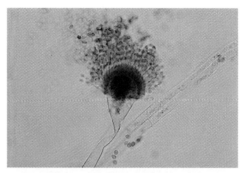

Color Figure 2 *Aspergillus* species, a common fungus found in the environment can cause serious infection in the immunocompromised patient.

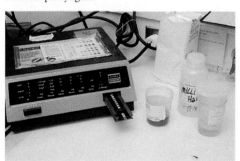

Color Figure 3 Urine sample tested for chemical substance using a chemistry instrument.

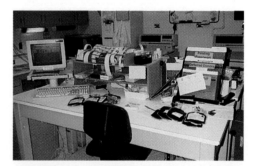

Color Figure 4 Immunohematology section, showing the area where units of blood are processed and labeled.

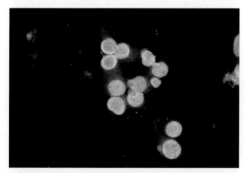

Color Figure 5 One of the methods used to demonstrate antigen-antibody reactions is immunofluorescence technique. Antinuclear antibodies usually detected in patients with systemic lupus erythomatosus are shown.

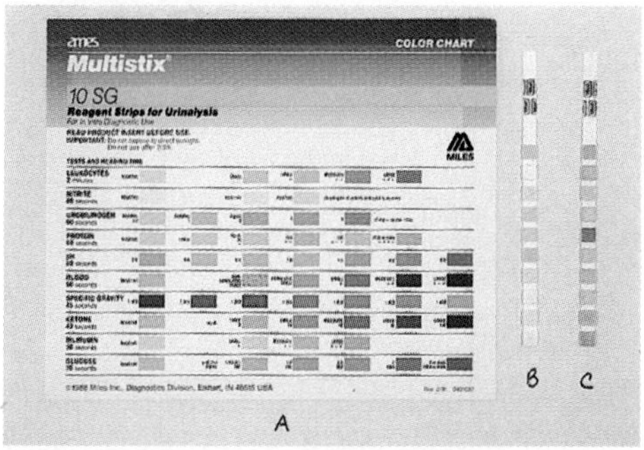

Color Figure 6 Macroscopic examination of urine by chemical methods. *A*, Ames Multisix 10 SG Color Chart used to determine results by comparing changes in color and/or intensity. *B*, Unused Ames Multistix 10 SG reagent test strip. *C*, Used Ames Multistix 10 SG reagent test strip. Note changes in color on each pad. (Permission granted by Bayer Diagnostics, Tarrytown, New York).

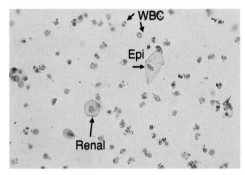

Color Figure 7 Renal tubular epithelial cells, squamous epithelial cell, white blood cells (leukocytes). Sedi-stain, ×400.

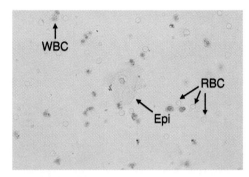

Color Figure 8 Squamous epithelial cell, degenerating white blood cells, red blood cells (erythrocytes). Sedi-stain, ×400.

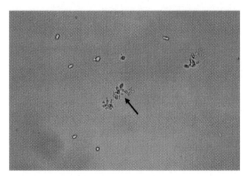

Color Figure 9 Yeast. Note budding forms present. Unstained, ×400.

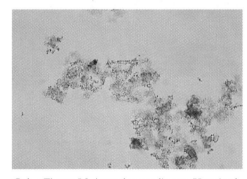

Color Figure 10 Amorphous sediment. Unstained, ×400.

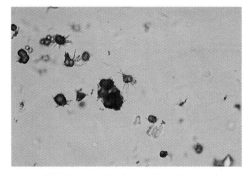

Color Figure 11 Ammonium biurate crystals. Unstained, ×400.

Color Figure 12 Calcium oxalate crystals. Unstained, ×400.

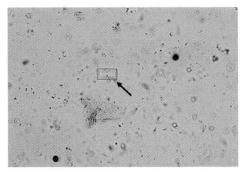

Color Figure 13 Triple phosphate crystal. Note the presence of white blood cells, a folded squamous epithelial cell, bacteria, and amorphous sediment. Sedi-stain, ×400.

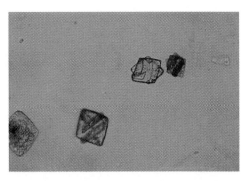

Color Figure 14 Uric acid. Unstained, ×400.

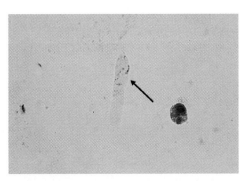

Color Figure 15 Hyaline cast with cellular debris attached to an otherwise clear and colorless cast. Also note a white blood cell attached to an old swollen WBC. Sedi-stain, ×400.

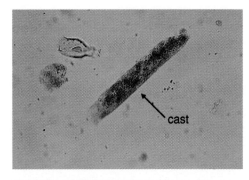

Color Figure 16 Cellular/granular cast. Also note folded squamous epithelial cell and swollen white blood cells. Sedi-stain, ×400.

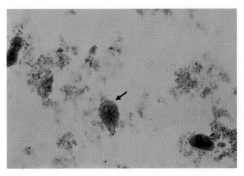

Color Figure 17 *Giardia lamblia* trophozoite. Fecal sample. Trichrome stain.

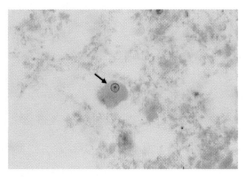

Color Figure 18 *Entamoeba histolytica*. Fecal sample. Trichrome stain.

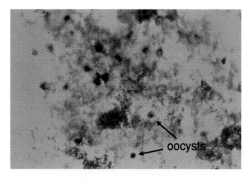

Color Figure 19 *Cryptosporidium parvum* oocysts. Fecal sample. Modified Kinyoun acid-fast stain.

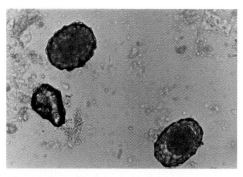

Color Figure 20 *Ascaris lumbricoides.* Fecal samples. Iodine stain.

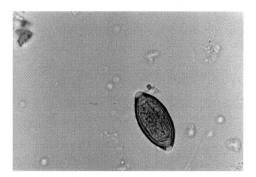

Color Figure 21 *Trichuris tricuria* ova. Fecal sample. Iodine stain.

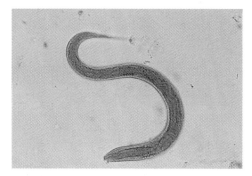

Color Figure 22 Hookworm larvae. Fecal sample. Iodine stain.

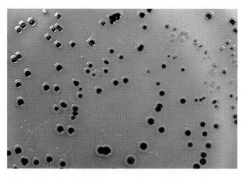

Color Figure 23 Black colonies of *Salmonella sp.* growing on Hektoen agar.

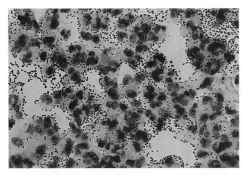

Color Figure 24 Cerebrospinal fluid (CSF) with numerous white blood cells and bacterial organisms typically seen in bacterial meningitis. Gram stain.

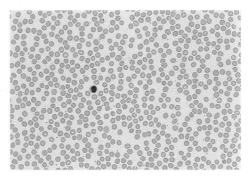

Color Figure 25 Normal erythrocytes. Peripheral blood; Wright-Giemsa stain.

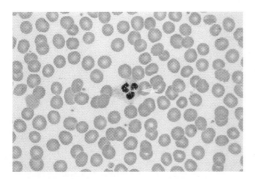

Color Figure 26 Segmented neutrophil. Peripheral blood; Wright-Giemsa stain.

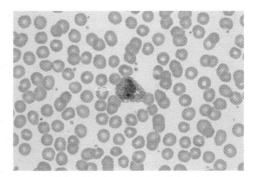

Color Figure 27 Eosinophil. Peripheral blood; Wright-Giemsa stain.

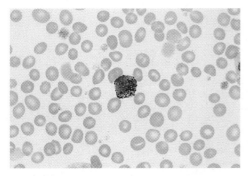

Color Figure 28 Basophil. Peripheral blood; Wright-Giemsa stain.

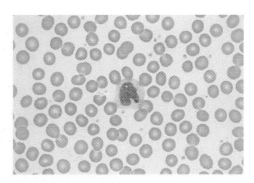

Color Figure 29 Monocyte. Peripheral blood; Wright-Giemsa stain.

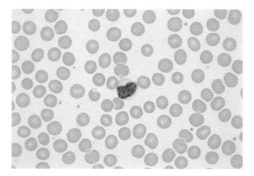

Color Figure 30 Lymphocyte. Peripheral blood; Wright-Giemsa stain.

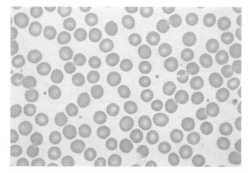

Color Figure 31 Normal platelets. Peripheral blood; Wright-Giemsa stain.

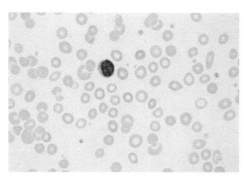

Color Figure 32 Hypochromic, microcyte erythrocytes in iron deficiency anemia. Peripheral blood; Wright-Giemsa stain.

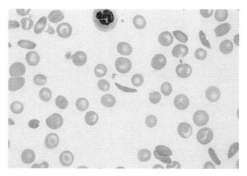

Color Figure 33 Sickle cell. Peripheral blood; Wright-Giemsa stain.

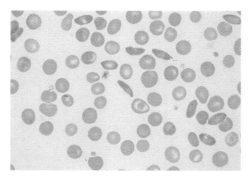

Color Figure 34 Sickle cells and target cells observed in sickle cell anemia. Peripheral blood; Wright-Giemsa stain.

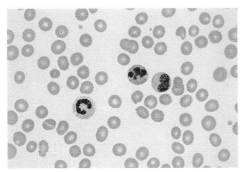
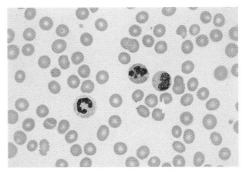

A   B

Color Figure 35 A, B Peripheral blood picture depicting a "shift-to-the-left". Notice the presence of a band neutrophil (*a*) and metamyelocyte (*b*). This picture may be associated with a bacterial infection. Wright-Giemsa stain.

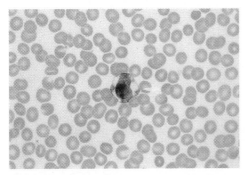
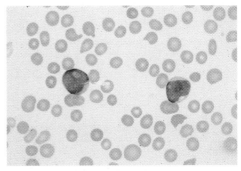

Color Figure 36 Reactive lymphocyte. Peripheral blood; Wright-Giemsa stain.

Color Figure 37 Myeloblasts in a bone marrow aspirate from a case of acute myeloblastic leukemia. Wright-Giemsa stain.

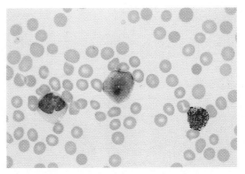

Color Figure 38 Increased numbers of neutrophil precursors and segmented neutrophils in the peripheral blood from a case of chronic myelogenous leukemia. Wright-Giemsa stain.

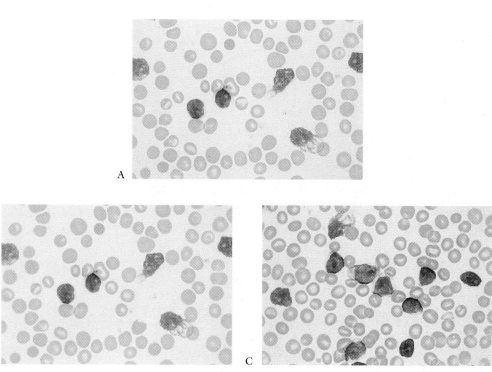

Color Figure 39 Malignant mature lymphocytes in chronic lymphocytic leukemia. *A*, The damaged cells are called smudge cells. *B*, They are characteristic of chronic lymphocytic leukemia. *C*, Peripheral blood; Wright-Giemsa stain.

PART I

General Information

CHAPTER 1

Introduction to the Profession

INTRODUCTION

HISTORY OF THE EDUCATION OF
CLINICAL LABORATORY
PERSONNEL
How Clinical Laboratory
    Science Evolved
Educational Programs

PROFESSIONALS WITHIN THE
CLINICAL LABORATORY
Clinical Laboratory
    Practitioners
Other Laboratory Practitioners
    Phlebotomist
    Cytotechnologist and
        histologic technician/
        histotechnologist
Categorical practitioner
Specialist
Cytogenetic technologist
Summary

CLINICAL DISCIPLINES IN THE
HOSPITAL LABORATORY

PLACES OF EMPLOYMENT

SKILLS NEEDED TO FUNCTION IN
THE CLINICAL LABORATORY

CERTIFICATION EXAMINATIONS
AND LICENSURE

PROFESSIONAL ORGANIZATIONS
American Society for Clinical
    Laboratory Science
American Medical
    Technologists
American Society of Clinical
    Pathologists–Associate
    Member Section
Other Professional
    Organizations

FUTURE OPPORTUNITIES
AND CHALLENGES

CHAPTER SUMMARY

Objectives

1. Describe the different designations of laboratory professionals, the major job functions, and the education required for entry into the profession.
2. List at least three organizations for laboratory professionals.
3. Describe several new or nontraditional roles for clinical laboratory science graduates.
4. Describe types of certification examinations available or required for clinical laboratory science professionals.

KEY TERMS

pathology	clinical laboratory	histotechnologist	cytogenetic
medical technology	technician	categorical practitioner	technologist
clinical laboratory	cytotechnologist	specialist	phlebotomist
scientist	histologic technician		

Introduction

The laboratory professional plays a vital role in the diagnosis and treatment of a patient. Results from laboratory tests may confirm or rule out a presumptive diagnosis of disease states such as leukemia, anemia, diabetes, or other chronic illness. Yet clinical laboratory science is one of the least understood health professions. Since clinical laboratory scientists require specialized equipment to perform testing on patient specimens and often work with hazardous materials, they are removed from the immediate vicinity of the patient. Therefore, these professionals are not as well known to the patient as the nurse or the physician. For example, patients recognize that someone comes to the bedside to draw their blood, but they are not aware of the variety of tests that may be performed on their blood sample. They may also not be aware of the impact the results have on the final diagnosis or treatment.

The public knows little about the rigorous education and training that are involved in preparing for this profession. Have you noticed what happens when you're asked "What degree are you getting?" and you answer "Clinical laboratory science." Do you get a funny look—the person wants to know "What's that?" Or perhaps someone asks, "Is that a special kind of nursing?" Or "I didn't' know you needed a degree to do that!"

This chapter is designed to provide an introduction to and overview of the complex field of laboratory medicine, including the history, the types of clinical laboratory practitioners, the educational requirements, and the professional opportunities available both within and outside the laboratory. The certification examinations practitioners may take and the professional organizations they may belong to are also presented.

HISTORY OF THE EDUCATION OF CLINICAL LABORATORY PERSONNEL

One cannot talk about the field of clinical laboratory science without also talking about the medical specialty of pathology. They are inexorably linked yet separate. Although the early laboratory practitioners may have been physicians, pathologists, or both, laboratory testing itself soon developed into a separate discipline. Today, clinical laboratory science has a body of knowledge separate from pathology. It has its own educational requirements and standards. However, the roots of the profession started with pathology.

HOW CLINICAL LABORATORY SCIENCE EVOLVED

Pathology *is broadly defined as the study of disease, including the cause, development, and consequences of the disease process.* Physicians as well as pathologists have utilized the laboratory and results of laboratory tests as a means of understanding and diagnosing disease. Probably no one can really say when and how the *clinical laboratory science* profession actually started. We know that there were early historical references to examination of body fluids around the time of Hippocrates. Pisse prophets of the Middle Ages had urine samples brought to them; they looked at the samples, compared their color and clarity with descriptions in a table, and gave a diagnosis. The development of the microscope was a major event that contributed to a medical practitioner's or scientist's ability to observe microscopic elements of body fluids and microorganisms not visible to the unaided eye. This particularly helped in the understanding of blood cells and microorganisms.

During the 19th century, Robert Koch's discoveries about tuberculosis and the development of his hypothesis concerning transmission of disease led to growth in the discipline of microbiology. In the early 20th century, the discipline of pathology emerged and flourished. At this point laboratory findings became even more important to the diagnosis of a patient's underlying condition. The physician was the first to perform many laboratory tests—but soon the volume of tests done on a patient, as well as the amount of information about testing itself, became too much for the clinician alone. Testing was delegated to assistants.

The 1920s saw the first large-scale employment of assistants to pathologists. Apprenticeship to the pathologist became a form of training, although there were no set curricula, no standards for training, and no designated supervision of apprentices. As time went on, and the need for testing increased, the need for formal and standardized training was recognized. In 1928, the American Society of Clinical Pathologists (ASCP) formed a registry of laboratory technicians. This later evolved into what is now recognized as the *ASCP Board of Registry.* The purpose of this body was to establish minimum standards of education and technical qualifications, classify levels of technicians based on their education and training, register schools that offered acceptable courses of training, and issue certificates of registration to individuals who met minimum qualifications. At that time, a formal examination could be taken by qualified individuals to assure the quality of the applicant's experience, but it was not required. Those individuals with a baccalaureate degree and 1 year of experience in a recognized laboratory were given the designation of *medical technologists* (MTs), while someone with a high school degree, 1 year of basic science coursework, and 6 months' experience in a recognized laboratory was designated as a *medical laboratory technician* (MLT). *The term* **medical technology,** *introduced to describe the practice domain of laboratory personnel, is the study and practice of diagnostic medicine.*

A final level of involvement between pathology and clinical laboratory science was in the inspection of schools that offered clinical laboratory training. This was brought about by cooperation of the ASCP Board of Registry and the American Medical Association's Council of Medical Education and Hospitals. (The latter organization later changed its name to the Council of Medical Education.) The first list of approved schools was issued in 1933, and several years later the minimum standards of accreditation of programs to educate medical technologists was published.

During the 1930s, Dr. Kano of the ASCP Board of Registry conducted a series of surveys concerning the status of training programs for medical technologists. Results led to the development of the first set of "Essentials" for medical technology education programs. These *Essentials* have evolved into the guidelines that provide the requirements for accreditation. An agency known as the National Accrediting Agency for Clinical Laboratory Science (NAACLS) has responsibility for maintaining and updating these Essentials to keep pace with the changes in the field and to assure that programs provide the educational experiences to produce graduates who can function in the ever-changing health care field. Essentials cover a range of topics from the level of instruction and examinations to credentials of instructors and budgetary support for programs.

EDUCATIONAL PROGRAMS

As with many other medical professions, education of laboratory practitioners evolved from on-the-job training to formal education programs. During the early period of formal medical technology education, the training programs were primarily based in the hospital. Later, academic programs were established in university settings. Another change that has come about over the last several years is in the terminology, reflecting the broadened function of the laboratory profession. The new term *clinical laboratory science* identifies the expanded responsibilities, career opportunities, and role of the laboratory practitioner. Medical technology programs, particularly those in university settings, have changed the titles of their programs to "Program in Clinical Laboratory Science" or "Department of Clinical Laboratory Sciences". A graduate with a baccalaureate degree is now called a **clinical laboratory scientist** (CLS), while one with an associate degree is now referred to as a **clinical laboratory technician** (CLT). Both the "clinical (CLS and CLT) and the "medical" (MT and MLT) designations are currently used in most publications and documents.

There are multiple educational program formats for the clinical laboratory scientist (medical technologist). All have the common requirements of a baccalaureate degree and supervised clinical laboratory experience, but the program structures vary. CLS/MT programs may offer 3 + 1, 4 + 1, 2 + 2, or integrated curricula. A brief description of each type follows.

A *3 + 1 program* is based in a college or university that offers the basic science and general education requirements. The student takes these courses during the first 3 years in the program. In the last year, students spend 52 weeks at a hospital affiliated with the university. During this time they receive formal instruction in clinical laboratory science and acquire practical laboratory experience.

In the *4 + 1 program,* the student must already have a baccalaureate degree in a discipline such as biology to apply. This format is usually found in hospital-based programs that offer a year of training that includes lectures and practical experience in each of the clinical disciplines. The student receives a postbaccalaureate certificate upon successful completion of this program.

In a *2 + 2 program,* the student takes the required science prerequisites and general education during the freshman and sophomore years (preprofessional courses). Students then make a formal application to the next 2 years of the curriculum (professional phase). During these 2 years, the student takes clinical laboratory science lectures and laboratory courses and completes the program with laboratory experience in a clinical setting.

The *integrated program* is somewhat similar to the 2 + 2 program. The difference is that students in an integrated program take CLS courses throughout the first 3 years along with basic science and general education courses. During their senior year, students complete the program with didactic courses and clinical practicums. One advantage of this format is that students can decide early on in their academic career whether the profession is what they want without losing a significant number of semester hours. Students who successfully complete any of these programs are eligible to take the national certification examination.

Clinical laboratory technician/medical laboratory technician programs are most often based in a community college or junior college and lead to an associate degree. The first year of study is spent in science and general education courses and the second is spent in clinical practicums. There are a few 1-year certificate programs that are frequently based in a technical institute or hospital. Upon graduation, the CLT/MLT student is also eligible to take the appropriate national certification examination.

PROFESSIONALS WITHIN THE CLINICAL LABORATORY

Medical technology is a relatively young profession that started formally educating practitioners in the 1920s. Up until that time, most laboratory testing was done either by the physician or by an apprentice who was trained on the job. The much broader term *clinical laboratory science* has since been adopted by many in the profession. However, regardless of the terminology, the student in laboratory medicine is educated and trained in the four major disciplines of the clinical laboratory—hematology, chemistry, microbiology, and immunohematology.

CLINICAL LABORATORY PRACTITIONERS

Clinical laboratory practitioners (CLS/MTs or CLT/MLTs) perform tests that analyze blood, urine, tissue, or other body specimens. They use complex instrumentation, sophisticated techniques, and specialized knowledge to provide critical data for diagnosis, treatment planning, and preventive health care. For example, if a patient complains of a sore throat, the physician takes a sample from the throat with a swab and this sample is sent to the clinical laboratory. The CLS/CLT determines what may be causing this patient's illness by examining the organisms that grew from the sample. The physician then decides what course of treatment is appropriate. Another example is a stroke patient or heart attack patient who is on anticoagulant therapy. A blood sample must be drawn and analyzed to make sure that there is not too much or too little of the anticoagulant in the patient's blood. The results from the laboratory test performed by the CLS/CLT will determine how the patient's therapy is adjusted.

CLTs often perform routine testing on specimens, perform quality control tasks, calibrate instruments and perform preventive maintenance, and report normal test results. In some instances they may perform nonroutine or complex testing, but that is usually reserved as a task for the CLS. The CLS has much more theoretical knowledge, technical expertise, and management background. CLSs may handle routine testing and tasks that a CLT does, but also are capable of handling abnormal samples or more difficult and complex tests. In addition, the CLS may be responsible for supervising the CLT, writing procedure manuals, implementing new testing protocols, evaluating quality control data, teaching CLT or CLS students, and participating in the development of test protocols.

In addition to the major role that clinical laboratory practitioners have in diagnosing disease and monitoring therapy, they may also work with other health care professionals, including the physician, to provide information for establishing appropriate, cost-effective testing protocols for suspected diagnoses. This allied health profession is constantly changing and advancing as new technology evolves. This technology provides better methods for diagnostic testing and interpretation as well as providing new areas in which the laboratory professional can work.

OTHER LABORATORY PRACTITIONERS

Phlebotomist

A **phlebotomist** is a specially trained person who is responsible for drawing blood from patients. The phlebotomist is a high school graduate who may be trained on the job or who goes through a phlebotomy training program. These programs may be sponsored by a hospital or community college and take as little time as 2 months or as long as 1 year to complete. After completion of the program, phlebotomists may sit for an examination that allows them to use specific credentials [PB (ASCP) from the ASCP Board of Registry or CLPlb from the National Certification Agency] after their names. Other examinations are offered by the American Society of Phlebotomy Technicians. In this changing era of health care, the phlebotomist may be given expanded responsibilities, including specimen processing or in some cases simple laboratory testing such as the macroscopic analysis of a urine specimen.

Cytotechnologist and Histologic Technician/Histotechnologist

While most clinical laboratory practitioners are trained in all major disciplines of the clinical laboratory, practitioners such as the cytotechnologist and histotechnologist are single-discipline laboratory personnel. Both the field of cytology and that of histology have as their focus the science of the cell—its makeup, its normal or abnormal form, and its normal or abnormal function. The tissue specimens which these professionals prepare and screen provide clues to disease, illness, or malignancy in the body.

The **cytotechnologist** is the laboratory practitioner who examines human specimens for detection of cancer cells or other diseases. The most common specimen they examine is the genital smear for cervical cancer (Papanicolaou, or Pap, smear), but other body fluids or tissues are also examined for abnormal changes in color, size, or shape that provide clues to a disease process. The cytotechnologist works closely with the pathologist to arrive at a final diagnosis. The cytotechnologist has a baccalaureate degree with a strong science background. A 1-year postbaccalaureate program in a hospital provides the specialized training. Cytotechnologists learn to perform special chemical stains and techniques as well as determine differences among inflammatory, viral, and malignant changes in cells.

The histologic technician (HT) and histotechnologist (HTL) are somewhat analogous to the CLT and CLS. **Histologic technicians** routinely prepare, process, and stain biopsy and tissue specimens for microscopic examination by a pathologist. Special equipment such as the microtome allows the HT to cut very thin slices of tissue so that single cell layers can be seen. Special stains applied to the slides make cellular detail clearer or demonstrate organisms or specific components such as connective tissue.

Histotechnologists perform all aspects of a job that HTs do but also perform more complex processing, staining, or identification procedures. They may initiate or develop new procedures, evaluate quality control data, or work with electron microscopy.

There is a 12-month training program for a student to become a histologic technician. Coursework includes classes in anatomy, biology, chemistry, laboratory mathematics, medical ethics, and terminology. Although programs will accept student with a high school diploma, the professional society recommends that student complete an associate degree before entering the clinical HT program. Histotechnology students must have a baccalaureate degree with 30 hours in chemistry and biology to be accepted into the 1-year clinical program. The majority of clinical practicum programs for either the HT or HTL are associated with a hospital. Upon successful completion of the clinical experience, students may sit for national examinations.

CATEGORICAL PRACTITIONER

Some laboratories employ laboratory personnel who are educated and trained in only one laboratory discipline and therefore can only work in that particular area of the clinical or reference laboratory. These individuals are referred to as **categorical practitioners**. Individuals who already possess a baccalaureate degree in a science major may apply for categorical training. Two categories commonly pursued by individuals with a degree are microbiology and chemistry. Courses in the general microbiology or chemistry curriculum, however, do not concentrate on human pathogens or on the chemical constituents of the human body, which is the focus of the clinical laboratory. Therefore, applicants for categorical training must complete specific courses and training in a clinical laboratory science program to acquire the background knowledge and skills necessary to practice in the clinical laboratory.

SPECIALIST

A **specialist** is a CLS/MT who has worked for a number of years in a specific discipline and who has extensive knowledge and experience in this area. The CLS who would like to become a specialist in a particular discipline may take an exam to demonstrate expertise in the discipline. The successful completion of the examination allows the CLS to use credentials indicating the specialty area. For example, a CLS with a baccalaureate degree who has several years of experience working in the blood bank and who has completed an extra year of structured courses and training in the field of transfusion medicine is qualified to take the Specialist in Blood Bank (SBB) examination offered by the ASCP. Passing the examination allows the CLS to use the SBB (ASCP) initials behind his or her name. Specialists in microbiology, chemistry, and hematology have extensive experience and knowledge in their specific disciplines. Cytotechnologists may also acquire a specialist certification with advanced education and training.

CYTOGENETIC TECHNOLOGIST

A closely allied field into which clinical laboratory scientists may gravitate is that of cytogenetics. Cytogenetic technology is a highly complex area of the clinical laboratory that provides diagnosis of inherited and acquired chromosomal disorders. These disorders may range from leukemia or solid tumors to the underlying chromosomal changes in children with birth defects. **Cytogenetic technologists** culture cells from tissue and body fluid in order to obtain chromosomes for analysis. Although the procedures in the cytogenetics laboratory are labor intensive and demand patience and attention to detail, they are varied. Cytogenetic technologists must master the art of cell culture, chromosome banding and analysis, and photography and darkroom skills. Computer imaging has become a major part of this field. Most cytogenetic technology programs offer either a baccalaureate degree or a postbaccalaureate certificate. Course work includes chemistry, genetics, biology, cell biology, and a clinical practicum.

SUMMARY

All of the practitioners described above are laboratory professionals. Each has a slightly different background and training, yet each contributes significantly to the welfare of the patient. Without these health care professionals, diagnosis and treatment of a disease or clinical condition would be much more difficult, time consuming, and expensive. Perhaps it could not be done at all.

CLINICAL DISCIPLINES IN THE HOSPITAL LABORATORY

The areas of the laboratory in which the CLS or CLT works are generally divided into hematology, hemostasis (coagulation), chemistry, urinalysis, serology (immunology), immunohematology (blood bank), and microbiology, which may include virology, parasitology, mycology, and/or mycobacteriology. Although these areas are explained in detail in Chapter 3, the general testing performed in each is described here.

In the *hematology* section, blood from the patient is tested for the amount of hemoglobin and the number of leukocytes, erythrocytes, and platelets. The morphology of each cell type is described. This information will help diagnose anemia, leukemia, or other diseases involving the blood cells. In *hemostasis*, the plasma is tested to detect problems with clotting and bleeding. In patients with diseases such as hemophilia, there is a defect in one of the plasma constituents that allows blood to clot. Tests done in the hemostasis laboratory can help detect this defect.

The *chemistry* section is responsible for performing tests that determine levels of blood constituents such as glucose or protein, detect elevations in enzymes characteristic of heart attacks or liver disease, or measure ions such as sodium and potassium that control the electrolyte balance in the body. Often *urinalysis* is also performed in the chemistry section. Results of urinalysis may suggest the presence of a urinary tract infection, kidney disease, or diabetes mellitus.

In *microbiology*, bacteria that may be present in body fluids such as urine and blood or in specimens from infected wounds are grown on special media and identified through the use of biochemicals. In addition to identification of these organisms, the microbiology laboratory also identifies which antimicrobial agents might be useful in fighting the infection. Cultures for fungal and yeast infections as well as for the organisms responsible for tuberculosis are also performed in some laboratories. Examination of stool specimens for the presence of parasites is a routine test in many laboratories.

In *serology*, the serum is tested for the presence of antibodies to specific viral, fungal, or bacterial agents. Results from tests such as the rubella or hepatitis tests determine whether a patient currently has a specific disease or is immune to it. In the *blood bank*, a patient's blood type is determined and the blood is tested against potential donor blood to make sure that there will be no problems with a transfusion. In addition, specific blood components such as platelets are prepared for transfusion to patients who are undergoing chemotherapy and require these cells to prevent uncontrolled bleeding.

Prior to the development of automated laboratory instrumentation, practitioners performed laboratory tests manually, one test at a time. Today, laboratory instruments in chemistry and hematology are designed to perform up to 60 tests in just a few minutes. In microbiology, the identification of many organisms is performed by automated equipment. Most laboratories are now equipped with complex instruments that are interfaced with laboratory information systems (LIS) for data collection and patient reporting. Nevertheless, a practitioner is still needed to monitor the instrument and to review and validate the results.

A risk factor in the profession is that laboratory personnel are also exposed to many hazards—acids, noxious odors, and blood-borne pathogens such as hepatitis B and human immunodeficiency virus (HIV). In recent years, risks of occupational hazards have decreased because of the regulations imposed by the Occupational Safety and Health Administration (OSHA) and other government agencies. However, the final responsibility for safety rests with the clinical laboratory professional, who is always responsible for following safety policies and procedures to decrease exposure to these hazards.

PLACES OF EMPLOYMENT

The most common place for the laboratory professional to work is in the *hospital*, but there are many opportunities for CLSs/CLTs to apply their knowledge and training. Table 1–1

Table 1–1 ■ Career Opportunities for Clinical Laboratory Scientists

Traditional Roles	*Nontraditional/Newer Roles*
Hospital clinical laboratory	Infection control
Traditional disciplines	POC testing
Hematology	Quality assurance
Hemostasis	Special laboratories
Urinalysis	Fertility
Serology	Cytogenetics
Microbiology	Transplant/antigen matching
Blood bank	Forensics
Toxicology	Flow cytometry
Chemistry	Veterinary laboratory
	Industrial laboratory
Research (hospital medical center)	Corporate research and development
	New product development
Reference laboratory	Consultant to physician office laboratories
	Laboratory inspector
	Public health laboratory
Sales/technical representative	Laboratory marketing
Laboratory administration	Hospital administration
	Manager of group practice laboratory
	Lab/hospital information systems
CLS educator	Patient educator
	Patient case manager

shows the traditional roles of the CLS and also outlines some of the different career opportunities that are now available to graduates.

The CLS or CLT may work in a *reference laboratory* that is not associated with a hospital. In these facilities, a large number and variety of tests are performed on specimens that come from other laboratories or clinics or from many parts of the city or country. Some of these tests are routinely requested tests such as a complete blood count (CBC) or glucose level. In addition, special tests done in only a few laboratories throughout the country may be sent to reference laboratories. The CLS or CLT who enjoys patient contact may work in the laboratory of a *medical clinic* or in a *physician's office* laboratory. Here, they perform a limited number and variety of tests but get the opportunity to interact with patients, nurses, and the physician.

Public health laboratories are another employment site for the CLS, categorical practitioner, or specialist. The focus of these laboratories is the identification and tracking of diseases that are a risk to the public's health. This may involve identification of organisms spread by fecal contamination of water or by insects. For example, if there is a suspected outbreak of food poisoning, the public health lab would help identify *Salmonella* or *Shigella* species that are common causative agents. These laboratories also serve as reference laboratories for hospitals, perform tests to detect antibodies against uncommon organisms such as the agent that causes Lyme disease, and confirm the presence of rabies in animals. Public health laboratories may receive water, milk, and environmental samples for detection of chemicals, bacteria, or other agents that may be a source of harm to the public.

Some CLSs have an interest in *research*. There are opportunities in medical research laboratories, industrial laboratories, and laboratories that develop equipment or test kits/reagents for clinical laboratory use. The background and knowledge of the clinical lab that the CLS possesses proves invaluable in developing new products. They provide input on all product aspects from an experienced user's point of view. Cytogenetic technologists may also work in research laboratories where cytogenetic techniques can be applied to basic science research.

CLSs also work in less traditional work settings such as in *veterinary offices*, in laboratories of large *marine amusement parks*, in *forensics laboratories* associated with the medical examiner or state police, or in *industrial testing* or *food testing* laboratories. Many have developed their own *consulting* businesses to help small physician office laboratories adhere to rigorous inspection and accreditation requirements. Some have become *coordinators* for large multisite clinical studies. Others have become *inspectors, educators,* or *laboratory managers.* The emphasis on meeting federal and accrediting agency requirements has created a need for those with knowledge of the laboratory to be inspectors. The focus on safety and protection of workers from hazardous materials has given some CLSs the opportunity to enter the field of *occupational safety* or *infection control.*

Some laboratory personnel leave the laboratory environment and move into the *corporate* world. They may go into sales or become a technical representative who trains personnel to use the corporation's equipment or troubleshoots equipment problems. Some may become interested in marketing. Those with an interest in computers may work for companies selling/installing laboratory or hospital information systems or may be the laboratory specialist in computer systems. HTs and HTLs work in laboratories of firms that manufacture or process chemical or pharmaceutical products. Cytotechnologists may be employed in hospitals, private reference laboratories, or research facilities. A few may find positions in education or industry.

Graduates of CLS programs may choose to get *advanced degrees* in a scientific discipline, in management, or in education. Some also go on to medical or dental school. The broad, general scientific background of the CLS is an excellent knowledge base for any of these professional programs.

SKILLS NEEDED TO FUNCTION IN THE CLINICAL LABORATORY

A mixture of technical, organizational, and interpersonal and communication skills is needed to work in the clinical laboratory. Clinical laboratory professionals must be able to organize, and prioritize; to perform technical tasks accurately and precisely, and, perhaps most importantly, work under stress. Although CLS/CLTs are not usually in direct contact with patients in the hospital, they are an integral part of the comprehensive health care team. They need to be able to effectively communicate with clinicians, nurses, and other personnel. In some settings they must also interact with patients.

CERTIFICATION EXAMINATIONS AND LICENSURE

There are several different examinations available to the graduate of an accredited MT/CLS or MLT/CLT program. Table 1–2 shows the general categories of laboratory professional and the education needed to be able to take the national certification or registry examination for a given professional area.

The *ASCP Board of Registry* has been in existence the longest time and offers all levels of examinations, including technician, technologist, categorical, and specialist. Examinations are administered by computer-assisted testing. If an individual successfully passes the examination, credentialing initials for the category [e.g., MT (ASCP)] are placed after the individual's name. For many years, the Board of Registry has not required practitioners to retake the exam or show proof of continuing education credits to maintain their creden-

Table 1–2 ■ **Categories of Clinical Laboratory Personnel and Education Required To Sit for National Examinations**

Designation	Degree	Education Source
CLT/MLT	Associate	Community college
CLS/MT	Baccalaureate	University/college
	Postbaccalaureate certificate	Hospital program
Cytotechnologist	Postbaccalaureate certificate	Hospital program
Histologic technician	Certificate	Hospital program
Histotechnologist	Certificate	College or hospital program
Cytogenetic technologist	Postbaccalaureate certificate	University
Categorical practitioner	Postbaccalaureate certificate	University
Specialist	Examination (eligibility determined by experience/education)	

tials. However, proposals of voluntary re-examination or proof of continuing education to maintain credentials are now being examined by the ASCP.

The other type of examination is the certification examination offered by the *National Certification Agency for Medical Laboratory Personnel* (NCA). The new graduate must take the initial exam and then every 2 years show evidence of obtaining a specific number of continuing education credits or take the examination again to be recertified. This requirement helps assure the ongoing competency of the laboratory professional. At this time the NCA has fewer certification exams than the ASCP, but it is adding categories. In addition, this examination is not yet computerized.

The *American Medical Technologists* (AMT) organization also offers medical technologist and medical technician examinations. The eligibility requirements for the exams include provisions for those with a baccalaureate degree as well as those who are at the MLT level and who have the required work experience. There are requirements for revalidation of certificates issued by the AMT.

The *International Society for Clinical Laboratory Technology* (ISCLT) certifies registered medical technologists (RMTs) or registered laboratory technicians (RLTs). The requirements for certification are varied and include academic coursework, technical training, and work experience.

Licensure of health care professionals protects the public by controlling who may practice in a specific discipline. State licensure examinations for CLSs and CLTs are required in some states. A few states require licensure for HTs and HTLs. These licensure examinations are developed by a state agency and professionals must pass the examination to be able to practice in that state. In contrast to the fact that all states require licensure examinations for physicians and nurses, there are a limited number of states that require licensure for CLSs. Although there are only 10 states with personnel licensure at the moment, there are many more states trying to get state licensure legislation passed. Some states may have reciprocal arrangements with other states. In this way licensure in one state allows a CLS or CLT to practice in other states with licensure without having to retake the examination.

PROFESSIONAL ORGANIZATIONS

Although membership in a professional organization may not seem particularly important to a student, it is the link to learning and career opportunities. The organizations provide a chance to develop leadership skills, participate in continuing education courses, and network with other professionals from throughout the country. Exciting opportunities to direct the course of the profession they have chosen exist for those who take leadership positions within the state, local, or national organization. A short description of each of the major organizations follows.

AMERICAN SOCIETY FOR CLINICAL LABORATORY SCIENCE

The American Society for Clinical Laboratory Science (ASCLS; formerly the American Society for Medical Technology, or ASMT), founded in 1932, is the umbrella organization for all clinical laboratory scientists. Its mission is to promote the clinical laboratory science profession and to provide service to those who practice the profession. To that end, it sponsors continuing education programs for all practitioners in the scientific disciplines, as well as laboratory administrators, consultants, and educators. Each state has a constituent society, and many states have local districts to which members belong. Membership in the national organization provides membership at the state and local level.

AMERICAN MEDICAL TECHNOLOGISTS

American Medical Technologists is an organization that has its own examination and continuing education program. The organization meets at a national level, and states also have meetings at which the focus is continuing education.

AMERICAN SOCIETY OF CLINICAL PATHOLOGISTS–ASSOCIATE MEMBER SECTION

The Associate Member Section (AMS) is an affiliate of the ASCP that allows membership for nonphysicians, including medical technologists, technicians, Ph.D. clinical scientists, and students. Its mission is to provide high-quality educational products and continuing education activities. Educational programs are held in numerous parts of the country. Teleconferences and other forms of continuing education are also offered to all segments of the profession.

OTHER PROFESSIONAL ORGANIZATIONS

The *International Society of Clinical Laboratory Technology* is the parent organization for those with ISCLT certification and meets yearly for continuing education activities. The *Association of Genetic Technologists* is primarily composed of cytogenetic technologists but is also open to molecular technologists and biochemical geneticists. This organization provides opportunities for continuing education as well as journal publications. The *National Society for Histotechnology* provides continuing education, publications, and promotion of knowledge in histotechnology.

Other organizations to which a clinical laboratory scientist may belong are focused on specialty areas. These organizations have members who are physicians and Ph.D. scientists as well as specialists. The most widely known of these include the *American Association of Blood Banks* (AABB), *American Society for Microbiology* (ASM), *American Association for Clinical Chemistry* (AACC), and *Clinical Laboratory Management Association* (CLMA).

FUTURE OPPORTUNITIES AND CHALLENGES

The traditional practice of medicine is changing with the advent of increased federal legislation as well as new mergers and alliances between and among hospitals, reference laboratories, home health care agencies, and major medical suppliers. There is a change in philosophy in the delivery of health care—from using health care dollars and facilities in treating the sick to concentrating efforts in preventive medicine and wellness testing. In the hospital, the focus in caring for patients is to shorten their hospital stay. Point-of-care (POC) testing, that is, performing the test at the patient's bedside, has provided rapid identification of critical parameters so that change in treatment can be started as soon as possible and the patient can be released. The adaptation of the corporate concept of teams has allowed hospitals to implement laboratory teams with no supervisor. The team members are also less specialized in a discipline and more able to perform testing in multiple areas within the laboratory.

In the laboratory, the advent of DNA probes and polymerized chain reaction technology provides new methods of diagnosing diseases that traditionally were almost impossible to confirm by laboratory results. There is increased automation and computerized systems for reporting data (LIS). As automation and robotics testing have become less complicated, monitoring of quality assurance has become more important to assure valid results.

CHAPTER SUMMARY

The profession of clinical laboratory science is a young one that has its roots in pathology but has acquired a unique body of knowledge and practice. The educational program required to practice in the field is rigorous, with a strong science background. The clinical training requires the student to become proficient not only in technical skills but also in interpersonal communication skills and the ability to function in a stressful environment. The traditional location for practice in a hospital laboratory has changed with expanded opportunities in industry, research, and nontraditional sites.

CHAPTER 2

Introduction to Medical Terminology

INTRODUCTION

GENERAL TERMS FOR BODY DIRECTION

MEDICAL TERMINOLOGY
Breaking Down Medical Terms
Construction of Medical Terms
Prefixes and Suffixes

EXERCISES IN CONSTRUCTING MEDICAL TERMS

Cardiovascular System
    Heart and blood vessels
    Blood cells
Respiratory System
Digestive System
The Liver
Renal System
Musculoskeletal System
Neurologic System, Including
    the Brain
Reproductive System

CHAPTER SUMMARY

REVIEW QUESTIONS

Objectives

1. *Explain the meaning of the more common prefixes and suffixes used in medical terminology.*

2. *Given a medical term, break it down into prefix, root word, and suffix and give the meaning.*

3. *Given a condition, create the medical term that would be used to describe it.*

KEY TERMS

anatomic position	dorsal	umbilical region	sacral vertebrae
transverse plane	ventral	hypogastric region	coccyx
inferior	cranial cavity	hypochondriac region	root term
superior	thoracic cavity	lumbar region	prefix
sagittal plane	abdominal cavity	inguinal region	suffix
frontal plane	pelvic cavity	cervical vertebrae	
anterior	quadrant	thoracic vertebrae	
posterior	epigastric region	lumbar vertebrae	

Introduction

Your first classes in clinical laboratory science may be similar to traveling to another country where you may not be able to speak or understand the native language—you are reading and hearing words that you think you will never learn. However, if you stay long enough, study the language, or both, you can soon communicate using basic words and phrases. If you keep learning, listening to, and speaking the language, you will soon be fluent.

Just as with a foreign language, you will soon master these new medical terms by learning some of the Greek or Latin terms that form their bases and by practicing. You will find that many medical terms have identical suffixes or prefixes, and that words referring to a specific part of the body share a common root word. This will make it easier for you to learn how to decipher terms you may not initially recognize.

This chapter serves to introduce you to common terms used in the medical field. Obviously not every medical term can be included, but the information and exercises should provide you with an understanding of how to analyze terms you do not know so that you can understand their meaning. You should also have a medical dictionary to enable you to find terms that you cannot decipher or do not understand.

The chapter starts with the terms used to describe the relationship of body parts among and to each other. Then core words and the prefixes and suffixes most commonly used are discussed. Finally, there are exercises in constructing words by using the different body systems to identify key words for that system.

GENERAL TERMS FOR BODY DIRECTION

Many times organs or parts of the body are described by relating their position to other organs or to a specific body position. The terms for describing body direction are derived from the **anatomic position**—*a figure of a person standing erect, facing you with arms at the sides and palms forward.* Note that when the terms "right" and "left" are used, they are always referring to the figure's or patient's right and left.

Figure 2–1 shows the transverse, sagittal, and frontal planes of the body. In the **transverse plane** of the body, the organs/body parts are said to be either **inferior** to (below) or **superior** to (above) the plane. In this example, the heart is superior to the intestinal tract. The **sagittal plane** is the plane that divides the body in a vertical manner. If the plane goes directly though the center (midline) of the body, it is called *midsagittal* and divides the body into a right and left side. The **frontal plane** divides the body into **anterior** and **posterior** aspects. If you are facing the figure of the person, the face is anterior and the back is posterior. Now take that same figure with the same plane and place it face down. In this position, the back is referred to as the **dorsal** surface and the abdomen is on the **ventral** surface.

Figures 2–2*A* and 2–2*B* show the major body cavities—cranial, thoracic, abdominal (celiac), and pelvic, as well as the designations—dorsal, ventral, and abdominopelvic. The **cranial cavity** houses the brain and, together with the *spinal cavity*, forms the *dorsal cavity*. The brain itself is in the area sometimes referred to as the *cephalic cavity*. The **thoracic cavity** houses the heart, trachea, lungs, and major blood vessels supplying those organs. The esophagus and part of the digestive tract lie in this cavity. The **abdominal cavity** contains the major organs such as the stomach, kidneys, intestinal tract, liver, spleen, and pancreas as well as the ovaries and uterus. Organs such as the bladder and uterus lie below the abdominal cavity in the **pelvic cavity.**

The abdominal cavity is the largest cavity in the body and is divided into quadrants. Figure 2–3 shows the four **quadrants** of the *abdominopelvic cavity.* These terms are used when describing clinical symptoms or the location of organs. For example, the liver is in the right upper quadrant; the pancreas and spleen are in the left upper quadrant; the appendix is in the right lower quadrant.

Figure 2–4 shows the major anatomic regions of the abdomen. These regions can be divided into the three down the center of the abdomen—the **epigastric,** the **umbilical,** and the **hypogastric**—and the three along each side of the abdomen—the **hypochrondriac,** the **lumbar,** and the **inguinal** (right and left for each)—for a total of nine regions. The epigastric region is the central region below the sternum, the umbilical region is the central region around the navel, and the hypogastric region is below the navel. The hypochrondriac regions are the lateral regions, which include the lower ribs; the lumbar are the middle lateral regions; and the inguinal regions are the groin regions.

The spinal column extends down the back, and vertebral regions are described as seen in Figure 2–5. The **cervical** vertebrae (C1 to C7), or neck, are at the top and are the connection with the cranium. The next region downward is the **thoracic** (vertebrae T1 to T12). This region of the back corresponds to the thoracic cavity. The **lumbar** region, or "small of the back" (vertebrae L1 to L5), and the **sacral** region (five fused vertebrae) are the final portions at the top of buttocks. The **coccyx** (three to four fused vertebral remnants), commonly referred to as the tailbone, is at the very end of the spinal column.

Injuries to the spinal column often have serious consequences. The further up the spinal column that an injury occurs, the more of the body that is affected. For example, someone who fractures a vertebra in the cervical area is often left a quadriplegic (all four limbs are affected by paralysis), whereas someone who fractures a vertebra in the lumbar region may be a paraplegic (only the lower part of the body and the legs are paralyzed).

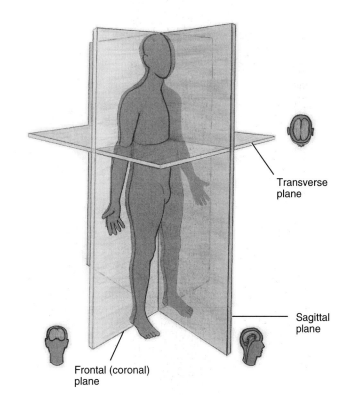

FIGURE 2-1

The planes of the body. (From Applegate, E.J.: The Anatomy and Physiology Learning System. Philadelphia. W.B. Saunders, 1995, with permission.)

Transverse plane

Sagittal plane

Frontal (coronal) plane

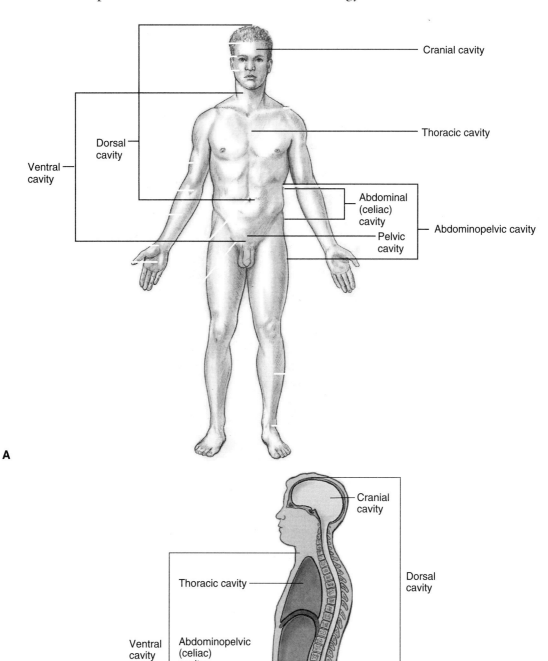

Cranial cavity

Thoracic cavity

Dorsal cavity

Ventral cavity

Abdominal (celiac) cavity

Pelvic cavity

Abdominopelvic cavity

A

Cranial cavity

Dorsal cavity

Thoracic cavity

Ventral cavity

Abdominopelvic (celiac) cavity

Abdominal cavity

Pelvic cavity

B

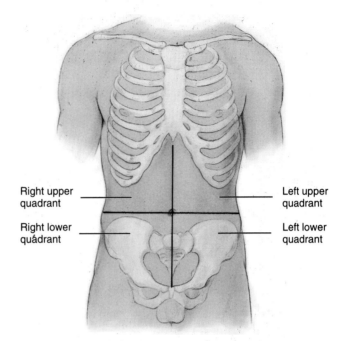

FIGURE 2-3

The four quadrants of the abdomen.
(From Applegate, E.J.: The Anatomy and Physiology Learning System. Philadelphia, W.B. Saunders, 1995, with permission.)

Right upper quadrant

Left upper quadrant

Right lower quadrant

Left lower quadrant

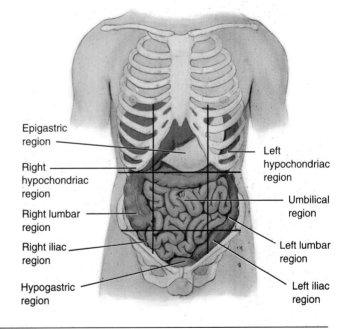

FIGURE 2-4

The abdominopelvic regions.
(From Applegate, E.J.: The Anatomy and Physiology Learning System. Philadelphia, W.B. Saunders, 1995, with permission.)

Epigastric region

Right hypochondriac region

Right lumbar region

Right iliac region

Hypogastric region

Left hypochondriac region

Umbilical region

Left lumbar region

Left iliac region

FIGURE 2-2

The major body cavities. *A*, Viewed from the front. *B*, Viewed from the side.
(Modified from Applegate, E.J.: The Anatomy and Physiology Learning System. Philadelphia, W.B. Saunders, 1995, with permission.)

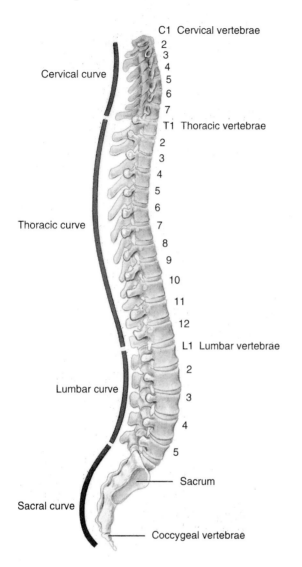

C1 Cervical vertebrae
2
3
4
5
6
7
T1 Thoracic vertebrae
2
3
4
5
6
7
8
9
10
11
12
L1 Lumbar vertebrae
2
3
4
5

Cervical curve

Thoracic curve

Lumbar curve

Sacral curve

Sacrum

Coccygeal vertebrae

FIGURE 2-5

The spinal column with the vertebral regions indicated: cervical, thoracic, lumbar, sacral, and coccygeal (coccyx). (From Applegate, E.J.: The Anatomy and Physiology Learning System. Philadelphia, W.B. Saunders, 1995, with permission.)

MEDICAL TERMINOLOGY

In this section, the breaking down of terms into common components, the construction of medical terms, and the use of prefixes and suffixes are discussed.

BREAKING DOWN MEDICAL TERMS

Medical words can be broken down into parts. Just as in English words, there is always a **root term.** Table 2–1 gives the Latin terms used as root words for the major body systems

Table 2–1 ■ Root Terms for Organs, Organ Systems, and Structures

blood vessels	vaso-
bones	osteo-
brain	encephalo-
chest	thoraco-
eyes	oculo-
female reproductive organs	gyneco-
genital	genito-
heart	cardio-
heart and vessels	cardiovasculo-
intestine	entero-
joint	arthro-
kidneys	nephro-
liver	hepato-
lungs	pneumo-/pulmono-
lymphatic	lympho-
meninges	meningo-
mouth	oro-
muscles	myo-
nerves	neuro-
nose	naso-
skin	dermato-
stomach	gastro-
teeth	dento-
urinary	uro-

and organs. There may also be a prefix, a suffix, or both. The **prefix** will appear at the beginning of the word, and the **suffix** at the end of the word. The prefix or suffix is a syllable, or perhaps only a few letters, added to the root term that will alter its meaning. The root is usually combined with the prefix or suffix by a combining letter (vowel).

Example 2–1   What does the term "myocardial" refer to?
First divide the term into its parts:

myo	cardi	al
prefix	root	suffix

Now define each separately

- The prefix *myo-* refers to muscle
- The root term *cardio-* pertains to the heart
- The suffix *-al* means "pertaining to"

Finally, put them together starting at the suffix end and read backward: *pertaining to + heart + muscle* means that the term "myocardial" refers to the heart muscle. So, for example, *myocardial injury* is damage to the heart muscle.

Example 2–2   What does the term "electrocardiogram" mean?

electro	cardi	o	gram
prefix	root	combining vowel	suffix

- The prefix *electro-* means "electrical"
- The root word *-cardio-* refers to the heart
- The suffix *-gram* refers to reading/recording

Reading the definition from the suffix backward to the prefix, *recording + heart + electrical* means that an *electrocardiogram* is the recording of the heart's electrical impulses.

Example 2–3   A "dermatologist" would deal with what specialty area? Notice there is no prefix in this word, just a root word and a suffix:

dermat	o	logist
root	combining vowel	suffix

- The root word *derma-* refers to the skin
- The suffix *-logist* means "person who studies"

A *dermatologist*, therefore, is a specialist who studies conditions and diseases that involve the skin.

Example 2–4   The term "appendectomy" describes what procedure?

append	*ectomy*
root	suffix

- The root word *append-* means "relating to the appendix"
- The suffix *-ectomy* refers to removal

Reading from suffix to root word, the term "appendectomy" means the *removal of the appendix.*

CONSTRUCTION OF MEDICAL TERMS

Often you may need to come up with the scientific or medical term for a common phrase or a short description of a condition. For example, you may need to know the term for a physician who specializes in the diseases and conditions of the brain and nervous system. The root word pertaining to the brain/nervous system is *neuro-*; the suffix for specialist is *-logist*. Therefore, a *neurologist* is a physician who specializes in diseases of the brain and nervous system.

If someone has been diagnosed with bacteria in the blood, the medical term would be derived from the term for bacteria (*bacter-*) and the suffix *-emia*, pertaining to the presence of a substance in the blood. Therefore, the word used to describe the condition of bacteria in the blood is *bacteremia*. However, if the bacteria were present in the urine, the word would be *bacteriuria*. In this case, the suffix *-ur* refers to urine and the suffix *-ia* refers to a condition.

There are also common terms that describe diseases or conditions that can be applied to any organ or body system. For example, in the terms "atrophy" and "hypertrophy,"

- The root word *troph-* pertains to nutrition
- The prefix *a-* means "without"
- The prefix *hyper-* means "excessive" or "above normal"

Therefore, muscle that has *atrophied* has wasted away. For example, someone who has paralysis of the legs would have atrophied calf and thigh muscles because they are not used and do not get proper nutrients. Muscle that has *hypertrophied*, in contrast, has enlarged beyond its usual or normal size due to excess use. In patients with congestive heart failure, the heart must work beyond its usual capacity in order to pump blood. Over a period of time it becomes larger; we say that the heart muscle has hypertrophied.

PREFIXES AND SUFFIXES

Another part of constructing a medical term is to learn the common suffixes and prefixes. Table 2–2 gives a list of the most common prefixes. Table 2–3 gives the most common suf-

Table 2–2 ■ Common Prefixes for Medical Terms

Prefixes as opposites

a-, an-	without	con-	with
ad-	toward	ab-	away from
ante-, pre-, pro-	before	post-	after
endo-	inside	ecto-, exo-	outside
hetero-	different	homo-	same
hyper-	more than	hypo-	less than
inter-	between	peri-, circum-	around
macro-	big	micro-	small
super-	above, excessive	infra-, sub-	below
tachy-	fast	brady-	slow

Other Prefixes

angi-	blood vessel	leuko-	white
anti-	against	meta-	change
auto-	self	neo-	new
bi-	two	path-	disease
epi-	upon	pedi-	children
erythro-	red	poly-	many
ex-	from	re-	back
hemi-	half	trans-	across, through
in-, intra-	inside	uni-, mono-	one
iso-	equal		

fixes. There are many other prefixes and suffixes, but the ones in these tables are those that you will probably encounter most frequently in your clinical laboratory studies. Note that some prefixes are paired with the term that gives an opposite meaning when used with a root word. For example, the prefix *ante-* means "before" and is paired with the prefix *post-*, which means "after." Also notice that there are several prefixes that have similar meanings.

Table 2–3 ■ Common Suffixes for Medical Terms

-algia	pain
-cyte	cell
-ectomy	removal
-emia	blood condition
-genic	cause, origin, production
-gram	record of
-graphy	way/method of recording
-ic, -al, -ac, -ium	pertaining to
-ism, -ia	condition of
-itis	inflammation, infection
-logist	person who specializes
-logy	study of
-lysis	breakdown
-megaly	enlarge
-oid	resembling
-oma	tumor
-osis	state of, caused by
-pathy	pertaining to disease
-penia	decrease, reduction
-plasia	form
-plasty	repair
-scopy	viewing, examination
-stasis	stop/control the flow
-tomy	incision of
-toxic	poison

EXERCISES IN CONSTRUCTING MEDICAL TERMS

In this section the specific organ systems of the body are used to help demonstrate how medical terms describe conditions or procedures. These exercises will help you construct terms or define the meaning of terms.

For the following exercises, read the paragraph and then find the terms in the paragraph that fit the given definition.

CARDIOVASCULAR SYSTEM

The first system is the cardiovascular system—the heart and blood vessels. The blood cells are also included with this group of words. Root words referring to this system include *cardio-* (heart), *athero-* (vessel), and *-cyte* (cell).

Heart and Blood Vessels

George was a 55-year-old obese man who was admitted to the emergency room with severe chest pains. The physician suspected a myocardial infarction and ordered an electrocardiogram (ECG). The results of the ECG showed ischemia to the myocardium. The patient did have atherosclerosis. There was no myocarditis suspected. The patient required cardiac by-pass surgery to increase the vasculature of the heart.

Find the word that means

Method of recording the heart's action	_____
Heart muscle	_____
Inflammation of the heart muscle	_____
Pertaining to the blood vessels	_____

Blood Cells

A 6-year-old girl was taken to her pediatrician because she was tired all the time and bruised easily. The physician ordered a complete blood count (CBC), and the clinical laboratory technician performed a phlebotomy. Results of the CBC showed the presence of leukemia. Her leukocyte count was elevated and her erythrocyte count demonstrated anemia.

Find the word that means

A disease of the white cells	_____
White blood cells	_____
Red blood cells	_____
A condition of too few red cells	_____
Procedure to draw blood	_____

RESPIRATORY SYSTEM

Root words referring to this system include *pneumo-* (lung).

A 75-year-old man was admitted with suspected pneumothorax due to an auto accident. He was hyperventilating and cyanotic. The cardiothoracic surgeon decided to do a tracheotomy first. Once the patient was breathing regularly, he was taken to the ward. While in the hospital, he required a bronchiolar lavage, a bronchoscopy, and a biopsy. The pleural fluid showed no cells. He developed pneumonia.

Find the word that means

Air in the chest   _____

Specialist in heart/lung disease   _____

Opening in the trachea   _____

Infection in the lungs   _____

DIGESTIVE SYSTEM

Root words referring to this system include *gastro-* (stomach) and *entero-* (intestine).

A patient with a history of gastric ulcers was admitted for a partial gastrectomy. The gastroenterologist who first saw him suspected that the man might also have acute enteritis due to the presence of a pathogenic bacteria. The biopsy of the stomach obtained during gastroscopy showed hyperemia, ulcerations with bleeding, and possible carcinoma.

Find the words that mean

Removal of the stomach   _____

Infection in the intestinal tract   _____

Visualization of the stomach   _____

Specialist of stomach/intestinal tract   _____

Increased blood flow   _____

For the next set of body systems or organs, give the root words listed and the meaning for the italicized terms. If you cannot construct the term, then use your medical dictionary to look up the meaning.

THE LIVER

A patient was seen by his physician for *yellow color of the skin, enlargement of the liver*, and *enlargement of the spleen*. The physician suspected *inflammation of the liver* due to a viral agent. When blood was drawn for laboratory testing, the serum appeared icteric. Results of the laboratory tests showed that the patient most likely had hepatitis B viral infection.

Root word for liver   _____

Construct the medical term that means

Yellow color of the skin   _____

Enlargement of the liver   _____

Enlargement of the spleen   _____

Inflammation of the liver   _____

RENAL SYSTEM

A 65-year-old man with a history of diabetes mellitus complained to his physician that he had *pain on urination*, was *going to the bathroom frequently*, and had *blood in his urine*. The physician first examined the bladder using a *lighted instrument that allowed him to see inside the bladder*. There was evidence of a bacterial infection and the physician ordered a culture. The culture grew *Escherichia coli*, a common bacterium of the intestinal tract. However, the antibiotics prescribed by the *kidney specialist* did not work and the patient developed an *infection of the kidney itself*. The results of the urinalysis demonstrated the presence of glycosuria, proteinuria, hematuria, and pyuria.

Root word for kidney   _____

Construct the medical term that means

Pain on urination   _____

Going to the bathroom frequently _____

Blood in the urine   _____

Instrument to see inside the bladder _____

Kidney specialist   _____

Infection of the kidney itself   _____

MUSCULOSKELETAL SYSTEM

An 18-year-old girl was injured in a motorcyle accident and suffered many broken bones, including a compound fracture of the femur. She had the bone surgically set by a *bone specialist* but developed an *infection of the bone*. The injuries also caused an *inflammation of the muscles* and *muscle pain*.

Root word for muscle   _____

Root word for bone   _____

Construct the medical term that means

Bone specialist   _____

Infection of the bone   _____

Inflammation of the muscles _____

Muscle pain   _____

NEUROLOGIC SYSTEM, INCLUDING THE BRAIN

A patient with suspected *inflammation of the covering of the brain* was *afraid of or sensitive to bright light.* The physician performed a spinal puncture and withdrew some spinal fluid for analysis. The cell count showed *increased numbers of white blood cells*, elevated protein, and decreased glucose, consistent with a bacterial etiology. The culture and bacterial antigen test were negative.

Root word for brain   _____

Root word for covering of brain   _____

Construct the medical term that means

Inflammation of the covering of the brain   _____

Afraid of or sensitive to bright light   _____

Increased numbers of white blood cells   _____

REPRODUCTIVE SYSTEM

A 23-year-old man complained to his physician of a purulent discharge from his penis. He also had *pain on urination* and *inflammation of the urethra.* He asked if he might have *inflammation of the prostate* or even syphilis.

Construct the medical term that means

Pain on urination   _____

Inflammation of the urethra   _____

Inflammation of the prostate   _____

Disciplines in Laboratory Medicine and Applications to Functions of the Body Systems

CHAPTER

3

INTRODUCTION

HEMATOLOGY
Complete Blood Count
Other Frequently Requested
  Tests
Flow Cytometry
Coagulation Studies

MICROBIOLOGY
Mycobacteriology
Mycology
Virology
Parasitology

CLINICAL CHEMISTRY

URINALYSIS

IMMUNOHEMATOLOGY
Blood Donor Processing
Compatibility Testing
Component Therapy
Prenatal Testing
Histocompatibility Testing

IMMUNOLOGY

CHAPTER SUMMARY

REVIEW QUESTIONS

Objectives

1. Discuss the specific functions of the hematology, microbiology, clinical chemistry, and immunohematology areas of the clinical laboratory.
2. Describe the components of a complete blood count.
3. Discuss the importance of performing a complete blood count.
4. Describe the different procedures performed in a coagulation section of a hematology laboratory.
5. Name the different specialized areas in a microbiology laboratory and describe the procedures performed at each area.
6. List the tests performed in the clinical chemistry laboratory that are essential in the treatment of life-threatening situations.
7. Discuss compatibility testing in the immunohematology laboratory and explain why this test is critical in patient care.
8. Describe blood donor processing and component preparation.
9. List the most common infections and diseases that are tested for in the immunology laboratory.

KEY TERMS

hematology	normal bacterial flora	toxicology	prenatal testing
complete blood count	mycobacteriology	electrophoresis	histocompatibility
differential	mycology	urinalysis	testing
flow cytometry	virology	immunohematology	immunology
coagulation studies	parasitology	compatibility testing	
microbiology	clinical chemistry	component therapy	

Introduction

The clinical and laboratory diagnosis of disease is a very dynamic and interactive process. When the patient presents to the clinician with signs and symptoms of disease, the clinician makes a presumptive diagnosis based on physical examination and history. Because

35

the clinical signs and symptoms may not always be overt and most often are nonspecific, the clinician requests laboratory tests to confirm or reject the presumptive diagnosis. Depending on the diagnosis, clinical samples such as blood, urine, and other body fluids are collected for analysis. These samples are sent to the different areas in the laboratory, depending on the disease condition. These areas include microbiology, clinical chemistry, hematology, and immunohematology. For example, microbiologic cultures are performed if an infectious disease is suspected. Blood samples collected from a patient suspected of having a heart attack are sent to the chemistry department for testing for analytes indicative of a heart attack. If a patient is believed to be anemic or suspected of having leukemia, the blood sample is analyzed in the hematology department. When a patient is bleeding because of trauma or ulcers or must undergo surgery, compatibility tests to prepare blood for transfusion are performed in the immunohematology section.

Clinical laboratory science is the study and practice of diagnostic medicine. The primary function of the clinical laboratory scientist (CLS) is to perform procedures that analyze blood and other body fluids. With the use of automated instruments and computerized information systems, the practitioner provides clinicians with information critical to the diagnosis of illness, and monitors therapy and prognosis of the disease. This chapter discusses the different areas and disciplines in the clinical laboratory that facilitate this main function.

Table 3–1 shows the most common tests performed in each section of the clinical laboratory. Each area in the laboratory has a specific function and role in the diagnosis of a wide variety of illnesses. In each of these major areas of the laboratory, there are subspecialty areas where special tests are performed. The following sections describe the role and functions of the major areas of the laboratory and the tests performed at each respective subspecialty section.

HEMATOLOGY

Hematology *is the study of blood.* Blood is composed of approximately 35 to 45% formed elements and 55 to 65% plasma (the liquid portion). The formed elements are blood cells, while plasma is made up of primarily water, with small amounts of salts, proteins, and carbohydrates. It also contains coagulation factors such as factor VIII. The main function of blood is to carry nutrients and oxygen to tissues and organs throughout the body and to collect metabolic waste products for elimination. Blood cells also function as an immune defense against bacteria, viruses, fungi, and parasites.

Red blood cells (RBCs; erythrocytes) contain hemoglobin (Hgb), the constituent that makes blood appear red. This is also the component that carries oxygen to the organ sys-

Table 3-1 ■ Examples of Commonly Requested Laboratory Tests

Clinical Discipline	Panels/Test Profiles	Clinical Condition/Purpose
Hematology	Complete blood count (CBC)	Anemia
	Platelet count	Infection
	Reticulocyte count	Leukemia
		Thrombocytopenia
		Leukemia
Flow Cytometry	Lymphocyte phenotype	Leukemia/lymphoma
	Autoimmune profile	
	Prothrombin time	Autoimmune diseases
Coagulation	Activated partial	Anticoagulant therapy
	thromboplastin time	Coagulation factor deficiency
Chemistry	Glucose level	Diabetes assessment
	Electrolyte panel	Dehydration
	Blood urea nitrogen level	Kidney function
Microbiology	Bacterial culture	Bacterial infection
	Ova and parasites exam	Parasitic infection
	Mycology culture	Fungal infection
Immunohematology	Compatibility testing	Blood transfusion
	Blood type and Rh status	Donor and patient blood type and processing

tems and tissue cells to keep them alive. *Anemia* results when there is a deficiency in the number of erythrocytes or in the amount of hemoglobin present. There are five types of white blood cells (WBCs, leukocytes): neutrophils (polymorphonuclear leukocytes, or PMNs), lymphocytes, monocytes, eosinophils, and basophils. Each type has a specific function in protecting the body against infection. For example, neutrophils respond primarily to bacterial infections while lymphocytes respond to viral infections. Therefore, an increase in either neutrophils or lymphocytes may presumptively indicate an invading organism. Overproduction of leukocytes, especially immature leukocytes, from the bone marrow and their release into the peripheral system is called *leukemia*. There are several types of leukemia, depending on which cell type is affected.

COMPLETE BLOOD COUNT

When the physician requests a **complete blood count** (CBC), the CLS takes a sample of blood from the patient to the hematology section of the laboratory. A CBC includes erythrocyte (RBC), leukocyte (WBC), hemoglobin (Hgb), hematocrit (Hct), and platelet counts. The CLS also prepares a blood smear for microscopic examination by placing a small drop of blood on a microscope glass slide and spreading the drop into a thin smear. The purpose of the microscopic examination of the blood smear is to identify and quantitate the different types of leukocytes, such as neutrophils, lymphocytes, monocytes, eosinophils, and basophils. The CBC is the test used to screen for blood disorders such as anemia and leukemia, and serves as an indicator for infections.

Because of the abundant and varied information that results from a CBC, it is probably the most commonly requested test in the clinical laboratory. In most clinical laboratories, regardless of size, a CBC is performed using an automated instrument. Automated blood cell counters have been available for the past 30 years. Newer, more sophisticated technology has provided more features and expanded capabilities. In addition to performing erythrocyte, leukocyte, and platelet counts, measuring hemoglobin, and calculating hematocrit, the cell counter differentiates each leukocyte based on cell size and nuclear and cytoplasmic characteristics. This **differential** is a task a CLS traditionally performed manually using a microscope.

OTHER FREQUENTLY REQUESTED TESTS

Other tests that are frequently performed in the hematology laboratory include reticulocyte count to evaluate erythropoietic activity of the bone marrow. Another test is erythrocyte sedimentation rate (ESR) which is used to identify and monitor inflammation. Body fluids such as cerebrospinal fluid (CSF), pleural fluid (from the lungs), peritoneal fluid (from the abdomen), and synovial fluid (from the joints) are examined for the presence and numbers of inflammatory cells or malignant cells. Clinical laboratory practitioners in the hematology section also assist pathologists and other clinicians in preparing *bone marrow smears*. Bone marrow is a substance found within the bones that contains precursor cells and immature erythrocytes, leukocytes, and platelets. When a patient is suspected of having severe anemia or leukemia, bone marrow biopsy and aspiration are performed to confirm or reject this suspicion. A pathologist or the physician performs the biopsy and aspiration procedure while the hematology practitioner prepares the sample for processing. Bone marrow smears are stained and examined for abnormal changes in leukocytes, erythrocytes, and platelets.

FLOW CYTOMETRY

Flow cytometry is one of the newest technological innovations in the hematology laboratory. A flow cytometer is an instrument that not only count cells but also helps differentiate cell types based on how cells scatter a laser light beam. Using a panel of fluorescent-labeled antibodies, a patient's lymphocytes may be categorized into two major types, B lymphocytes or T lymphocytes and further delineated into a specific stage of development. This is essential in accurate differentiation of the different types of leukemia and to provide appropriate therapy for the patient.

COAGULATION STUDIES

Depending on size and organization of the hospital laboratory, coagulation testing may be performed in the hematology department or in a separate section called coagulation or hemostasis. **Coagulation studies** are performed to diagnose bleeding or clotting disorders. Screening tests for coagulation status are critical in patients who will undergo a surgical procedure. Coagulation studies are also essential in monitoring patients undergoing anticoagulant therapy. Anticoagulants, or "blood thinners," are given to patients who have suffered a heart attack or stroke, to prevent blood from clotting again. *Prothrombin time* (PT) and *activated partial thromboplastin time* (APTT) are the two tests performed to monitor the dosage of anticoagulant given to the patient. If the dose is too high, the patient may spontaneously bleed; if the dose is too low, the clotting problem may recur.

Special coagulation studies are tests performed to detect deficiencies in coagulation factors, or poorly functioning or abnormally low numbers of platelets. Other anomalies of the blood vessels and coagulation system are also tested in this area. Coagulation factor VIII, or antihemophilia factor, deficiency is the factor deficiency most people are familiar with. Hemophiliacs lack this clotting factor and therefore are at high risk for bleeding episodes. Coagulation testing is performed by semiautomated or fully automated instruments.

MICROBIOLOGY

The **microbiology** section of the laboratory performs tests and procedures that will isolate and identify causative agents of infectious diseases. The majority of culture and identification studies for bacterial species are performed in the bacteriology section. Parasites, fungi, mycobacteria, and viruses are isolated and identified in the respective subspecialty areas. In bacteriology, culture and identification studies of organisms that cause common bacterial infections, such as streptococcal pharyngitis, bacterial pneumonia, urinary tract infections, and bacteremia, are performed.

To recover and isolate the suspected pathogens, the microbiologist uses several types of culture media. Culture media such as sheep blood agar (Color Figure 1) and chocolate agar support most of the common bacterial species. Certain types of media, such as MacConkey agar, contain nutrients that will provide the growth requirements for the pathogens but will inhibit certain bacterial species, while others may contain chemical substances that will help distinguish certain groups of organisms, usually the pathogens, from non-pathogenic species. These different types of culture media are particularly useful in working with samples that come from body sites (e.g., the respiratory tract or gastrointestinal tract) that are colonized with normal bacterial flora. **Normal bacterial flora** *are organisms that exist indigenously at certain body sites in healthy individuals.* These organisms, under normal conditions, do not cause disease; rather, they serve as a protective mechanism against potentially harmful species. Distinguishing the normal indigenous flora from the true pathogens is challenging for the clinical laboratory practitioner.

Once the potential pathogen is isolated, biochemical tests are set up to identify the species. Currently, automated instruments for identification are commonly used in most laboratories. In addition to identifying the bacterial organism, *antibiotic susceptibility stud-*

ies are also performed on each bacterial species. Antibiotic susceptibility studies determine which antibiotics would be most effective in killing or suppressing the growth and multiplication of the identified pathogen. It usually takes 24 to 48 hours to complete identification and susceptibility testing of suspected pathogens.

MYCOBACTERIOLOGY

There are some organisms that are difficult to recover using routine culture media. Bacterial species such as *Mycobacterium tuberculosis*, a very fastidious and slow-growing organism, require special nutritional and other growth factors for recovery. The **mycobacteriology** section receives samples specifically to isolate *Mycobacterium* species. Using conventional methods of isolation, it takes mycobacteria approximately 2 to 3 weeks to produce colonies. It is for this reason that molecular biotechniques such as DNA probes have been very useful for early detection and diagnosis. All work to detect these organisms must be perfomed under biologic safety cabinet (Fig. 3–1).

MYCOLOGY

The **mycology** section of the clinical laboratory is where fungi (Color Figure 2) are identified. Fungal agents have different nutritional and environmental requirements as well. In addition, isolation of these agents is extremely hazardous. Therefore, all microbiologic work must be performed under biologic safety cabinets (Fig. 3–1).

VIROLOGY

Isolation and identification of pathogenic viral agents is done in the **virology** section. Identification of viruses requires the use of tissue cells. Viruses that are difficult to culture require immunologic methods for identification. For example, herpes simplex, the virus that causes "fever blisters" or "cold sores," grows readily in tissue culture but hepatitis viruses do not. Therefore, diagnosis of viral hepatitis is best done by using hepatitis markers. With immunologic methodology, antibodies produced by the patient are detected using the specific hepatitis marker (antigen).

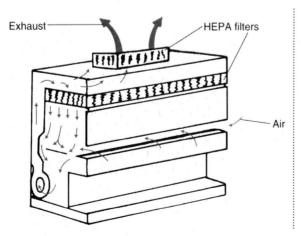

Exhaust — HEPA filters — Air

FIGURE 3-1

Class II biologic safety cabinet. This is the most common type of biologic safety hood used in most microbiology laboratories. The cabinet is equipped with high-efficiency particulate air (HEPA) filters, which filter the air drawn into the cabinet. (From Miller, D.A.: Control of microorganisms. *In* Mahon, C.R., and Manuselis, G., Jr. [eds.]: Textbook of Diagnostic Microbiology, Philadelphia, W.B. Saunders, 1995, with permission.)

PARASITOLOGY

Parasitology, the identification of parasites such as tapeworms, pinworms, and protozoans, is also performed in the microbiology laboratory. Protozoans such as *Entamoeba histolytica* and *Giardia lamblia* are not uncommon findings in patients with diarrheal illness. *Taenia saginata* (beef tapeworm) and *Enterobius vermicularis* (pinworm) are other parasites that are identified in the parasitology laboratory. Unless the facility is large enough to justify a parasitology section, this task is performed in the bacteriology section.

CLINICAL CHEMISTRY

In the **clinical chemistry** section, clinical laboratory practitioners perform biochemical analyses of body fluids using highly complex, most often fully automated instrumentation. Body fluids tested in this area include serum, urine, CSF, amniotic fluid, pleural fluid, and synovial fluid. Common tests performed on serum, urine, and CSF include serum glucose and total protein concentrations. Other analytes tested for in the serum are electrolytes such as sodium (Na^+), potassium (K^+), and chloride (Cl^-), and carbon dioxide (CO_2). Blood urea nitrogen, creatinine, liver enzyme, and cardiac enzyme levels are also commonly requested tests.

Serum glucose level is determined to diagnose and monitor diabetes. Elevated levels as well as low levels of glucose are life threatening if the patient does not receive the appropriate intervention. The presence of glucose in urine provides a similar diagnostic and monitoring tool.

Proteins serve numerous bodily functions. Exploring each function in detail is beyond the scope of this chapter. Table 3–2 lists the major functions of proteins. Measuring total serum protein concentrations provides valuable information regarding disease processes in major organ systems. Low levels (*hypoproteinemia*) as well as high levels (*hyperproteinemia*) are indicative of pathologic conditions, some of which can be serious. An example of a decreased level of proteins is found in renal disease, in which proteins are lost by excretion through the kidneys. Proteins are not usually detected in the urine; therefore, loss of plasma proteins through the kidneys results in *proteinuria* (proteins in the urine). Dehydration that results from excessive vomiting and diarrhea may produce an increased level of plasma proteins. Conditions such as multiple myeloma produce highly elevated protein concentrations.

An increase in total protein in the CSF indicates the presence of inflammatory cells such as PMNs and debris of damaged tissue commonly associated with bacterial meningitis. In this type of infection, the total protein level in the CSF is elevated while the glucose level is usually decreased as a result of the bacterial utilization of glucose in the fluid.

Chemical analyses of body fluids in the clinical chemistry laboratory have been performed routinely by automated analyzers since 1957. The first autoanalyzer, developed by Technicon, dominated the market during the early years of automated instrumentation in the clinical laboratory. Several decades later, one could visit a clinical chemistry section and find a wide variety of analyzers manufactured by numerous companies. Today, fully automated computerized instruments are used to analyze hundreds of tests on clinical samples.

There are areas in the clinical chemistry laboratory that perform special procedures, such as toxicology and electrophoresis. The **toxicology** section is the area where samples are

Table 3–2 ■ Major Functions of Proteins

- Nourish tissues
- Maintain water distribution between cells and tissues, interstitial compartments and blood vessels
- Act as buffer to maintain pH
- Transport metabolic substances
- Act as receptors for hormones
- Serve as immune defense
- Catalyze biochemical reactions
- Participate in the hemostasis and coagulation of blood
- Contribute in the connective-tissue structure

Modified from Lindsey, B.J.: Amino acids and proteins. *In* Bishop, M., Duben-Engelkirk, Jr., and Fody, E. (eds.): Clinical Chemistry: Principles, Procedures, Correlations, 3rd ed. Philadelphia, Lippincott-Raven, 1996, p. 179, with permission.

tested either for the presence of drugs of abuse or to monitor levels of therapeutic drugs. In **electrophoresis,** serum samples are placed on a special gel medium. An electrical current is passed through the gel to separate the different serum protein components. These special tests are usually available in large institutions; in smaller hospital laboratories, these tests are frequently sent to a reference laboratory.

URINALYSIS

The urinalysis section of the laboratory is most often a part of a larger department such as hematology or chemistry. Clinical laboratory practitioners perform testing on urine samples to detect disorders such as urinary tract infections or damage to the kidneys. Urine testing also is used to screen for and monitor diabetes and phenylketonuria, an inborn error of metabolism that can result in mental retardation.

There are several parts to a routine **urinalysis**. First, the physical characteristics of the urine are determined and described. Is the urine clear, hazy, or cloudy? What is the color of the urine sample submitted? Normal urine color is yellow. Intact erythrocytes make the urine appear hazy red; and when the erythrocytes are hemolyzed, the urine appear may appear clear red or amber. The specific gravity, which measures the amount of solutes in the urine, is also determined. Next, the urine specimen is tested for significant chemical substances that would indicate the presence of disease by using a plastic strip that contains pads impregnated with chemicals. The chemical substances tested for include glucose, blood, proteins, pH, ketones, bilirubin, urobilinogen, nitrites, and leukocyte esterase (Color Figure 3).

After the urine is tested chemically, it is centrifuged so that sediment is collected. The sediment is examined microscopically for erythrocytes, leukocytes, epithelial cells, crystals, and other structures such as casts, yeasts, bacteria, and parasites. When present in significant numbers, these structures may indicate the presence of infection or other kidney disorder. The clinical laboratory practitioner also differentiates these structures from common artifacts such as cloth fiber, hair, and talc powder.

IMMUNOHEMATOLOGY

The immunohematology laboratory and the blood donor center are responsible for ensuring that the blood supply will not jeopardize public health and safety. **Immunohematology** consists of the donor processing area, transfusion services, and special testing areas such as those involved in hemolytic disease of the newborn. The immunohematology or blood bank department, because of the critical nature of its role and function in medical care, is probably one of the most stressful areas in the laboratory in which to work. Clinical laboratory practitioners in blood banks must be able to handle the challenges and problem-solving activities common in this area of practice.

BLOOD DONOR PROCESSING

Before a unit of blood is transfused into a patient, several tests must be performed on the unit to make certain that (1) the transfused blood will benefit the patient and (2) the transfused blood will not cause any harm to the patient. The process begins when a potential blood donor comes to the blood center to donate blood. To guard the safety of both donor and potential recipient, a medical history is taken prior to blood collection. The donor's blood pressure, temperature, pulse rate, and hemoglobin are determined to ensure that it is safe for the donor to donate blood.

Once the blood is taken, the clinical laboratory practitioner performs numerous tests on the unit of blood before it is released for patient transfusion. First, the blood type is determined. Blood is typed according to the *ABO groups* A, B, AB, and O. The blood is also tested for the presence of *Rh factor*; if it is present, the blood is labeled as Rh positive (Rh$^+$); if it is not present, the blood is labeled Rh negative (Rh$^-$). In addition, the donor blood is tested for the presence of erythrocyte antibodies that may endanger the recipient if the blood is transfused. Other tests performed are those that determine the presence of antibodies to infectious agents such as hepatitis viruses, human immunodeficiency virus (HIV), and cytomegalovirus. Tests for the sexually transmitted disease syphilis are also done. After all these tests are completed, the unit of blood is appropriately labeled (Color Figure 4).

COMPATIBILITY TESTING

When a patient requires a unit of blood for transfusion, a tube of blood is drawn from the patient for compatibility testing. **Compatibility testing** *is performed to determine if the* *donor's blood can be safely transfused into the patient (recipient).* The test involves mixing a small amount of the patient's serum with a small amount of the erythrocytes from the donor's unit. The blood bank technologist, in performing the test, looks for clumping (*agglutination*), which would indicate that the donor's blood is "incompatible" with the recipient's and may cause a transfusion reaction if the blood is infused. A compatible unit is one in which the patient's serum does not cause clumping with the donor's erythrocytes.

Every procedure performed in the blood bank is executed with utmost care and competency. Simple clerical errors in the blood bank may cost a patient's life. Correct patient and donor unit identification must be maintained throughout the process. When a unit of blood is released for transfusion, incorrect identification of either the patient or the donor unit may result in a catastrophic or even fatal event.

COMPONENT THERAPY

There are cases when a patient may need only a specific part or component of blood. For example, a patient with a low platelet count (platelets are essential in clotting) may only require a platelet component transfusion, while another patient may require only the erythrocyte component. Providing patients with a specific blood component is referred to as **component therapy**.

A single unit of blood can be separated and processed into the following components: erythrocytes, platelets, plasma (liquid portion), and coagulation factor VIII, or antihemophilia factor. This process of separating whole blood into several different components, each of which may benefit a different patient is a major responsibility of the blood bank section.

PRENATAL TESTING

In addition to preparing blood or blood components for transfusion, clinical laboratory practitioners also perform tests on pregnant women. This **prenatal** or maternal **testing** is done to determine if the mother's serum contains antibodies against antigens she may not possess but her fetus does. Antibody production may have been stimulated when fetal cells entered the mother's circulation during delivery of a previous pregnancy. When fetal cells contain antigens that the mother's cells lack, the fetal cells behave like foreign bodies that stimulate the mother's immune system to produce antibodies against the foreign antigen. During a subsequent pregnancy, the antibodies circulating in the mother's blood, when exposed to the same antigen, will begin to destroy the fetal cells; hence, without the appropriate therapy, the fetus may become very ill or be stillborn. Therefore, prenatal testing provides information that will determine if the fetus requires immediate medical intervention.

HISTOCOMPATIBILITY TESTING

The blood bank is also now involved in testing for human leukocyte antigens (HLAs) and antibodies. HLAs are antigens present on the surface of nucleated cells (leukocytes, platelets, and most tissue cells). Detecting HLA antibodies in a patient who is a candidate for organ or tissue transplantation and determining HLA antigens in donor organs or tissues is called **histocompatibility testing.** Rejection of the donor tissue in transplant patients if HLA antibodies are present is immediate and very severe.

IMMUNOLOGY

The study of the immune system is called **immunology**. The immunology section of the laboratory is responsible for performing tests that help determine the immune status of an individual and aid in the diagnosis of infectious diseases and in the quantitation of serum components such as immunoglobulins. Immunologic methods are based on antigen-antibody reactions (Color Figure 5). Immunologic techniques such as immunodiffusion assays are used to measure the amount of serum proteins, such as immunoglobulins, albumin, and acute-phase proteins.

The primary function of the immune system is to recognize foreign materials that enter the body and to defend the body from these materials. Foreign materials that may invade the human body include bacterial organisms, viruses, parasites, and fungi as well as transplanted organs or tissues. The protective or immune defenses of the body include physical barriers, such as intact skin and mucous membrane surfaces; secretions that contain antimicrobial substances, such as tears and lysozyme; leukocytes, such as lymphocytes and monocytes; inflammatory cells (macrophages and phagocytes); and antibodies produced against specific antigenic substances. When the function of the immune system is disrupted or suppressed, the host becomes more highly susceptible to infectious diseases (*immunocompromised*) than individuals with intact immune systems (*immunocompetent*).

Deficiencies of the immune system are numerous and are either *hereditary* (inborn) or *acquired* (by contact with foreign material). An example of hereditary or congenital immunodeficiency is agammaglobulinemia, a condition in which the body does not produce immunoglobulins (antibodies). The primary function of immunoglobulins is to combine with antigens and neutralize toxins or viruses. Inability to produce immunoglobulins predisposes the body to infectious disease because it does not have a mechanism to protect it. The five distinct classes of immunoglobulins (Igs) are IgG, IgM, IgA, IgD, and IgE. These immunoglobulins differ from each other in characteristics and in functions. An increased level of a particular class is associated with certain disorders or diseases. Decreased levels can be seen in congenital or acquired disorders.

The diagnosis of infectious diseases is sometimes supplemented with immunologic studies for the presence of antibodies to bacterial cell antigens. For example, brucellosis, a disease common to domestic animals but transmissible to humans, is often detected by the presence of *Brucella* species antibodies in the patient's serum. This is important in the diagnosis of this particular life-threatening infection because *Brucella* organisms are slow-growing bacteria. Early detection of the antibodies provides a presumptive diagnosis; therefore, appropriate therapy is immediately prescribed by the clinician. Infectious diseases due to viruses, unusual organisms, and other difficult-to-culture types of infectious agents may be detected by immunologic methods. Examples are infectious mononucleosis, syphilis, hepatitis, HIV, and rheumatoid arthritis.

Another function of the immunology section is to determine the functional ability of leukocytes, such as lymphocytes, monocytes, and PMNs. There are instances in which there may be enough circulating leukocytes but the cells are damaged or nonfunctional.

Immunology is a clinical discipline that is continuously being explored. New technology, methods, and assays are constantly being developed and introduced. Sophisticated instrumentation and applications of molecular technology will continue to be developed to detect minute quantities of serum components.

CHAPTER SUMMARY

The wide range of services performed by clinical laboratory practitioners enable the clinician to establish diagnosis and initiate appropriate therapy and intervention. Practitioners in the major areas in a clinical laboratory, namely, clinical chemistry, hematology, microbiology, and immunohematology perform specific functions and role in the diagnosis of disease states. They run a wide variety of tests in each area using complex instrumentation and technology. With the knowledge and training that clinical laboratory scientists receive, they become integral members of the health care team.

Review Questions

1. What are the different specialized areas in a microbiology laboratory?

2. Glucose testing is performed in which area of the clinical laboratory?

3. What is compatibility testing? How is this test used in the immunohematology laboratory?

4. What tests are performed in the hematology section? Why are these tests important?

BIBLIOGRAPHY

Anderson, S., and Cockayne, S.: Clinical Chemistry: Concepts and Applications. Philadelphia, W.B. Saunders, 1993.

Clerc, J.: An Introduction to Clinical Laboratory Science. St. Louis, C.V. Mosby, 1992.

Lindsey, B.J.: Amino acids and proteins. *In* Bishop, M., Duben-Engelkirk, Jr., and Fody, E. (eds.): Clinical Chemistry: Principles, Procedures, Correlations, 3rd ed. Philadelphia, Lippincott-Raven, 1996, p. 179.

Mahon, C.R., and Manuselis Jr, G.: Textbook of Diagnostic Microbiology. Philadelphia, W.B. Saunders, 1995.

McKenzie, S.B.: Textbook of Hematology, 2nd ed. Baltimore, Williams & Wilkins, 1996.

Turgeon, M.L.: Fundamentals of Immunohematology: Theory and Technique. Philadelphia, Lea & Febiger, 1989.

Turgeon, M.L.: Immunology and Serology in Laboratory Medicine. St. Louis, C.V. Mosby, 1990.

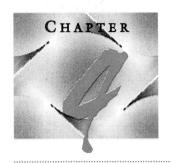

CHAPTER 4

Laboratory Mathematics

INTRODUCTION

MEASUREMENT SYSTEMS
The Metric System
Conversions
    Conversion of standard lab
        units to Système
        Internationale d'Unités
Temperature

SOLUTIONS AND DILUTIONS

EXPRESSIONS OF CONCENTRATION
Molarity
    Traditional method
    Quick and simple method
Normality
Percent Concentration
    Complex problems
Osmolarity
Specific Gravity

pH AND ACID-BASE
RELATIONSHIPS
pH
A Quick Word about
    Logarithms
Acid-Base Relationships

PHOTOMETRY CALCULATIONS
Photometry
Standard Curve

BASIC STATISTICS
Mean, Mode, Median,
    and Range
Standard Deviation
Coefficient of Variation

CHAPTER SUMMARY

REVIEW QUESTIONS

Objectives

1. Define the metric system and the units used to perform metric measurements.

2. Convert temperatures between the three scales of temperature measurement.

3. Convert given metric units to SI units.

4. State the components of a solution and use appropriate calculations to perform dilutions.

5. Express units of concentration in various meaningful ways.

6. Calculate normality, molarity, specific gravity, and percent concentration of various compounds or solutions given appropriate data.

7. Understand the concept of pH and be able to calculate a pH value given appropriate data.

8. Understand the concept of the acid-base relationship and the formula used to calculate pH using acid and base concentrations.

9. Explain the mathematical basis of photometric determinations used to measure unknown concentrations of substances in human blood.

10. State Beer's law and calculate unknown concentrations using formulas derived from Beer's law.

11. Plot a standard curve given appropriate data.

12. Use statistical formulas to calculate mean, mode, median, standard deviation, and coefficient of variation.

13. Apply statistical analysis to laboratory quality control assessment and prepare a Levey-Jennings chart.

KEY TERMS

SI units	mole	Henderson-Hasselbalch	mean
solution	normality	equation	mode
solute	equivalent weight	photometry	median
solvent	osmolarity	transmittance	range
simple dilution	osmolal gap	absorbance	variance
serial dilution	specific gravity	Beer's Law	standard deviation
molarity	pH	standard curve	coefficient of variation

Introduction

In the clinical laboratory, the clinical laboratory scientist and clinical laboratory technician are expected to perform procedures that will involve mathematical calculations in their preparations of reagents, samples, and solutions. Therefore, it is important that the laboratory practitioner is knowledgeable of metric measurements and other mathematical skills to calculate concentrations, use statistical formulas, and assess the validity of laboratory data.

Some of the concepts this chapter covers include the application of the metric system and the formulas to convert units in the metric measurements. It demonstrates how to calculate normality, molarity, and concentration of solutions, and explains the concept of acid-base balance, Beer's law, and the mathematical basis of photometric determinations. Mathematical applications in the clinical laboratory are explored.

MEASUREMENT SYSTEMS

THE METRIC SYSTEM

In the clinical pathology laboratory, as in most biologic labs, measurements of volume, mass, or length are reported in metric system units. Patient test results are typically reported with a value and a metric unit of measurement; as an example, a glucose value would be reported as 110 milligrams per deciliter of glucose, more commonly written as 110 mg/dl. In this case, the number describes the numeric value or amount, while the units denote a physical measure of mass in a specific volume. Prefixes are used that describe a unit multiple of "110" and are attached to a standard measurement name. In the clinical laboratory, these measurement names describe physical measures of substance mass or concentration. Volume is measured in liters, mass in grams, and length in meters. Table 4–1 contains examples of prefixes attached to units of measure most commonly used in the clinical laboratory.

Multiple	Prefix	Mass	Length	Volume
1,000	Kilo	Kilogram (kg)	Kilometer (km)	Kiloliter (kl)
1	none	Gram (gm or g)	Meter (m)	Liter (l or L)
$1/10\ (10^{-1})$	Deci	Decigram (dg)	Decimeter (dm)	Deciliter (dl)
$1/100\ (10^{-2})$	Centi	Centigram (cg)	Centimeter (cm)	Centiliter (cl)
$1/1,000\ (10^{-3})$	Milli	Milligram (mg)	Millimeter (mm)	Milliliter (ml)
$1/1,000,000\ (10^{-6})$	Micro	Microgram (μg)	Micrometer (μm)	Microliter (μl)
$1/1,000,000,000$	Nano	Nanogram (ng)	Nanometer (nm)	Nanoliter (nl)
$1/1,000,000,000,000$	Pico	Picogram (pg)	Picometer (pm)	Picoliter (pl)

Table 4–1 ■ **Examples of Prefixes for Units of Measure**

CONVERSIONS

The most simple method of converting measurements from one unit to another is to determine a conversion factor between the two units. The advantage of using the metric system is that the mathematical units are derived by multiplying or dividing by some power of 10. The prefixes of each unit should be noted and converted into an exponent of 10, then the exponent of the desired unit can be subtracted from the exponent of the existing unit. Ten to the power of this number becomes the conversion factor; this is then written as a whole number, and then multiplied times the value in the existing units to obtain the desired units.

Example 4–1 How many milliliters (10^{-3}) are in 57 deciliters (10^{-1})? The desired units are milliliters, and the existing units are deciliters.

$$-1 - (-3) = 2 = 10^2 = 100$$
$$100 \times 57\ dl = 5,700\ ml$$

Or, constructing an equation relating deciliters (10) to milliliters (1,000):

$$\frac{57}{10} = \frac{x}{1,000}$$
$$57,000 = 10x$$
$$5,700 = x$$

Therefore, 5,700 mls are in 57 dls.

Conversion of Standard Lab Units to Système Internationale d'Unités

In an attempt to standardize concentration units of measure in clinical laboratories worldwide, a special system of unit measurement was devised in the 1960s. Unfortunately, these units, referred to as *Système Internationale d'Unités* or **SI units,** have not been widely accepted in this country because of the recalcitrance of the medical community to change (analogous to the difficulty in the adoption of the metric system in our society). SI units of concentration are reported as milliequivalents per liter (mEq/l), so the equivalent weight of a substance must initially be determined prior to conversion of standard units of concentration to SI units. The equation used to convert milligrams per deciliter to milliequivalents per liter is expressed as follows:

$$mEq/l = \frac{mg/l}{Eq} \quad or \quad \frac{mg/100\ ml \times 10}{Eq} \quad or \quad \frac{mg/dl \times 10}{Eq}$$

where Eq refers to the equivalent weight of a substance.

Example 4–2   Calculate the SI units for 16 mg/dl magnesium. The equivalent weight of magnesium is 24.

$$mEq/l = \frac{16 \times 10}{24}$$

Therefore, 16 mg/dl magnesium is equal to 6.7 mEq/l.

For compounds such as cholesterol, the formula weight of the substance must be determined before calculating the SI unit value. For ease in calculating SI units from conventional units, "conversion factors" for most substances examined in a patient's blood have been derived from the equivalent weight formula shown previously.

TEMPERATURE

Most often, in the clinical laboratory, the *Celsius* (incorrectly referred to as the centigrade) scale of temperature measurement is used. Two other scales exist, the *Fahrenheit* and the *Kelvin*. The Kelvin (K) and the Celsius (C) scales are divided into similar units of degrees, with the difference between the two being the set of the zero point. The Fahrenheit (F) scale is divided into units (degrees) of a different size with a different zero setting from the Kelvin and Celsius scales. The zero of the Celsius scale is set at the freezing point of water, the zero of the Kelvin scale is the theoretical temperature at which no more heat can be lost from a thermodynamic reaction (absolute zero), and the zero of the Fahrenheit scale is set at the point where the temperature of a mixture of water and table salt can go no lower.

To convert Celsius temperatures to Kelvin degrees, simply add 273 to the Celsius temperature. Subtract 273 from the Kelvin temperature to obtain degrees Celsius. Unfortunately, it is not as simple to convert Fahrenheit to Celsius and vice versa, since 1° C is equal to 1.8° F, or 1° F equals 0.556° C, and both zero set points are different! To convert to Fahrenheit degrees, multiply the Celsius degrees times 1.8 and add 32 to the product. To determine Celsius degrees, subtract 32 from the Fahrenheit degrees and multiply the result by 0.556.

Example   Convert 43 Celsius degrees to Fahrenheit degrees.

Fahrenheit degrees = (43°C × 1.8) + 32 = 109.4°F

SOLUTIONS AND DILUTIONS

In today's clinical laboratory, solutions are typically purchased from a vendor in a final ready-to-use concentration with no additional preparation required. However, certain manual procedures in the clinical laboratory and most procedures in the research laboratory require the manual preparation of solutions of a specific concentration. This section is designed to aid the laboratory scientist in understanding the terminology, process, and calculations used in making such solutions.

Solutions *are mixtures of solutes and solvents. A* **solute** *is the substance that is dissolved, and a* **solvent,** *sometimes referred to as a diluent, is the dissolving substance,* typically a liquid. However, in certain solutions, such as a mixture of alcohol and water, it may be unclear which is the solute and which is the solvent.

Solutions are typically described as parts of solute in parts of solvent. Designations such as milligrams of solute per liter of solvent, grams per deciliter, or milliliters per milliliter are descriptions of *concentration.*

A concentrated solution that contains a large amount of solute in a small amount of solvent is referred to as a *"stock"* solution. When a solution of lesser concentration is required, the stock solution is diluted to make what is referred to as a *"working"* solution. To reduce the concentration of solute in a solution, a simple dilution is required. *A* **simple dilution** *is defined as the number of parts of material being diluted in the total number of parts.* For example, making a 1:10 or 1/10 (read as 1 to 10 or 1 in 10) dilution of a stock solution of 9% saline means adding 1 part saline to 9 parts of water for a total of 10 parts. The 9% stock solution has been diluted 10 times, producing a 0.9% working solution of saline.

Dilution of patient serum must be done if a measured substance is extremely elevated. For example, a patient's triglyceride concentration may be too high to be in a chemistry analyzer's linearity range, and a dilution of the patient specimen is required. It is critical to remember that, if a 1:5 dilution of patient serum is prepared (i.e., 1 part serum in 4 parts saline), the triglyceride value from the analyzer must be multiplied by a factor of 5 to obtain the correct triglyceride concentration.

Simple dilutions are stated as 1 to something. For example, 1 to 10 or 1 to 3, also written as 1:10 and 1:3 or 1/10 and 1/3, are typical dilution statements. However, in some cases, the dilution is not stated in this manner. For example, a dilution of 4 parts of a substance in 25 parts of another is stated as 4:29 (4 + 25 = 29). To convert 4:29 to a 1:x dilution, a simple calculation is required and is set up in this fashion:

$$\frac{4}{29} = \frac{1}{x}$$
$$4x = 29$$
$$x = 7.25$$

Therefore, a 4:29 dilution is stated as a 1:7.25 dilution.

Serologic analyses, particularly antibody titers, require the use of serial dilutions to allow visualization of an endpoint in antigen and antibody reactions. *A* **serial dilution** *is a series of simple dilutions in which the dilution factor (the total parts) is exactly the same in each step.* In preparing a serial dilution, a series of test tubes is set up with exactly the same amount of diluent in each tube. Serum is then added to the first tube in an amount that yields a particular dilution. For example, if 0.5 ml of diluent is added to each test tube in the series and 0.5 ml of serum is placed in the first tube and carefully mixed, a dilution of 1:2 is obtained (0.5 ml diluent + 0.5 ml serum = 0.5:1.0 or 1:2). To the second test tube containing 0.5 ml of diluent, 0.5 ml of the solution from the first tube is added and mixed, yielding a second 1:2 dilution. Now the serum has been diluted twice. To calculate the dilution of serum in the second test tube, multiply the dilution of the first tube (1:2) by the dilution of the second tube (1:2). This equation can be stated as $1/2 \times 1/2 = 1/4$, or a 1:4 dilution. Continuing with this example, 0.5 ml of the solution in the second test tube is added to the third tube containing 0.5 ml diluent and mixed, making another 1:2 dilution. The serum dilution in the third test tube is calculated by multiplying $1/2 \times 1/2 \times 1/2$, equaling 1/8 or a dilution of 1:8. Dilutions can be made and calculated in this manner in any number of test tubes. Of course, serial dilutions are not always 1:2 dilutions. Any dilution factor may be used, such as 5 or 10. To determine the dilution in the last tube of the series, multiply each dilution by the previous dilution (such as $\frac{1}{5} \times \frac{1}{5} \times \frac{1}{5}$ and so on until all tubes have been counted).

EXPRESSIONS OF CONCENTRATION

MOLARITY

Another method of describing the concentration of a solute within a solution is through the determination of the relative number of reactant particles (the solute) involved in a reaction mixture (the solution). This number is referred to as the **molarity** of the solute within the solution, and it describes the number of moles of solute in a specific amount of solution. *A* **mole** *of a substance is the molecular weight of that substance and contains* 6.02×10^{23} *particles.* A mole is referred to as the *gram molecular weight* of a substance. For example, a mole of sodium is equal to the molecular weight of sodium, or 23 g; therefore, 23 is the gram molecular weight of sodium. A mole of a compound (such as sodium hydroxide, NaOH) is the total of the molecular weights of each substance within the compound and is referred to as the *formula weight*. For example, the formula weight of NaOH is the molecular weight of sodium (23 g) plus the molecular weight of oxygen (16 g) plus the molecular weight of hydrogen (1 g), equal to 40 g, the gram molecular weight of NaOH. Therefore, 1 mole of NaOH is equal to 40 g. The gram molecular weight of a substance expressed in milligrams is equal to a millimole (mmol).

Molarity (M) is expressed as the number of moles per liter of solution (mol/l). The designations "M" and "mol/l" are often used interchangeably. The term "1-molar solution" is defined as 1 mole of a substance in 1 liter of solution; likewise, a 2-molar solution is defined as 2 moles of a substance in 1 liter of solution. To prepare a 1-molar solution of NaOH, 40 g of solid NaOH is added to a 1-liter volumetric flask containing a solvent (typically water or buffer). Once the NaOH is added, more solvent is added to the flask until the liquid meniscus reaches the calibrating mark on the neck of the flask (referred to as "diluted up to..."). Once the solid has dissolved in totality, the solution is referred to as a "1-molar solution of NaOH in buffer" and is written "1M NaOH in buffer" or "1 mol/l NaOH in buffer."

To determine what amount of solute must be added to a solvent to make a solution of a specific molarity, or to determine the molarity of a solution containing a given amount of solute and solvent, a calculation must be performed. There is a "quick and simple" method that can be used to calculate molarity problems. However, the traditional method should be reviewed by all laboratory practitioners to gain a full understanding of what is involved in the calculation prior to learning the quick and simple method.

Traditional Method

In this calculation of molarity, one must initially determine what units of measurement are provided in the problem and then what units are needed in the final answer. Knowledge of the formula weight of the compound or substance involved is necessary. An equation is then used to solve the problem.

Example 4–3 How many grams of sodium chloride (NaCl) are needed to make 1 liter of a 2-mol/l (or 2M) solution?

- ■ What units of measurement are provided in the problem?   mol/l
- ■ What units of measurement are needed for the final answer?   g/l
- ■ What is the formula weight of NaCl?   Na (23 g) + Cl (35.5 g) = 58.5 g
- ■ How many grams of NaCl are in 1 mole of NaCl?   58.5 g/mol

$$\frac{58.5 \text{ g NaCl}}{\text{mole}} \times \frac{2 \text{ mole}}{\text{liter}} = \frac{58.5 \text{ g} \times 2 \text{ mole}}{\text{mole} \times \text{liter}} = 117.0 \text{ g/l}$$

Therefore, 117 g of NaCl in 1 liter of solvent are required to prepare a 2-mol/l solution.

Example 4–4 What is the molarity of a solution that contains 32 g of NaOH in 300 ml of buffer?

- ■ What units of measurement are provided in the problem?   g/ml
- ■ What units of measurement are needed for the final answer?   mol/l
- ■ What is the formula weight of NaOH?   Na (23 g) + O (16 g) + H (1 g) = 40 g
- ■ How many grams of NaOH are in 1 mole of NaOH?   40 g/mol
- ■ What is the conversion factor needed to convert milliliters to liters?   1,000 ml/1 liter

$$\frac{32 \text{ g NaOH}}{300 \text{ ml buffer}} \times \frac{1000 \text{ ml}}{1 \text{ liter}} \times \frac{1 \text{ mole}}{40 \text{ g}} = \frac{32 \text{ g} \times 1000 \text{ ml} \times 1 \text{ mole}}{300 \text{ ml} \times 1 \text{ liter} \times 40 \text{ g}} = 2.7 \text{ mol/l}$$

Therefore, 32 g of NaOH in 300 ml of buffer has a molarity of 2.7 mol/l.

Quick and Simple Method

This calculation achieves an answer similar to that of the traditional method without the need for units placement. The equation used is

$$M = \frac{g/l}{MW}$$

where M is moles per liter, or molarity, and MW is the molecular weight of the compound in question. This equation can be used to solve Examples 4–3 and 4–4 using the quick and simple method. Example 4–3 calculated the number of grams of sodium chloride (NaCl) needed to make 1 liter of a 2-mol/l (or 2M) solution. Using the new equation,

$$2 = \frac{g/l}{58.5} = 2 \times 58.5 = 117 \text{ g/l}$$

Therefore, 117 g of NaCl are needed to make 1 liter of a 2M solution of NaCl.

    Example 4–4 calculated the molarity of a solution that contains 32 g of NaOH in 300 ml of buffer. Using the new equation,

$$M = \frac{32/0.3}{40} = \frac{106.7}{40} = 2.7M$$

Therefore, 32 g of NaOH in 300 ml of buffer gives a 2.7 m/l solution. In this problem, the amount of buffer is 300 ml, which is written as 0.3 liters. It is important to always use the *liter* amount when entering the grams per liter value in this formula.

Example 4–5   How many grams of NaCl are required to prepare 250 ml of 6-mol/l NaCl?

$$6M = \frac{g/0.250}{58.5} \quad or \quad 6 \times 58.5 \times 0.250 = g \quad or \quad 87.75 \text{ g}$$

Therefore, 87.75 g of NaCl are needed to prepare 250 ml of a 6-mol/l solution of NaCl.

NORMALITY

Whereas molarity is based upon the molecular weight of a substance, **normality** is based upon the equivalent weight of a substance. *An **equivalent weight** (Eq) of a substance is the mass of that substance that will replace (or combine with) one mole of hydrogen.* Equivalent weight (also referred to as "gram equivalent weight") is calculated by dividing the gram molecular weight of a substance by the valence, or the number of hydrogens that it can replace or combine with. If a substance is monovalent, the gram equivalent weight is equal to the gram molecular weight; however, if a substance is polyvalent, the equivalent weight is less than the molecular weight. For example, NaCl, when dissociated, forms one Na^+ ion and one Cl^- ion. One mole of Cl^- will combine with one mole of H^+ in a chemical reaction, so NaCl has an equivalent weight equal to 1 mole of NaCl. One mole of NaCl is equal to 58.5 g, and one equivalent weight of NaCl is equal to 58.5 g. If K_2SO_4 is placed in a solvent, it will dissociate into two K^+ ions and one SO_4 ion, and this SO_4 ion can combine with two moles of hydrogen. In this case, K_2SO_4 has an equivalent weight equal to 0.5 mole of K_2SO_4 because two hydrogen ions will combine with one SO_4 ion (equivalent weight is equal to the gram molecular weight divided by the number of hydrogens that it can combine with or replace). One mole of K_2SO_4 is equal to 168 g, and 0.5 mole of K_2SO_4 is equal to 84 g, so one equivalent weight of K_2SO_4 is equal to 84 g. Equivalent weights expressed in milligrams are referred to as *milliequivalents (mEq).*

Normality (N) is expressed as the number of equivalent weights per liter of solution (Eq/L). The term "1-normal solution" is defined as one equivalent weight of a substance in 1 liter of solution; likewise, a 12-normal solution is defined as 12 equivalent weights of a substance in 1 liter of solution. To prepare a 1-normal solution of NaCl, for example, it is necessary to first determine the equivalent weight of the compound. Because only one hydrogen ion will combine with a Cl^- ion, the equivalent weight is equal to the gram molecular weight (58.5 g), and therefore 58.5 g of NaCl added to 1 liter of solvent will produce a 1N or 1 Eq/l solution of NaCl. Preparation of a 1-normal solution of K_2SO_4 requires determination of the equivalent weight of the compound. In the case of this compound, SO_4 will combine with two hydrogen ions, so the equivalent weight is equal to one half of the gram molecular weight. Therefore, adding 84 g of K_2SO_4 to 1 liter of solvent will produce a 1N solution of K_2SO_4.

To determine what amount of solute must be added to a solvent to make a solution of a specific normality, a calculation similar to those used in the determination of molarity is used. The traditional method of calculating normality problems is similar to the calculation for molarity problems except that it is critical to determine the equivalent weight of the substance in question prior to setting up the equation. The quick and simple method can be used to calculate normality problems as well, although equivalent weight must be determined first. The formula for calculating normality is

$$N = \frac{g/l}{Eq/l}$$

Only this method of normality calculation is examined here.

Example 4–6 How many grams of HCl are required to make a 6N solution of HCl in 1 liter of buffer?

- ■ Gram molecular weight of HCl = 35 g
- ■ Equivalent weight of HCl = 35 g

$$6N = \frac{g/l}{35\ g} \quad or \quad 6 \times 35 = 210\ g/l$$

Therefore, 210 g of HCl must be placed in 1 liter of buffer to make a 6N solution of HCl.

Example 4–7 What is the normality of a solution containing 50 g of NaOH in 300 ml of buffer?

- ■ Gram molecular weight of NaOH = 40 g
- ■ Equivalent weight of NaOH = 40 g

$$N = \frac{50\ g/0.300\ liter}{40\ g} = \frac{166.7}{40} = 4.2\ Eq/l$$

Example 4–8   What is the normality of a solution containing 80 g of H_2SO_4 in 450 ml of buffer?

- Gram molecular weight of H_2SO_4 = 98 g
- Equivalent weight of H_2SO_4 = 49 g

$$N = \frac{80 \text{ g}/0.450 \text{ liter}}{49 \text{ g}} = \frac{177}{49} = 3.6 \text{ Eq/l}$$

PERCENT CONCENTRATION

Concentration can be expressed as a percentage, or parts of solute per 100 parts of solvent. When a concentration is described as parts of a solid in 100 parts of a liquid, it is expressed as *weight per volume (w/v)*. An example of a weight per volume description would be "grams per deciliter," a typical description of analyte concentration in a patient's blood. In the clinical and research laboratory, this is the most commonly used description of percent concentration. If a liquid solute is added to a liquid solvent, it is described as a *volume per volume (v/v)* comparison. In contrast to molarity and normality, percent concentration is not dependent on the molecular or equivalent weight of the compound in question, but only on the weight or volume of a substance in 100 parts of the dissolving medium.

In calculating percent solution problems, the first step is to determine the amount of solute per 100 parts of solvent. For example, a 5% solution of NaOH in buffer contains 5 g of solid NaCl in 100 ml of buffer, a 20% solution would contain 20 g per 100 ml, and a 0.1% solution would contain 0.1 g, or 100 mg, per 100 ml of buffer. To determine how much solute to add to a solvent to obtain a given percentage solution of specified volume, a simple ratio equation is used.

Example 4–9   Make 350 ml of an 8% solution of NaOH in buffer.

$$\frac{8}{100} = \frac{x}{350} \quad or \quad 2,800 = 100x \quad or \quad x = 28$$

Therefore, 28 g of NaOH must be diluted up to 350 ml of buffer to obtain an 8% solution.

Example 4–10   What is the percent concentration of a solution that contains 90 g of NaOH in 750 ml of buffer?

$$\frac{90}{750} = \frac{x}{100} \quad or \quad 750x = 9,000 \quad or \quad x = 12$$

Therefore, 90 g of NaOH in 750 ml of buffer is a 12% solution.

When a solution of lesser concentration must be made from a solution of greater concentration, a different calculation than the one discussed previously must be used. Instead of a ratio equation, an inverse proportion calculation must be performed in which the volume of one solution multiplied by the concentration of that solution is equal to the volume of a second solution multiplied by the concentration of that solution. Written in notation: $V_1 \times C_1 = V_2 \times C_2$, in which V is volume and C is concentration. It is important to remember that the units (of both volume and concentration) on both sides of the equation must be the same.

Example 4–11 Fifty milliliters of a 7% solution of HCl is needed and only a 37% solution of HCl is available.

$$50 \times 7 = V \times 37 \quad or \quad 350 = V \times 37 \quad or \quad 9.5 = V$$

Therefore, 9.5 ml of 37% HCl is diluted up to 50 ml to make 50 ml of a 7% solution.

Complex Problems

In the laboratory, it is sometimes necessary to make a working solution described by a particular unit concentration from a concentrated stock solution that is given in a different unit concentration. For example, it may be that a solution of 10% NaOH must be made from a concentrated stock solution of 12N NaOH. These kinds of calculations are relatively simple provided the proper units are used in the equation. Percent solutions are always given in parts per 100 parts, molarity is always described in moles per 1,000 ml, and normality is described as equivalents per 1,000 ml. Once the equation is set up, solving the problem is straightforward.

Example 4–12 Prepare 500 ml of a 25% working solution of NaOH in water from a stock solution of 12N NaOH.

$$\frac{25}{100} = \frac{x}{500} \quad or \quad 100x = 12,500 \quad or \quad x = 125$$

Therefore, 125 ml of 12N NaOH diluted up to 500 ml of water equals a 25% solution.

Example 4–13 Prepare 500 ml of a 0.3-mol/l solution of HCl in water from a stock solution of 25% HCl. Molarity must first be changed to a percentage in order to calculate this problem. The formula for calculation of molarity is

$$M = \frac{g/l}{MW} \quad or \quad \frac{g/100 \text{ ml} \times 10}{MW} \quad or \quad \frac{\% \times 10}{MW}$$

Thus

$$0.3 \text{ mol/l} = \frac{x \times 10}{36.5} \quad or \quad 0.3 \times 36.5 = x \times 10 \quad or \quad 10.95 = x \times 10 \quad or \quad x = 1.95$$

Therefore, 0.3 mol/l = 1.95%. Using the equivalent formula $V_1 \times C_1 = V_2 \times C_2$ and the percent concentration for C,

$$500 \times 1.95 = V_2 \times 25$$
$$975 = V_2 \times 25$$
$$39 = V_2$$

Therefore, 39 ml of the 25% stock HCl solution diluted up to 500 ml with water will equal a 0.3-mol/l solution of HCl.

OSMOLARITY

Osmolarity *describes the number of moles of particles per kilogram of solvent and depends on the number of particles, not the kind of particles, present.* It is denoted as osmoles per kilogram

(Osm/kg), and an *osmole* is the amount of a substance that dissociates to produce 1 mole of particles in a solution. In the analysis of body fluids, the term "milliosmole" (mOsm) is typically used. As an example, when NaCl is added to water, it breaks down to Na^+ and Cl^- ions, so 1.0 mole of NaCl equals 2 Osm (or 1.0 mmol of NaCl equals 2 mOsm).

In urine, the solutes are varied depending upon which pass through the renal tubule wall and which are secreted by the tubules. Solutes in serum vary as well, and an important relationship between calculated serum osmolarity and measured osmolarity exists when the presence of an unusual solute is suspected. The formula for calculating serum osmolarity (mOsm/kg) is as follows:

$$[2 \times \text{Na concentration (mEq/L)}] + \frac{\text{glucose concentration (mg/dl)}}{18} + \frac{\text{BUN (mg/dl)}}{2.8}$$

where BUN is the blood urea nitrogen level. If the difference between the measured osmolarity (using vapor-pressure depression or freezing-point depression) and the calculated osmolarity is greater than zero, this is an indication that an abnormal concentration of some unmeasured substance is contributing to an elevated serum osmolarity. The difference between the two is referred to as the **osmolal gap.**

Urine osmolarity ranges from 275 to 900 mOsm/kg while serum osmolarity ranges from 275 to 300 mOsm/kg.

SPECIFIC GRAVITY

In the laboratory, specific gravity is used both in the description of concentrated solutions (typically acids) and in the determination of the amount of solutes present in urine. **Specific gravity** is a description of *density,* which is an expression of the amount of mass per volume; therefore, specific gravity measurements depend on the number of solutes present as well as the mass of the solutes in a given volume. To determine specific gravity, the mass of a substance is compared to the mass of an equal volume of pure water at 4° C. Because water has a mass of 1 g/ml, specific gravity is the mass in grams of 1 ml of a substance.

In the case of concentrated solvents, the specific gravity is noted on the container with a value referred to as *percent purity.* The specific gravity value is a statement of mass in grams per milliliter and the percent purity value tells how much of this 1-ml mass is actually the solute used to make up the solution. For example, a container of HCl has a specific gravity of 1.19 and a 53% purity. This means that there are 1.19 g of mass in 1 ml of the solution and 53% of the 1.19 g is HCl. The next step is to determine how much of the 1.19 g of mass is actually HCl. The equation is set up as follows:

$$1.19 \text{ g/ml} \times 0.53 = 0.63 \text{ g of HCl/ml of solution}$$

To determine how many milliliters of solution contains 1.0 g of HCl, a ratio equation is set up:

$$\frac{0.63 \text{ g}}{1 \text{ ml}} = \frac{1 \text{ g}}{x \text{ ml}} \quad or \quad 0.63x = 1 \quad or \quad x = 1.58 \text{ ml}$$

Therefore, 1.58 ml of solution contains 1 g of HCl.

In urine, specific gravity is related to osmolality. However, because the solutes in urine, such as urea, protein, glucose, and NaCl, differ in mass (but not necessarily in number of particles per mole), the specific gravity is affected more than the osmolality when these solutes are present in abnormal concentrations. Normal urine specific gravity ranges from 1.002 to 1.035 g/ml.

pH AND ACID–BASE RELATIONSHIPS

Because of the wide availability of accurate and precise pH meters and blood gas analyzers, it is unnecessary to devote a great deal of time to the calculation of these parameters. However, a brief review of the formulas used to derive these values is given.

pH

Molecules are formed by the interaction of positively and negatively charged ions through the formation of ionic bonds. When certain compounds or molecules are dissociated in water (or another solvent), they contribute either hydrogen (H^+) ions or hydroxyl (OH^-) ions to the solution. Those that contribute H^+ ions are referred to as *acids*, those that contribute OH^- ions are called *bases*, and those molecules that contribute neither are called *salts*. An example of an acid would be H_2SO_4, which dissociates into two H^+ ions and a sulfate ion. A base such as NaOH breaks apart into a sodium ion and an OH^- ion. Salts such as NaCl or $MgSO_4$ dissociate into their component ions without contributing either a H^+ ion or an OH^- ion to the solution. When a solution is referred to as "acidic," it contains many free H^+ ions; in other words, it has a high H^+ ion concentration. A solution containing more OH^- than H^+ ions is referred to as a "basic" or "alkaline" solution and has a high OH^- concentration. The *pH ("potential of hydrogen") scale* was formulated to express the degree of acidity or alkalinity of a solution.

pH is an expression of the H^+ ion concentration in a solution. It is typically defined as the negative logarithm of the hydrogen ion concentration, and the pH scale uses the numbers 0 to 14 to describe the acidity or alkalinity of a solution. The scale of 0 to 14 is derived from the fact that, in an aqueous solution, the concentration of hydrogen ions multiplied by the concentration of hydroxyl ions always equals 1×10^{-14}. The equation used to determine the pH of a solution is stated as $pH = -\log[H^+]$. As the hydrogen ion concentration decreases, the pH value increases. A 1-molar solution of hydrogen ion (a 10^{-14}-molar solution of hydroxyl ion) is equal to a pH of 0, and a 1-molar solution of hydroxyl ion (a 10^{-14}-molar solution of hydrogen ion) is equal to a pH of 14. A 0.1-molar hydrogen ion concentration is equal to a pH of 1. Therefore, a change of one pH unit on the pH scale is equal to a 10-fold decrease (or increase) of hydrogen ion concentration. A solution with a pH of 7.0 is considered neutral.

A QUICK WORD ABOUT LOGARITHMS

So, what is a logarithm? *There are two types of logarithms,* **common logarithms** (*log or log₁₀*) using a base 10 and **natural logarithms** *(ln) using a base e* = 2.718. . . . A logarithm of a number x is simply the exponent to which the designated base (10 or e) must be raised in order to equal that number. Logarithms are composed of two parts, a character and a mantissa. For example, in $\log_{10} 50 = 1.699$, the character is 1 and the mantissa is 0.699. Because logarithms are exponents, the logarithm of the product of two numbers is the sum of the logarithms of the numbers: $\log xy = \log x + \log y$. Therefore, $\log_{10} 50 = \log (5 \times 10)$ $= \log 5 + \log 10$; the log of 5 (0.699) added to the log of 10 (1.0) = 1.699. Large numbers are first put in exponential form: $\log_{10} 56,800,000 = \log (5.68 \times 10^7) = \log 5.68 +$ $\log 10^7$. The log of 5.68 is 0.7543 and the log of 10^7 is 7.0; therefore the answer equals 7.7543. Numbers less than 1 will produce a negative logarithm, such as $\log_{10} 0.000367 =$ $\log (3.67 \times 10^{-4}) = \log 3.67 + \log 10^{-4} = 0.5647 - 4 = -3.4353$. Log values are found in basic logarithm tables.

ACID-BASE RELATIONSHIPS

In human blood, normal pH lies in the range of 7.35 to 7.45, which is equivalent to a hydrogen ion concentration of approximately 4.0×10^{-8} mol/l. To maintain this pH, the blood contains several buffer systems that act in concert to respond to alterations in pH. The bicarbonate buffer system consists of water, carbon dioxide (CO_2), carbonic acid (H_2CO_3), bicarbonate (HCO_3^-), and protons (H^+), and the relationship between these components is written:

$$H_2O + CO_2 \leftrightarrow H_2CO_3 \leftrightarrow H^+ + HCO_3^-$$

Removal of CO_2 from the body is the primary function of this buffer system. During normal cellular metabolism, CO_2 is formed in the tissues and combines with water to form H_2CO_3, which is quickly broken down into H^+ and HCO_3^-. A second buffer system, hemoglobin, accepts the proton and becomes deoxyhemoglobin (HHb). HHb moves to the lungs, where the proton is removed and oxygen is again attached to the hemoglobin to form oxyhemoglobin. In the lungs, the extra protons are scooped up by the bicarbonate buffer system to combine with HCO_3^- and form H_2CO_3, which breaks down into CO_2 and water. The CO_2 is then exhaled.

"Blood gases" that are directly measured include P_{CO_2}, P_{O_2}, and pH. Other parameters, including oxygen saturation, oxygen content, total CO_2, bicarbonate, and base excess, are calculated using the values obtained by direct measurement of blood gases. In the determination of the acid-base status of whole blood, a special equation relates the concentration of base (HCO_3^-) and the concentration of acid (H_2CO_3) in the blood to blood pH. The **Henderson-Hasselbalch equation** states this as

$$pH = pK + \log \frac{[HCO_3^-]}{[H_2CO_3]}$$

where pK is the pH of the bicarbonate–carbonic acid buffer system at which protonated and nonprotonated species are equal. In human plasma, the pK is equal to 6.1, and in whole blood the pK equals 6.3 (due to the presence of erythrocytes).

Because not all of the components of blood gas analysis are measured directly, the Henderson-Hasselbalch equation is programmed into blood gas analyzers to determine the concentration of bicarbonate in the blood. P_{CO_2} as well as pH values can be determined and placed into this equation to give a measurement of the bicarbonate value. Nomograms are also available to determine bicarbonate level in whole blood.

PHOTOMETRY CALCULATIONS

In spite of the sophistication of laboratory instrumentation, most analyzers depend on basic principles such as photometry, immunology, flow cytometry, and potentiometry to perform complicated procedures. Although the principles of these reactions are not discussed here, the basic mathematical formulas used in photometry determinations are presented.

PHOTOMETRY

Photometry *is the measurement of light.* In a laboratory situation where the concentration of a substance is of interest, light of a specific intensity (referred to as incident light, l_o) is directed through a solution and is absorbed by the molecules in that solution. Some light, however, passes through the solution, and the intensity of this light (intensity of transmitted light, l_s) is measured by a photometer. This can be written as a formula: *the intensity of transmitted light divided by the intensity of incident light is equal to* **transmittance** *(T), or* $l_s/l_o = T.$ *Only* transmittance, in relation to concentration, can be photometrically determined. In a chemical analysis, the transmittance of an unknown solution is compared to the transmittance of a reference sample, or "blank." The blank contains the same solvent as the unknown solution but not the substance of interest, so the transmittance of this blank is measured at 100, meaning 100% of the light passing into the solution is transmitted through it. Increased substance concentration will cause the transmittance of a solution to vary inversely and logarithmically.

    The amount of light absorbed by the solution is called the **absorbance** *of that solution and is equal to the concentration of a substance in solution multiplied by the length of the path that the light must pass through multiplied by the molar absorptivity of the substance of interest.* This statement is referred to as **Beer's Law** and is written mathematically as $A = abc$, where A is the absorbance (absorbance has no units), a is the absorptivity of a substance (a constant expressed in millimolars) at a given wavelength, b is the length of the light path in centimeters (typically 1 cm), and c is the concentration (in grams per deciliter). The formula can be rearranged to determine the value of any variable in the equation, for example, the concentration: $c = A/ab$. As opposed to transmittance, the absorbance changes in a linear fashion in *direct* proportion to the concentration of a substance in solution. Beer's law forms the basis for quantitative absorption photometric analysis. The following examples illustrate the relationship of concentration to absorbance.

Example 4–14   The absorbance of a glucose solution has been determined to be 0.311 using the hexokinase G6PD method. What is the concentration of this solution? The cuvette has a 1-cm light path and the absorptivity of NADH is 0.622 mM.

$$A = abc, \quad or \quad c = A/ab$$
$$c = 0.311/(0.622 \times 1)$$
$$c = 0.5 \text{ mM}$$

Because only transmitted light can be photometrically measured, absorbance must be calculated. By determining the percentage of light that has been transmitted through a solution (%T), the amount of absorbed light may be determined. Since the %T varies inversely and logarithmically with concentration, the absorbance is equal to the negative log of T or log $1/T$. This is equal to $2 - \log \%T$. Using this calculation, it can be observed that, if the %T of a solution is 100, the absorbance is 0; if the %T is 0, the absorbance is 1.0. The following example illustrates the relationship of absorbance to %T.

Example 4–15   The transmittance of a solution is 25%T compared to the blank reading of 100. What is the absorbance of this solution?

$$A = 2 - \log \%T$$
$$A = 2 - \log 25$$
$$\log 25 = 1.3979$$
$$A = 2 - 1.3979$$
$$A = 0.6021$$

STANDARD CURVE

In the determination of a concentration of a substance in solution, the absorbance of standard solutions is measured and plotted against the known concentration of the standards. The resulting graph is referred to as a **standard curve.** Concentration of an unknown solution is determined by using this plot. Typical clinical analyzers calculate this information in their computers and output the information as a patient result.

A typical standard curve plots the absorbance value on the y axis and the standard concentrations on the x axis. A linear relationship should be observed between the absorbance and concentration. Figure 4–1 shows a standard curve of absorbance versus glucose standard concentration.

If the absorbance values are linear in relationship to concentration, Beer's law can be utilized to determine the concentration of an unknown when standards of known concentration are used in the analysis. Once the absorbance of the standards (std) and unknown (unk) are known, the concentration of the unknown can be calculated. The formula is based upon Beer's law and is stated as follows:

$$\frac{\text{Absorbance}_{unk}}{\text{Absorbance}_{std}} \times \text{Concentration}_{std} = \text{Concentration}_{unk}$$

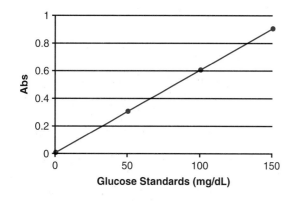

FIGURE 4-1

Example of a standard curve. Absorbance values are plotted on the y axis and the standard concentrations are on the x axis.

For example, if the concentration of a glucose standard is 50 mg/dl and the absorbance value is determined to be 0.19, and the absorbance of an unknown specimen is determined to be 0.135, the concentration of this unknown can be calculated as

$$\frac{0.135}{0.19} \times 50 \text{ mg/dl} = 35.5 \text{ mg/dl glucose}$$

Understanding this information is critical in understanding the operation of certain instrumentation that uses photometry as the basis for measuring analyte concentration.

BASIC STATISTICS

An important component of clinical or research analysis is gathering and interpreting data. These data must be statistically analyzed to demonstrate that they are significantly useful to those who require them for making diagnostic predictions, formulating hypotheses, or demonstrating trends. Statistical analysis includes various formulas applied to data for the purpose of describing the location and dispersion of those data compared to an average value. This type of analysis is referred to as *"descriptive" statistics*, and the formulas used are called *measures of central tendency*. *Inferential statistics* is analysis based upon statistical formulas that compare two or more groups of data and make inferences regarding a large population based on a small portion of that population. Although it is not in the scope of this text to explain all statistical formulas, those basic statistical analyses that are required to evaluate control values and have a bearing on quality control (and therefore on quality management) are presented.

MEAN, MODE, MEDIAN, AND RANGE

As mentioned, descriptive statistics describes data in relation to a central value, usually the average value in a set of values. *This average value is referred to as the* **mean** *value and is calculated by summing a set of values and dividing the sum by the number of values observed.* The formula for calculating the mean is written

$$\bar{x} = \frac{x_1 + x_2 + x_3 \ldots + x_n}{n}$$

where $\bar{x}$ (*x*-bar) is the mean, x is each individual value, and n is the number of values or observations. For example, consider the following group of values: 10, 9, 8, 9, 9, 10, 8, 7, 10, 10. To determine the mean or average value, first sum the values (90), then divide this sum by the number of values (10); the average is thus calculated to be 9. Therefore, the $\bar{x}$ for these data is 9.

Another way of describing data in relation to a central point is by determining the "mode" value of the data. *The* **mode** *is the value that occurs with the greatest frequency in a set of values.* Using the group of values given previously, it is observed that the value "10" occurs most often in the group; therefore, the mode of this set of data is 10. If the values 9 and 10 occurred with equal frequency, the two values are added together and divided by two to obtain a mode value of 9.5.

Similar to both mean and mode is the "median" value of a group of data. *The* **median** *is that value that occurs in the middle of a set of values when the values are arranged in increasing magnitude.* By "middle" it is meant that the same number of values lie above and below the central value. By arranging the above data in increasing magnitude (i.e., 7, 8, 8, 9, 9, 9, 10, 10, 10, 10), one can observe that there are actually two central values, both of which are 9. Therefore, the median value of this set is 9. If the two central values are not the same, they must be added together and divided by 2 to obtain the median value. The median is considered to be a more accurate description of the central tendency of a set of data points or values.

A simple statistic that describes data is referred to as the "range." *The **range** is a single number calculated by subtracting the lowest value in a group of values from the highest.* The range of the values given above would be 10 − 7, or 3. Range is used when preparing frequency histograms in a medical laboratory.

STANDARD DEVIATION

Standard deviation (*s* or SD) is the most commonly used descriptive statistic in the laboratory for describing the dispersion of data around a central value. Before calculating the standard deviation for a set of values, the mean must be determined. *The **variance** of the data illustrates how much the values vary from this mean, and the **standard deviation** is the square root of the variance.* When a set of observations is plotted on a frequency histogram with frequency (number of values observed) plotted on the *y* axis and actual values plotted on the *x* axis, most values are spread around the mean value. Some values, however, are farther away from the mean than others. If a curve were drawn to encompass all values, it would represent a "normal" curve or distribution, also referred to as a *Gaussian distribution.* In the laboratory, only certain values are acceptable, and those values are determined by calculating the standard deviation.

The formula for standard deviation is as follows:

$$s = \sqrt{\frac{\Sigma(\bar{x} - x_i)^2}{n - 1}}$$

where *s* is the standard deviation, Σ means "the sum of," $\bar{x}$ is the mean of the set of values, x_i is each individual value, and $n - 1$ is the number of observations minus 1. To calculate standard deviation, first subtract each individual value from the mean and then square the value. Add all of these squared values and divide by $n - 1$. Finally, determine the square root of this number; that will be the standard deviation. The standard deviation tells how much the data deviate (vary) from the mean.

In the clinical laboratory, control fluid is analyzed with each set of patient unknowns to assess the precision and integrity of analytic variables such as pipetting, equipment function, and reagent quality. Daily control values are analyzed statistically using mean and standard deviation and then are plotted on a *Levey-Jennings control chart* (Fig. 4–2). Typically, acceptable control values are considered to be those that lie within ±2 standard deviations from the mean. These limits include approximately 95% of the values obtained and are referred to as *95% confidence limits.* In other words, you are confident that the control results you obtain are accurate 95% of the time and are not obtained due to chance. If control values fall outside of these limits, specific actions must be initiated prior to the release of any

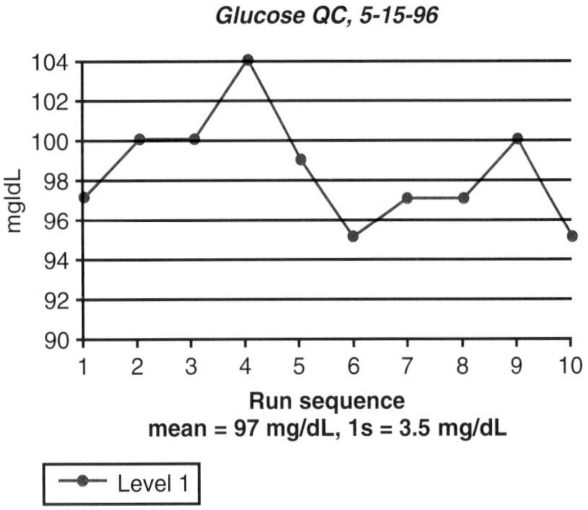

Glucose QC, 5-15-96

FIGURE 4-2

Example of a Levey-Jennings control chart showing glucose quality control (QC) values plotted over 10 days.

patient results, including equipment and reagent assessment, reanalysis of the control fluid, and contact with the equipment or reagent manufacturer.

COEFFICIENT OF VARIATION

Laboratory analyses produce results, and these results are expressed in values and units. For example, a patient's glucose value is 96 and the units reported by the lab are milligrams per deciliter. Many times it is important to compare two different data sets obtained by performing two different procedures and resulting in different units. An appropriate method of comparing different procedures is to compare how much the data in each set vary from their respective means. When comparing the relative variability of two different sets of values that are described by different units, it is best to use a statistic referred to as the "**coefficient of variation**" (CV). The CV is expressed as a percentage and is calculated using the standard deviation and the mean:

$$CV\% = \frac{\text{standard deviation}}{\text{mean}} \times 100\%$$

CHAPTER SUMMARY

Understanding laboratory mathematics is essential for working in any laboratory. The metric system is used exclusively in clinical and research laboratories and is the basis of any analytical measurement made in a clinical laboratory setting. Despite the prevalence of "kit" packaging of many reagents for use in analytical tests, it is wise to have a working knowledge of molarity and normality calculations in the event that substitutions must be made for kit components. Most reagents used in research laboratories, whether basic science or clinical, must be formulated from stock solutions or from dry chemicals. It is important as well to know how to prepare dilutions not only in the preparation of reagents but in analyzing patient samples.

Although automation has changed the clinical laboratory dramatically, requiring less of a laboratory scientist's time and effort in performing mathematical calculations, a basic knowledge of the background formulas involved in analytical measurements leads to an understanding of the principles involved in the measurement. Blood gas analysis and pH calculations are examples of this, as are the formulas involved in photometric measurements. Preparation of standard curves is rarely performed manually, yet use of a standard curve (the plot of standard calibrator values versus absorbance readings) is the method by which most analyzers determine analytical concentration of various substances in patient samples.

Finally, a most critical component of any laboratory are the quality control procedures used to assess performance. Again, many of these procedures are a component of automated systems, yet laboratorians must check the quality control of laboratory instrumentation to determine whether the assayed values are accurate and precise. A working knowledge of the terminology and calculations involved in quality control is essential for a laboratory scientist to produce quality results.

Review Questions

1. Convert 220 milliliters to deciliters.

2. How many milligrams equal 0.01 g?

3. Convert 75 Fahrenheit degrees to Celsius degrees.

4. Define "mole."

5. Calculate the molarity of each of the following:
   a.   60 g NaOH in total volume of 300 ml of water
   b.   112 g $BaSO_4$ in total volume of 700 ml of buffer

6. Determine the molarity, normality, and percent (w/v) for a solution containing 50 g of NaCl in 500 ml of distilled water.

7. How many milliliters of a 3% solution can be made if 6 g of solute are available?

8. What is the normality of a solution containing 100 g of H_2SO_4 in 450 ml of buffer?

9. Which one of the following is the formula for calculating the molarity of a substance in solution?
   a. $\dfrac{\text{number of grams of solute}}{\text{liter of solution}} \times$ the gram molecular weight
   b.   number of moles of solute $\times$ 100
   c.   gram equivalent weight of solute $\times$ 10
   d. $\dfrac{\text{gram equivalent weight of solute}}{\text{liter of solution}}$

10. Which one of the following is the formula for calculating the equivalent weight of a compound?
   a. $\dfrac{\text{gram molecular weight}}{\text{\# of replaceable hydrogens or valence}}$

b. gram molecular weight × # of hydrogens or valence

c. gram molecular weight + # of hydrogens or valence

d. gram molecular weight − # of hydrogens or valence

11. A photometric method calls for the use of 0.1 ml of serum, 5 ml of reagent, and 4.9 ml of water. What is the dilution of the serum in the final solution?

12. State the Henderson-Hasselbalch equation.

13. Calculate the protein concentration of a sample with an absorbance of 0.03 if the standard concentration is 4.0 g/dl and the absorbance of the standard is 0.018.

14. Calculate the coefficient of variation when 1 standard deviation (*s*) equals ±7 mg/dl and the mean = 89 mg/dl.

15. In a Gaussian (normal) distribution, the ±2*s* range includes what percentage of values (confidence limits)?

a. 95.5%

b. 99.7%

c. 68.3%

d. 31.6%

16. Given the following values—100, 120, 150, 140, 130—calculate the mean.

17. Which of the following is the formula for standard deviation?

a. square root of the mean

b. square root of $\dfrac{\text{(sum of squared differences)}}{n-1}$

c. $\dfrac{\text{(sum of squared differences)}}{n-1}$

d. square root of $\dfrac{\text{mean}}{\text{(sum of squared differences)}}$

18. The following values (in mg/dl) were obtained from a group sample of glucose measurements: 109, 102, 104, 97, 105, 98, 100, 96, 103, 97, 96, 97, 97, 104, 99, 105, 94, 95, 97, 100. Calculate the mean, mode, median, standard deviation, and CV.

PART II

Clinical Disciplines and Applications to Functions of the Body System

CHAPTER 5
The Musculoskeletal System

INTRODUCTION

ANATOMY AND FUNCTION OF THE
SKELETAL SYSTEM
**Subdivisions of the Skeletal
    System**
    Axial skeletal system
    Visceral skeletal system
    Appendicular skeletal system
**Structure and Chemistry of
    Bone**
Cellular Elements of Bone
**Hormonal Control of Skeletal
    Homeostasis**
Major Bone Diseases
    Rickets
    Osteomalacia
    Osteoporosis
    Bone tumors

THE MUSCULAR SYSTEM
**Microscopic Structure of the
    Muscle Cell**
    Skeletal muscle
    Cardiac muscle
    Smooth muscle
**Physiology of Muscle
    Contraction**
Skeletal Muscle Disorders

LABORATORY TESTS ASSOCIATED
WITH MUSCULOSKELETAL
DISORDERS

CHAPTER SUMMARY

REVIEW QUESTIONS

Objectives

1. Describe the anatomy of the musculoskeletal system.
2. Describe the structure and chemistry of bone.
3. Describe the functions of the skeletal system.
4. Describe the hormonal control of bone metabolism.
5. Describe the major bone diseases: ricketts, osteomalacia, and osteoporosis.
6. Describe the microscopic structure of skeletal muscle.
7. Describe the different types of muscle: skeletal muscle, cardiac muscle, and smooth muscle.
8. Describe the mechanism of muscle contraction.
9. Describe skeletal muscle disorders, such as muscular dystrophies.
10. Describe and correlate laboratory tests with musculoskeletal disorders.

KEY TERMS

musculoskeletal system	diaphysis	osteoclast	myofibrils
axial skeletal system	epiphyses	acid phosphatase	sarcoplasm
visceral skeletal system	metaphysis	lacunae	myoglobin
thoracic basket	cortical bone	rickets	type I fibers
sternum	cancellous (trabecular)	osteomalacia	type II fibers
costal cartilage	bone	osteoporosis	myopathy
appendicular skeletal	osteoblast	Klinefelter's syndrome	muscular dystrophy
system	alkaline phosphatase	multiple myeloma	isoenzyme
pelvic girdle	epiphyseal plate	cardiac muscle	lactate dehydrogenase
pectoral girdle	osteocyte	smooth muscle	creatine kinase
ligaments	canaliculi	striated muscle	

Introduction

The **musculoskeletal system** *is a mechanical system made up of bones (the skeleton) and several unique tissues and organs which produce various degrees of rigidity: the components include cartilage, ligament, tendon, and of course muscle, which has a very high degree of contractility.* The musculoskeletal system performs three major functions: movement (locomotion), support, and protection. The human body contains more than 430 muscles that can be classified into three main groups: cardiac, smooth, and striated. Cardiac muscles, as the name suggests, occur mostly in the walls of the heart; smooth muscles are found predominantly in the gastrointestinal tract and the walls of blood vessels; and striated (skeletal) muscles comprise about 40% of the total body weight and are usually associated with the skeleton.

A number of individual bones of different shapes and sizes are recruited in different combinations to provide three basic functions in the body. The function of locomotion is accomplished through the formation of movable joints in association with different muscle groups. Cartilage plates at the ends of the bones help to reduce friction, prevent bone erosion, and ensure smooth movement. The skeletal movements may take place in all directions, as in the ball-and-socket joints of the shoulders and the hips, the wrists, and the neck, or the movement could be restricted to only one plane, as in the knee. In addition to movement, the bones provide the architectural framework upon which the soft muscular tissues of the body are anchored. Therefore, they must be strong enough to carry the bulk of the body weight. Portions of the bones have also been modified to provide protection for the delicate parts of the body. For example, the skull protects the brain, the vertebral column protects the spinal cord, and the rib cage protects the heart, lungs, and liver during breathing and movement. The bone may also be seen as the predominant reservoir for minerals such as calcium and phosphate. Although the skeletal system appears to be relatively inert, it is actually well vascularized, and, through the action of hormones, the process of bone resorption (breakdown) and formation is used to regulate the mineral homeostasis for the body.

This chapter describes the structure and composition of the musculoskeletal system and the physiology of muscle contraction, and discusses how skeletal mineral homeostasis is controlled. Major bone and skeletal muscle disorders and the laboratory tests associated with some of the musculoskeletal diseases are discussed.

ANATOMY AND FUNCTION OF THE SKELETAL SYSTEM

SUBDIVISIONS OF THE SKELETAL SYSTEM

The human skeleton (Fig. 5–1) is made up of over 200 bones of different shapes and sizes that may be loosely divided into three subdivisions. These subdivisions are loosely made because they are based essentially on function, and in fact all three systems may perform similar functions (e.g., protection), only of a different type and at different locations in the body.

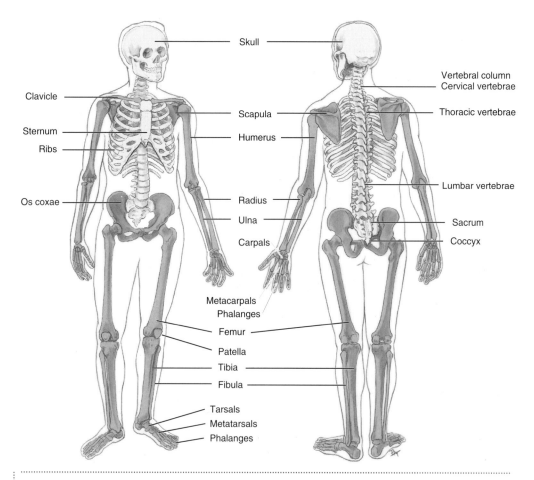

FIGURE 5-1

Bones of the human skeleton.
(From Applegate, E.J.: The Anatomy and Physiology Learning System. Philadelphia, W.B. Saunders, 1995, with permission.)

Axial Skeletal System

The first group is called the **axial skeletal system** *which comprises the vertebral column (the spine) and much of the skull* (Fig. 5–2*A*). The axial skeletal system provides protection for the central nervous system; the brain, for example, is sheltered in the *skull* and the spinal cord is protected by the *vertebral column*. The vertebral column also serves as a support for the trunk, and, although the vertebral column of a newborn child is relatively straight, the column becomes S-shaped in the adult. With this conformation, the vertebral column is able to absorb the shocks of walking on hard surfaces. As shown in Figure 5–2*B*, the vertebral

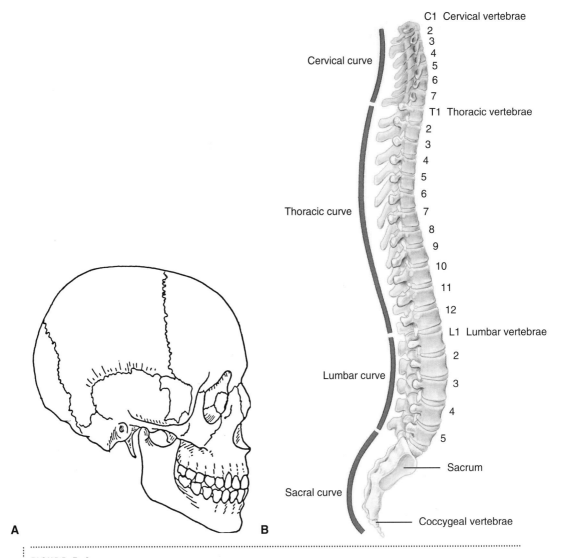

FIGURE 5-2

Axial skeletal system. *A*, Cranial bones. *B*, Vertebral bones.
(From Applegate, E.J.: The Anatomy and Physiology Learning System. Philadelphia, W.B.
Saunders, 1995, with permission.)

column has five structurally distinct segments: the *cervical* has 7 bones, the *thoracic* has 12, the *lumbar* has 5, the *sacral* has 5, and the *coccygeal*, or tailbone, segment contains 4 to 5 small bones. The individual bones in these segments have distinctive shapes and sizes that are adapted to providing firm anchoring holds for different types of muscle groups. The intervertebral discs, made up of cartilage, protect the ends of the individual bones from erosion as they rub against adjacent bones.

Visceral Skeletal System

The second subdivision of the skeleton is termed the **visceral skeletal system.** This is formed by the attachment of the vertebral column to the rib cage (or **thoracic basket**) with 24 ribs and a breastbone (or **sternum**). The first seven curved ribs are termed "true ribs" because they are attached to the sternum by **costal cartilages.** Of the remaining five ribs, three have their costal cartilages connected only to the cartilages above them and have no connection with the sternum. They are therefore described as "false ribs." The last two are termed "floating ribs," and their costal cartilages end in the muscles of the abdominal wall. The rib cage serves as a protective shield for the heart, lungs, and other vital organs in the chest. The small joints between the ribs and the vertebral column are made of ligament attachments that permit only a limited gliding motion during breathing and other activities.

Appendicular Skeletal System

The third collection of bones constitutes the **appendicular skeletal system**. This is composed of the hip **(pelvic)** and shoulder **(pectoral) girdles** and their attachment to the long bones of the upper arms (*humerus*) and thighs (*femur*) and cartilage of the limbs, respectively. The pelvic girdle, composed of three fused bones, is joined to the vertebral column by the *sacroiliac joint*. The pectoral girdle is composed of the shoulder blade (*scapula*) and the collar bone (*clavicle*). Unlike the upper arm and the thigh, which have only one long bone each, the forearm and the lower leg have two bones each. In the forearm are the *radius*, located on the thumb side, and the *ulna*, located toward the little finger. The bones in the lower leg are the *tibia* (the shinbone) and the *fibula*. The radius corresponds to the tibia and the ulna corresponds to the fibula.

   Ligaments *attach muscles across individual bones to form joints, which permit the musculoskeletal system as a whole to perform its function of locomotion*. The knee joint, for example, the largest in the body, is formed by the femur and tibia. The elbow joint is formed by the ulna and the humerus.

   The hand is capable of very complicated movements, and the thumb plays a very important role in providing the dexterity associated with the hand. The complex movements provided by the hand allow us to manipulate a variety of tools and items with consummate ease. The skeleton of the wrist (or *carpus*) consists of two rows of four bones, whereas the ankle (or *tarsus*) consists of seven bones.

STRUCTURE AND CHEMISTRY OF BONE

On the basis of shape, the major bones in the body may be classified as either as *long* or *flat*. The long bones (Fig. 5–3*A*) are found predominantly in the limbs, and visual inspection reveals distinct sections: *they consist of a shaft* **(diaphysis),** *two ends called the* **epiphyses,** *and the region where these two sections meet, called the* **metaphysis.** A cross section through the bone (Fig. 5-3*B*) at the level of the diaphysis reveals two major components: (1) compact **cortical bone,** which accounts for about 80% of the skeletal mass; and 2) **cancellous** or **trabecular bone,** which makes up the remaining 20%. Found in the shafts of the long bones, cortical bone has the texture of ivory and is arranged as a hollow cylinder that resists bending. Cancellous or trabecular bone is a spongy material that, in the long bones, is limited to the metaphyses. However, it may also be found in the bones of the vertebral column and in

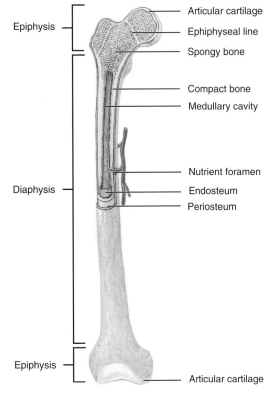

Epiphysis

Articular cartilage

Ephiphyseal line

Spongy bone

Compact bone

Medullary cavity

Nutrient foramen

Endosteum

Periosteum

Diaphysis

Epiphysis

Articular cartilage

A

FIGURE 5-3

Structure of the long bones. *A*, General features. *B*, Cortical and cancellous bone structures.
(From Applegate, E.J.: The Anatomy and Physiology Learning System. Philadelphia, W.B. Saunders, 1995, with permission.)

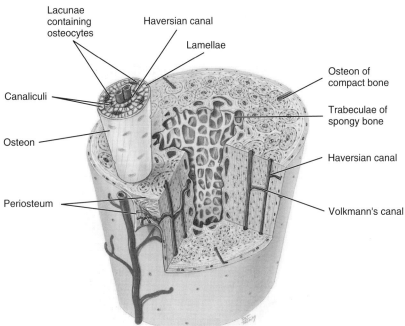

Lacunae containing osteocytes

Haversian canal

Lamellae

Osteon of compact bone

Trabeculae of spongy bone

Canaliculi

Osteon

Haversian canal

Periosteum

Volkmann's canal

B

most flat bones. Although cortical and cancellous bone have different morphologies, they have identical composition.

Bone may appear to be inert but, in fact, it is a mixture of living cellular elements and an extracellular matrix. The cells synthesize and secrete structural components, which are assembled into an organized meshwork constituting the extracellular matrix, which has about 35% organic and 65% inorganic components. The organic component is made up predominantly of *collagen*, an insoluble, rod-like, structured molecule with great tensile strength. Different types of collagen exist: type I accounts for about 90% of all collagens and is present in bones, tendons, ligaments, and skin; type II collagen is the predominant type found in cartilage; and type III collagen may be found predominantly in elastic tissues. About 10% of the noncollagen, organic component of the bone is made up of compounds, including glycoproteins and lipids, that participate in the important function of bone mineralization. Even though several other ions are present in varying amounts, the inorganic portion of the bone matrix is composed primarily of calcium and phosphate. Adequate amounts of both the bone matrix and the minerals are required to maintain a healthy bone structure.

CELLULAR ELEMENTS OF BONE

Three types of cells are involved in the formation and resorption (breakdown) of bone. These are the osteoblasts, the osteocytes, and the osteoclasts. *Active* **osteoblasts** *are cuboidal cells, about 20 μm in diameter, located at the bone-forming surfaces.* They have basophilic cytoplasm and well-developed Golgi apparatuses with an abundance of an enzyme called **alkaline phosphatase**. The extensive vascularization of the bone is the main reason why increases in bone alkaline phosphatase activity, observed during periods of increased bone formation or when there is a bone tumor, may be expressed quickly in the blood. For this reason, laboratory analysis of the serum alkaline phosphatase level is a valuable marker for the diagnosis of bone tumor. The osteoblasts are responsible for secreting the collagen fibers.

During periods of active growth, the epiphyses, specialized areas at the ends of each long bone, are separated from the shaft by actively growing cartilage called the **epiphyseal plate.** Growth takes place at this junction as the cartilage is transformed into new bone by the osteoblasts. Because the epiphyses of the various bones close in an orderly fashion and sequence, the normal age at which each bone closes is known. This information can be used to determine the bone age of an individual. Normally, the last of the epiphyses closes after puberty, but during periods of hormonal imbalances linear bone growth may cease earlier than normal. For example, decreased activity of the production of growth hormone may lead to stunted growth. In contrast, when epiphyseal closure is delayed, an abnormal height may be the result.

An inactive osteoblast has a flattened, fibroblast-like appearance that acts as a semipermeable membrane controlling the movement of ions across the surface of the bone. The osteoblasts eventually become surrounded by the collagen they secrete. After calcification, they are transformed into osteocytes. *A metabolically active* **osteocyte** *is a highly mobile multinucleated cell that can reach a diameter of about 100* μm, about five times the size of an osteoblast. These cells have well-developed Golgi apparatuses and endoplasmic reticulum and an extensive system of channels called **canaliculi** that connect the osteocytes with the surface osteoblasts. It is believed that ions and nutrients may flow through these channels.

The third class of cellular bone elements are the **osteoclasts,** *which are usually found at locations where bone breakdown is actively taking place.* The cytoplasm of the osteoclast contains significant quantities of lysosomal enzymes, predominantly **acid phosphatase.** The osteoclasts glide across the surface of previously formed bone and, as they do, bone erosion takes place, creating holes called **lacunae.** Although the osteoclasts account for a small portion of the total bone volume, they play a very important role in what is referred to as *bone remodeling*—the phenomenon of bone formation and erosion and of mineral homeostasis. Because the osteoclasts control the rate of bone resorption, and therefore the release of calcium, they are regarded as important players in the control of blood calcium levels.

HORMONAL CONTROL OF SKELETAL HOMEOSTASIS

The adult human body's calcium content of 1.1 kg of calcium (1.5 to 2% of body weight) is located predominantly in the skeletal system. Several hormones that influence bone mineralization act through the regulation of serum calcium and phosphate. There are two types of bone calcium reservoirs in the body. There is a readily exchangeable reservoir (about 1 mole) that is in equilibrium with serum calcium, and there is a larger, stable pool of about 250 moles of calcium that is not readily accessible. Three principal components regulate the amount of calcium released into the blood. Serum calcium levels are controlled by *parathyroid hormone* (PTH), which is produced in the parathyroid glands located in the neck region. This hormone increases serum calcium, primarily by mobilizing calcium from bone and enhancing calcium reabsorption by the kidney. *Vitamin D_3* increases blood calcium by increasing the uptake and absorption of calcium from the gastrointestinal tract and mobilizing calcium from the bone. *Calcitonin,* whose action is opposite to that of PTH, is a hormone secreted by the thyroid gland that stimulates a decrease in circulating levels of calcium. The relationship of PTH, vitamin D_3, and calcitonin is schematically represented in Figure 5–4.

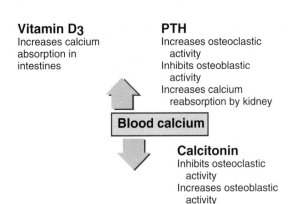

Vitamin D_3
Increases calcium
absorption in
intestines

PTH
Increases osteoclastic
    activity
Inhibits osteoblastic
    activity
Increases calcium
    reabsorption by kidney

Blood calcium

Calcitonin
Inhibits osteoclastic
    activity
Increases osteoblastic
    activity
Increases calcium
    excretion

FIGURE 5–4
The effects of PTH, calcitonin, and vitamin D_3 on blood levels.

MAJOR BONE DISEASES

Rickets

Rickets, *a disease of vitamin D nutritional deficiency, is a condition in which the bones become distorted and pliable, with increased susceptibility to fracture.* In the United States, the minimum requirement for vitamin D is approximately 2.5 μg (100 IU)/day in children and 10 μg (400 IU)/day in adults. Even though endogenous production is between 10 and 100 μg, cow milk and other similar foods are routinely fortified with vitamin D. Therefore, severe nutritional deficiency of vitamin D is a rare occurrence in the United States. Some of the factors that precipitate nutritional vitamin D deficiency include avoidance of vitamin D–fortified foods, especially for individuals who are lactose intolerant and therefore cannot digest milk. Inadequate exposure to light may also lead to a vitamin D deficiency because a significant portion of the need can be met by vitamin D_3 production in the skin under ultraviolet radiation.

The bone deformities seen in rickets are more pronounced if the vitamin D deficiency takes place during infancy or childhood. Congenital rickets occurs only in the children of mothers with severe vitamin D deficiency. After the first year of life, the deformities are most pronounced in the legs because of their rapid growth and the fact that the infant begins to walk and the bones in the legs must bear the body's weight. The result is the formation of bowleggedness or knock-knees, poor linear growth, and abnormal serum calcium, phosphate, and alkaline phosphatase levels. Moderate deformities that occur before the age of 4 may be adequately treated with vitamin D, but those that occur later may produce lasting deformity.

Osteomalacia

Osteomalacia *is a systemic bone disorder characterized by the loss of minerals, especially calcium, from the bone, resulting in softening of the bone.* Osteomalacia is essentially the adult version of childhood rickets, wherein the bones become weak and very susceptible to fracture. This may be caused by poor calcium intake, the inability to synthesize vitamin D, low sunlight exposure, or a metabolic disorder causing impaired absorption of these minerals. Sometimes, osteomalacia may be induced by a tumor (referred to as oncogenic), and laboratory results may reflect decreased blood levels of phosphates (*hypophosphatemia*) and increased urine phosphates (*hyperphosphaturia*). Because less than 5% of the adult bone mass is remodeled yearly, it appears that the defect in bone mineralization must be present for several years before a significant softening of the bone can occur. The clinical features of osteomalacia are less severe than those of rickets and are associated with pain when weight or pressure is applied to the affected bones.

Osteoporosis

Bone is continuously resorbed and formed during the process of remodeling. **Osteoporosis** *results when the progressive bone loss is sufficient to cause increased risk of fracture.* Although it is part of growing old, osteoporosis is also a condition that represents a disease state. In virtually all individuals, the bone mass begins to decline between the ages of 40 and 50 years. Although the cause of primary osteoporosis is still not well understood, there is a sexual component to the disease because the rate of bone loss is faster in women than in men and osteoporosis occurs more frequently in estrogen-deficient women. This has led to the descriptive term *postmenopausal osteoporosis,* such as that encountered after natural or surgical menopause (hysterectomy). It is believed that, during the estrogen-deficient state, the bones become more sensitive to the action of PTH, which causes the breakdown of bone to release calcium. Increased osteoporosis is also associated with other conditions of hypogonadism, such as in **Klinefelter's syndrome**. In this case, the increased bone loss may be due to the deficiency in gonadotropin production (and therefore reduced steroid production).

As a disease state, osteoporosis is usually characterized by a rapid loss of bone mass per unit volume. There is usually, however, no disturbance of the ratio of minerals to extracellular matrix in the remaining bone. Osteoporosis is by far the most common metabolic disease because bone remodeling is regulated by many factors, including hormones and nutrition. Hip fracture is the most serious complication of osteoporosis.

Bone Tumors

Tumors of the bone are infrequently encountered but, when they do occur, they are the most lethal cancer in humans. This is largely because they are able to spread widely and affect the bone marrow. Important examples of bone tumors include malignant tumors of the bone marrow (*myeloma* and *leukemia*) and of the osteoblastic cells. **Multiple myeloma** is the most important and most common syndrome. It is characterized by the invasion of the skeletal system by cancerous plasma cells, which secrete increased levels of complete or incomplete immnunoglobulins.

THE MUSCULAR SYSTEM

The human body contains more than 430 individual muscles and, as with the skeleton, they have been modified to perform various functions. The muscular system can be classified into three main groups: cardiac, smooth, and striated. **Cardiac muscles,** *as the name suggests, occur mostly in the walls of the heart;* **smooth muscles** *are found predominantly in the gastrointestinal tract, the bladder, and the walls of blood vessels; and* **striated** *(or skeletal)* **muscles** *are usually associated with the skeleton and comprise about 40% of the total body weight.* The muscle cell is a prime example of the process of adaptation of structure to function. The sizes of individual muscle cells and their cellular contents have been modified to suit their functions.

MICROSCOPIC STRUCTURE OF THE MUSCLE CELL

Structurally, the muscle is composed of muscle fibers: these are single, long, cylindrical, multinucleated cells with a diameter ranging from 10 to 100 μm. Skeletal muscles have an origin and an insertion point relative to the joint of motion, and the distance between these two points varies considerably among muscle groups. The length of a muscle fiber therefore varies considerably depending on where the joints of motion are located. Figure 5–5 is a diagrammatic representation of a skeletal muscle. Each muscle fiber is made up of a bundle of individual fibrils **(myofibrils),** which are themselves made up of individual thick and thin

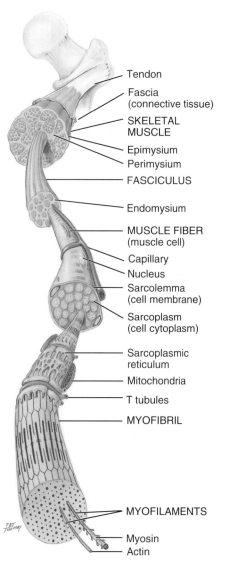

filaments of contractile proteins. Under the light microscope, myofibrils have a striated appearance created by alternating light and dark bands that run in the longitudinal and transverse directions. These bands were named after their effect on polarizing light. The dark *A (anisotropic) band* strongly rotates the plane of polarized light away from the eye, but the light *I (isotropic) band* has very little effect on polarized light. The dark A bands are bisected by the *H (Hensen's) zones* and the light I bands are bisected in the middle by the narrow dark *Z (zwischenscheibe) line*. The H zone, the center of which is the *M line*, is apparent in the center of the A band.

The myofibrillar material between two Z bands constitutes the *sarcomere*, which is embedded in the cytoplasm of the muscle cell, called the **sarcoplasm**. Electron microscopic examination and biochemical studies show that the sarcomere itself is made up of two sets of parallel and partly overlapping protein filaments. The A band contains only the thick filaments, which consist primarily of *myosin*; the thin filaments, which are attached to the Z line and extend across the I bands and partially into the A bands, contain principally *actin*. Composition analysis shows that skeletal muscle is about 75% water, 20% protein, and 5% inorganic salts (including high-energy phosphates such as ATP) and carbohydrates. The most abundant muscle proteins are *myosin* (52%), *actin* (23%), *tropomyosin* (15%), and *myoglobin*, which accounts for about 1% of the muscle protein mass. **Myoglobin** *is a protein that serves as an oxygen reservoir for the muscle cell by receiving oxygen from hemoglobin.* Along with the respiratory enzymes (the cytochromes), myoglobin gives muscle its characteristic red color. The sarcoplasm also contains lipid droplets and stored glucose in the form of glycogen particles.

Skeletal Muscle

The most distinctive characteristic of the skeletal muscle is its cross-striations. Muscle fibers may be classified on the basis of either their color or their metabolic and physiologic characteristics. On the basis of color, at least two types of fibers are found in skeletal muscles— *the red and white fibers.* The red fibers have a large amount of sarcoplasm that contains more nuclei and mitochondria, a greater content of myoglobin, and more lipid droplets than the white muscle fibers. Metabolically, the white muscle fibers have a lower respiratory and higher glycogenolytic capacity and a higher ATPase activity than the red fibers.

Cardiac Muscle

Cardiac muscle, as the name suggests, is found predominantly in the heart, where it contracts rhythmically in response to the pacemaker. Cardiac muscle is a specialized striated muscle resembling red skeletal muscle, except that cardiac muscle fibers are branched, producing irregularly shaped fibers and a more multicolored appearance. Despite the branching, the cardiac muscle fiber remains a separate cell surrounded by its distinct cell membrane, and the cells are arranged in parallel layers.

Smooth Muscle

Visually, the smooth muscle lacks cross-striations. Those that are found in places such as the hollow viscera may contain their own pacemakers but, unlike the cardiac muscles, smooth muscles may discharge irregularly. Other smooth muscle types, such as those found in the eye, may behave like skeletal muscle and be under voluntary control.

PHYSIOLOGY OF MUSCLE CONTRACTION

Since the production of motion is one of the fundamental functions of muscle, it is essential to understand this physiologic phenomenon. To produce motion, the muscle must contract, and this essentially involves the sliding back and forth of the staggered arrangement of the thin actin and thick myosin filaments described previously. The efficiency with which a particular muscle contracts, however, depends on the relative amount of biochemical factors such as myoglobin and mitochondria. These factors are used to classify muscle fibers.

The **type I fibers** *are characterized by slow contraction time and are resistant to fatigue.* They contain numerous mitochondria and increased amounts of myoglobin, features that are characteristic of the red fibers. The metabolism is mainly aerobic, and these fibers are best adapted for prolonged activity of low intensity. For example, muscle fibers in the buttocks, gluteal muscles attached to the hip, can undergo sustained contraction in order to maintain the upright posture. **Type II fibers** *twitch about two to three times faster than type I fibers, but they fatigue rather rapidly.* The muscle metabolism is essentially anaerobic, and the mitochondrial content is relatively sparse. These features are characteristics of white muscle fibers. An example of this type of contraction may be seen in some muscle cells of the fingers, which must contract less frequently and yet more rapidly when necessary.

SKELETAL MUSCLE DISORDERS

Disorders of skeletal muscle are termed **myopathies** *and may occur in a number of systemic diseases.* Damage to muscle cells may be caused by a direct invasion of microbiologic entities (e.g., staphyloccoci) or by the toxins they produce in subcutaneous abscesses (e.g., *Clostridium*) adjacent to the muscle fibers. Muscle weakness and atrophy may have a variety of origins. For example bedridden individuals may suffer atrophy of the muscle as a result of disuse, but muscle atrophy in general is a natural consequence of aging. It is characterized essentially by a reduction in the size of the myofibers and replacement of the muscle mass with fat cells. Muscular disorders, in particular, are characterized by regressive alterations in myofibers that lead to weakness in specific muscle groups.

One group of genetically determined disorders of the muscle is termed the **muscular dystrophies**. The time of onset is very important in their diagnosis. The most serious form is called *Duchenne muscular dystrophy.* A sex-linked recessive condition virtually limited to men, with women acting only as carriers, Duchenne muscular dystrophy appears early in life and may cause death by 20 years of age. The pathogenesis is still obscure, but the diagnosis is made when a child fails to sit up or walk at the time he is supposed to. There is difficulty in sitting and standing, and, as the disease progresses, there is weakness of the arms; eventually the individuals are restricted to wheelchairs. The *Becker* type, in contrast, is usually diagnosed during the second decade of life and is a milder form of the Duchenne type. The disorder is also characterized by increased serum levels of a variety of enzymes normally found within muscle cells, including creatine kinase and lactate dehydrogenase, suggesting a substantial injury to cells and abnormal permeability of the plasma membranes.

LABORATORY TESTS ASSOCIATED WITH MUSCULOSKELETAL DISORDERS

Tissues such as bone and muscle produce their specific functions because of the presence of a number of specific biochemical proteins and enzymes that their constituent cells possess. In healthy individuals, these compounds are well contained in the cells; in the event of metabolic disorders, when cell damage or necrosis takes place, these cellullar enzymes may leak into the blood. An elevated serum level of a cellular protein or enzyme may indicate that something is wrong but may not indicate which organ is involved. This is because many organs may contain the same class of enzymes. In some cases, a protein may be specific for a tissue. For example, myoglobin is found principally in the skeletal muscles, and therefore its presence in serum may be indicative of muscle trauma. In many cases, however, different organs may express slightly different forms of a large class of biochemical entities. In the enzyme class these are called **isoenzymes**. These isoenzymes are usually detected by electrophoretic separation.

An example of an enzyme that has tissue-specific isoenzymes and is used in the chemistry laboratory for diagnosis is **lactate dehydrogenase** (LD). Five isoenzymes (LD_1 to LD_5) exist and, because the different fractions may be found in varying quantities in different tissues, their quantification may be used for the diagnosis of myocardial infarction, liver congestion, acute hepatitis, or even breast cancer (in nipple discharge). The isoenzyme LD_1 is found predominantly in the cardiac muscle and, during normal conditions, serum levels of LD_2 are greater than those of LD_1. In the event of a heart attack, however, as a result of cardiac muscle damage, LD_1 levels increase in blood. Therefore, when serum levels of LD_1 become elevated relative to LD_2, this may be diagnostic of a myocardial infarction. This is usually called an *LD_1 / LD_2 flip*.

Another important enzyme is **creatine kinase** (CK), which has three isoenzymes (CK-MM, CK-MB, and CK-BB, referring to the location of its abundance—M for muscle and B for brain). These are also distributed in different quantities in heart muscle, the brain, and the lung. The myocardium has a relatively high concentration of CK-MB, and therefore the appearance of CK-MB in the blood is indicative of heart muscle damage. Sometimes a combination of tests, such as CK and LD isoenzymes or myoglobin and CK-MB, may be required to increase the accuracy of diagnosis of myocardial infarction.

CHAPTER SUMMARY

The muscular and skeletal systems each have hundreds of individual muscles and bones that have been adapted into a well-coordinated system to perform the functions of movement, support, and protection. Movement is made possible because the muscle and bones form efficient joints. The speed and duration of sustained movements is dependent on whether the muscle is made up of either red or type I fibers, which contract slowly and do not tire easily, or the type II white muscle fibers, which twitch rapidly and also fatigue easily. The skeleton has been modified to protect the very delicate parts of the body and to provide strong architectural support for the bulk of the body. It is estimated that the adult skeletal system is supplied by 200 to 400 ml of blood per minute, which brings nutrients and oxygen to millions of actively growing cells. The blood leaving the bone and muscles usually reveals defects in bone and muscle metabolism. Calcium, phosphate, and enzymes that are characteristic of damage to various tissues are quickly expressed in the blood and can be used for diagnosis.

Review Questions

1. What are the essential functions of the musculoskeletal system and how are the muscles and the bones adapted to perform these functions?

2. What consitutes a joint? What is the largest joint in the body?

3. What element in the musculoskeletal system may be considered an important determinant of blood calcium levels?

4. What is the significance of the measurement of CK and LD isoenzymes?

5. How many classes of muscles are there, and what criteria are used to classify them?

BIBLIOGRAPHY

Claarke, B.L., Wynne, A.G., Wilson, D.M., and Fitzpatrick, L.A.: Osteomalacia associated with adult Fanconi's syndrome: Clinical and diagnostic features. Clin Endocrinol *43*:479, 1995.

Delmas, P.D.: Biochemical markers of bone turnover. J Bone Miner Res *8*(suppl 2):S549, 1993.

Feldman, K.W., Marcuse, E.K., and Springer, D.A.: Nutritional rickets. Am Fam Physician *43*:1311, 1990.

Foreback, C.C.: Biochemical diagnosis of myocardial infraction. Henry Ford Hosp Med J *39*:159, 1991.

Hewison, M.: Tumor-induced osteomalacia. Curr Opin Rheumatol *6*:340, 1994.

Kairisto, V., Virtanen, A., Uusipaikka, E., Voipio-Pulkki, L.M., Nanto, V., Peltota, O., and Irjala, K.: Method for determining reference changes from patients' serial data: Example of cardiac enzymes. Clin Chem *39*:2296, 1993.

Kawamoto, M.: Breast cancer diagnosis by lactate dehydrogenase isoenzymes in nipple discharge. Cancer *73*:1836, 1994.

Marshall, T., Williams, J., and Williams, K.M.: Electrophoresis of serum isoenzymes and proteins following acute myocardial infarction. J Chromatogr *569*:323, 1991.

Miller, R.G., and Hoffman, E.P.: Molecular diagnosis and modern management of Duchenne muscular dystrophy. Neurol Clin *12*:699, 1994.

Parano, E., Pavone, L., Fiumara, A., Falsaperla, R., Trifiletti, R.R., and Dobyns, W.B.: Congenital muscular dystrophies: Clinical review and proposed classification. Pediatr Neurol *13*:97, 1995.

Young, G.P.: Myoglobin and creatine kinase-MB. Ann Emerg Med *28*:245, 1996.

The Cardiopulmonary System

INTRODUCTION

CIRCULATORY OR
CARDIOVASCULAR SYSTEM
Heart
Anatomy
Physiology
Vessels
Anatomy
Physiology
Blood
Composition

RESPIRATORY OR PULMONARY
SYSTEM
Anatomy
Upper respiratory tract
Lower respiratory tract
Physiology
Mechanics of breathing
Gas exchange in the lungs
Control of respiration
Respiration and the acid-base
balance

CONDITIONS OF CLINICAL
SIGNIFICANCE ASSOCIATED WITH
THE CARDIOPULMONARY SYSTEM
Heart and Vessels
Noninfectious conditions
Infectious conditions
Upper Respiratory System
Noninfectious conditions
Infectious conditions
Lower Respiratory System
Noninfectious conditions
Infectious conditions

LABORATORY TESTING ASSOCIATED
WITH THE CARDIOPULMONARY
SYSTEM

CHAPTER SUMMARY

REVIEW QUESTIONS

1. *Locate and identify the major components of the circulatory system and briefly describe their structure and function.*

2. *Briefly explain the cardiac cycle and the events that control the mechanical movements of the heart.*

3. *Trace the pathway of blood through the heart and distinguish between the pulmonary and systemic circulations.*

4. *Locate and identify the major components of the upper and lower respiratory tracts and describe their functions.*

5. *Identify the two sites where gas exchanges occur within the body and briefly explain the process by which these exchanges occur.*

6. *Describe the events that regulate respiration.*

7. *Define medical terminology related to the cardiopulmonary system.*

8. *Briefly discuss infectious and noninfectious diseases associated with the cardiopulmonary system.*

9. *Identify laboratory tests that are pertinent to the cardiopulmonary system.*

KEY TERMS

homeostasis	diastolic pressure	aneurysm	cyanosis
epicardium	plasma	circulatory shock	laryngitis
myocardium	erythrocyte	varicose veins	pneumonia
endocardium	leukocyte	phlebitis	bronchitis
artery	platelet	bacterial endocarditis	pleurisy
vein	respiration	allergic rhinitis	tuberculosis
capillary	partial pressure	influenza	blood gases
cardiac cycle	nervous regulation	tonsillitis	cardiac enzymes
arteriole	chemical regulation	emphysema	chemistry profile
venule	respiratory acidosis	cystic fibrosis	CBC with differential
blood pressure	respiratory alkalosis	pneumothorax	lipid profile
systolic pressure	myocardial infarction	hypoxia	microbial culture

Introduction

The ceaseless beating of the heart and the rhythmic rise and fall of the chest occur thousands of times daily without conscious decision on our part. The tireless efforts of the heart and lungs are often taken for granted, and they generally continue to operate unnoticed. However, the flutter of the heartbeat or an overextended stay under water may serve to remind us that we depend on the uninterrupted function of these organs for our very existence.

The cardiopulmonary system is a highly specialized network that includes two separate circuits working very closely with each other. First, the circulatory or cardiovascular system includes the heart, blood vessels, and blood. Second, the respiratory or pulmonary system includes the lungs, a series of airways leading to the lungs, and the chest structures responsible for the movement of air into and out of the lungs. Together, the primary function of these two circulations is to provide the necessary oxygen and nutrients to the cells and tissues of the body and to remove the waste products of cell metabolism. They also interact with the various other systems of the body to help maintain homeostasis. **Homeostasis** *is the state in which the internal environment of the body remains relatively stable, naturally maintaining survival by adapting appropriately to various situations.*

This chapter describes the anatomy and physiology of the cardiopulmonary system. It also illustrates its major functions and overall role in the maintenance of life. Conditions of significance related to the cardiopulmonary system are presented, and laboratory tests used for diagnosis of conditions related to the cardiopulmonary system are discussed.

CIRCULATORY OR CARDIOVASCULAR SYSTEM

The human body is composed of billions of customized and metabolically active cells that require constant nutrition and waste removal. The majority of cells within the body are fixed and immobile and are at a good distance from nutrient sources such as the digestive tract and sites of waste disposal such as the kidneys. As a result, the simple diffusion of nutrients used by unicellular organisms cannot sustain these cells. The circulatory or cardiovascular system provides a highly efficient and specialized means of connecting the food and oxygen sources to the cells and tissues of the body. The heart, a dual pump, provides a mechanism by which blood is moved through the vessels of two vascular circuits: the peripheral and the pulmonary circuits. Blood flows through a closed, circular network of blood vessels that extend between the heart and the peripheral and pulmonary tissues. With this network, no cell within the body is more than a few cell diameters from the transportation system. This section of the chapter examines each portion of the cardiovascular system.

HEART

The heart is the center of the cardiovascular system, and every tissue in the body depends on its continuous function. It is an extraordinary organ, with the strength to literally move hundreds of gallons of blood (about 1,800) per day through thousands of miles of vessels (approximately 60,000) without a moment of rest. The heart has both the capability to maintain our body's need for oxygen and nutrition under normal conditions and the incomparable ability to regulate blood flow as these needs change throughout the body.

Anatomy

The proportional size and weight of the heart disguise its remarkable strength and ability to endure. About the size of a clenched fist, the heart is a hollow, cone-shaped organ that weighs less than 1 lb in an average adult. It is located in the thoracic cavity between the lungs in an area known as the *mediastinum* (Fig. 6–1) and is covered by a protective sac known as the *pericardium* (see Figs. 6–2 and 6–3).

    External Anatomy.   The wall of the heart is composed of three layers: the epicardium, the myocardium, and the endocardium (Figs. 6–2 and 6–3). *The* **epicardium** *is the outermost cell layer.* It provides a smooth surface that helps prevent friction as the heart beats. *The* **myocardium** *is the middle layer and consists of bundles of cardiac muscle.* These bundles are arranged in such a way that, when the heart contracts, the internal chambers of

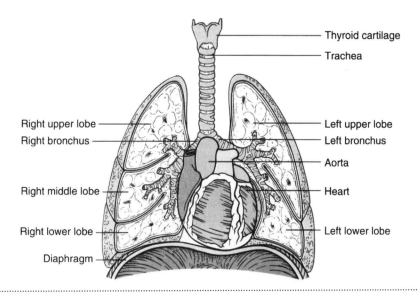

FIGURE 6-1

The location of the heart.
(From Frazier M.S., Drzymkowski, J.A., and Doty, S.J.: Essentials of Human Diseases and Conditions. Philadelphia, W.B. Saunders, 1996, with permission.)

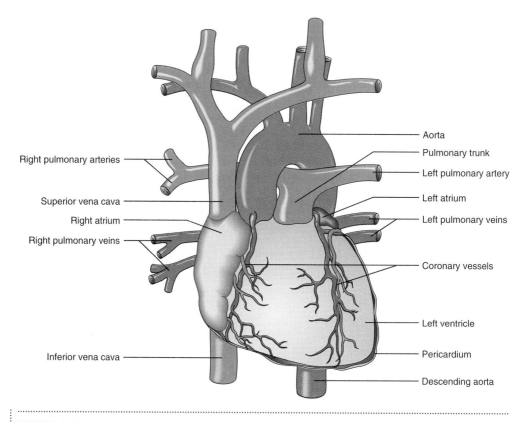

Right pulmonary arteries

Superior vena cava

Right atrium

Right pulmonary veins

Inferior vena cava

Aorta

Pulmonary trunk

Left pulmonary artery

Left atrium

Left pulmonary veins

Coronary vessels

Left ventricle

Pericardium

Descending aorta

FIGURE 6-2

External anatomy of the heart and associated great vessels.

the heart are compressed. This action forces the blood through the system. *The inner surface is called the* **endocardium** *and is continuous with the endothelium of the blood vessels associated with the heart.* It provides a smooth lining for the interior of the heart and also covers the valves.

Internal Anatomy.   The interior of the heart is hollow and is divided into four chambers (two *atria* and two *ventricles*) (see Fig. 6–3). The heart is a dual pump, serving two separate but interconnected vessel circuits. The right side is composed of the right atrium and the right ventricle. It is responsible for moving deoxygenated blood from the heart to the lungs and then to the left atrium, serving the pulmonary circuit. The left side, consisting of the left atrium and the left ventricle, receives newly oxygenated blood from the lungs and pumps it throughout the rest of the body and then to the right atrium. It services the peripheral or systemic circuit. Atrial and ventricular *septa* separate the right and left sides of the heart to prevent direct passage of blood from one side to the other. *Valves* separate the atrium from the ventricle on each side (tricuspid on the right and bicuspid on the left) and are designed to allow blood to flow in only one direction. These valves act as one-way gates and open and close only in response to the naturally occurring pressure differences in

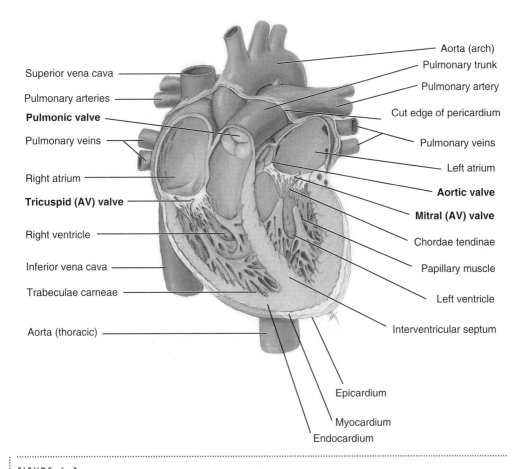

FIGURE 6-3

Internal anatomy of the heart.
(From Jarvis, C.: Physical Examination and Health Assessment. Philadelphia, W. B. Saunders, 1992, with permission.)

the heart. Also, a unidirectional semilunar valve guards the base of each large artery leaving the ventricles of the heart.

Associated Great Vessels. *There are three major types of blood vessels found within the body:* **arteries,** *which carry blood away from the heart;* **veins,** *which carry blood to the heart; and* **capillaries,** *which service the tissues.* Only the largest of the arteries and veins are directly associated with the heart. These are the aorta, superior and inferior venae cavae, pulmonary trunk, and pulmonary arteries and veins (see Fig. 6–2). The aorta is the main artery and rises upward from the left ventricle. It is responsible for transporting oxygenated blood from the heart into the various branches of the peripheral circuit. Deoxygenated blood is returned to the right atrium of the heart by the main veins in the body, the superior and inferior venae cavae. The pulmonary trunk emerges from the right ventricle, splits into the right and left pulmonary arteries, and carries blood from the heart to the lungs. The pulmonary veins bring oxygenated blood from the lungs to the left atrium of the heart to complete the pulmonary circuit. The blood supply for the heart itself is provided by the coronary vessels encircling the heart.

Physiology

The rhythm, speed, and strength with which the heart beats depends a great deal on one's health and relies on a combination of both mechanical and electrical events for proper function. With life depending on it (literally), the heart pumps blood to all tissues throughout the body.

Mechanical Events. As previously stated, the primary function of the heart is to transport blood to the various tissues in the body. One means of accomplishing this is with the use of a coordinated group of cardiac muscle reactions. The simultaneous contraction of both atria, followed very closely by the contraction of both ventricles, provides the mechanical force behind the movement of blood from the heart into the vessels. This precise sequence of events that keeps blood moving through the heart and vessels is known as the **cardiac cycle,** commonly referred to as a *heartbeat*. Each heartbeat consists of a period of contraction (called *systole*), in which blood is pumped from the heart, and a period of relaxation between the contractions of the atria or the ventricles (called *diastole*), in which the heart fills with blood. The normal heart beats approximately 70 times/min in the resting adult. This rate may fluctuate as the heart responds to stimuli such as exercise, stress, and medications. Since the cardiovascular system is closed and continuous, with no real beginning or end, we will arbitrarily trace the path of blood beginning with the right atrium (Fig. 6–4).

Dark, bluish-red, deoxygenated blood from the upper and lower portions of the body enters the right atrium via the superior and inferior venae cavae, respectively. There is also an additional opening into the right atrium that returns deoxygenated blood from the coronary vessel system that services the heart itself. As the atria contract, although very weakly, blood moves through the tricuspid valve and into the right ventricle. The right ventricle then contracts, the tricuspid valve closes, and blood exits the right ventricle via the pulmonary trunk. A semilunar valve prevents the backflow of blood into the ventricle. Blood then enters the lungs through the right and left pulmonary arteries. Carbon dioxide is exchanged for oxygen in the capillary beds of the lungs. The carbon dioxide is expelled into the air as we breathe. Bright, cherry-red, freshly oxygenated blood is then transported back to the left atrium of the heart by the right and left pulmonary veins, thus completing the *pulmonary circuit*.

The left atrium receives this blood and then pushes it through the bicuspid valve into the left ventricle. As the left ventricle contracts, the bicuspid valve closes to prevent backflow and the blood is forced out of the ventricle into the aorta. The contraction of the left ventricle must generate enough pressure to push the blood to every part of the body. The aortic semilunar valve protects the entrance of the aorta and prevents backflow of blood into the ventricle. From the aorta, blood flows into the systemic arteries that branch from it. These arteries continue to branch and eventually form the capillary beds, where the exchange of oxygen, nutrients, and metabolic by-products occurs between the blood and the various tissues of the body. Finally, the *systemic circuit* is complete when the deoxygenated blood returns again to the heart via the superior and inferior venae cavae.

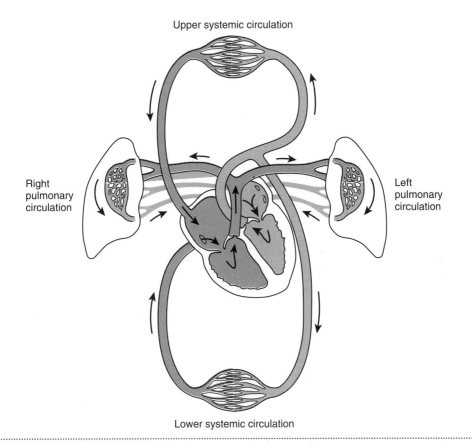

Upper systemic circulation

Right pulmonary circulation

Left pulmonary circulation

Lower systemic circulation

FIGURE 6-4

The path of blood through the circulatory system. The arrows indicate the direction of the flow.

Electrical Events. The cardiac cycle is a sequence of mechanical events regulated by electrical activity. Both mechanical and electrical events must work in harmony for the heart to perform as an effective pump. The arrangement of cardiac cells and the ease with which electrical messages can pass between cells enables the heart to accomplish its efficient pumping mechanism.

Unlike skeletal muscle, nerve impulses are not required to initiate the contraction of heart muscles. Certain cardiac muscle cells are self-excitatory and are able to repeatedly and rhythmically generate electrical impulses. These specialized cells have two important functions. They act as natural *pacemakers*, setting the rhythm for the entire heart. They also form the *conduction system*, which allows for the transmission of electrical impulses throughout the heart muscle. Signals from the nervous system, as well as hormones, such as epinephrine, do modify the heartbeat, but they are not responsible for the fundamental, faithful beating of the heart.

The spontaneous electrical impulses usually originate in the *sinoatrial (SA) node*, a group of specialized cells located in the right atrial wall (Fig. 6–5). The transmission of im-

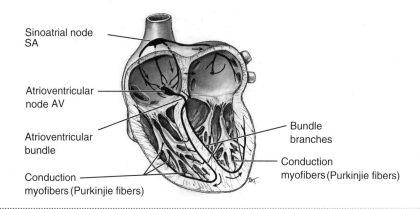

FIGURE 6-5

The conduction system of the heart.
(From Applegate, E.J.: The Anatomy and Physiology Learning System. Philadelphia, W. B. Saunders, 1995, with permission.)

pulses from the SA node to the rest of the atrial myocardium brings about atrial contraction. The impulse then spreads from the atrial fibers to the *atrioventricular (AV) node*, located in the center of the heart between the atria and the ventricles, and then to the atrioventricular (AV) bundle, or *bundle of His*. The AV bundle, located in the septum between the left and right ventricles, then transmits the signal along the left and right bundle branches and then along the Purkinje fibers (conduction myofibers). This activity brings about ventricular contraction. This conduction system coordinates the depolarization of the heart and ensures that the cardiac chambers contract in a coordinated manner, atria first and then ventricles.

While the heart generates and maintains its own beat, the rate at which this occurs may be altered in order to adapt to different situations. Heart rate may be increased in response to exercise, symphatetic nerve stimulation, hypoxia, hormonal influence, and some medications. The heart rate may be slowed by sleep, parasympathetic nerve stimulation, and some medications.

The electrical charges of the heart may be studied by placing several electrodes on the body's surface. Such a recording of the electrical activity of the heart is known as an *electrocardiogram* (ECG or EKG). A typical ECG consists of three distinct waves: the P wave, the QRS complex, and the T wave (Fig. 6–6). Each of these represents an electrical event within the heart. A discussion of the interpretation of ECGs is beyond the scope of this text, but it should be noted that ECGs are a vital tool in diagnosing cardiac disease.

VESSELS

The blood vessels of the body form the closed delivery system for blood that begins and ends with the heart. They are often compared to a plumbing system but, contrary to the inflexible pipes within a home, blood vessels are part of a dynamic system that reacts to the changing needs around them.

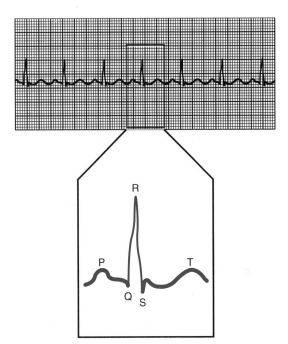

FIGURE 6-6

The electrocardiogram. The P wave represents atrial depolarization, or the transmission of the electrical impulse throughout the atrial myocardium. The QRS complex represents the depolarization of the ventricles as the electrical impulse is transmitted throughout the ventricular myocardium. The T wave represents the repolarization of the ventricles. (Repolarization of the atria is not represented by a separate wave because it is masked by the QRS wave.)

There are three major types of blood vessels: arteries, capillaries, and veins, each having a special purpose in the transit of blood throughout the body (Fig. 6–7). Arteries and veins act merely as conduits for moving blood away from and back to the heart. Only the capillaries come into intimate contact with the tissues.

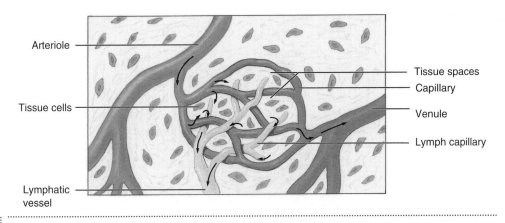

FIGURE 6-7

Vessels of the circulatory system.
(From Applegate, E.J.: The Anatomy and Physiology Learning System. Philadelphia, W.B. Saunders, 1995, with permission.)

Anatomy

Arteries.   Arteries are made up of strong, thick walls that contain large quantities of elastic tissue. This elasticity enables the arteries to expand and recoil, accommodating the change of blood volume and thus the pressure exerted on them by the heart. Large arteries are under high pressure and rapidly transport blood away from the heart and to the various capillary beds throughout the body. As the arteries move away from the heart and approach the capillary beds, they branch repeatedly, decreasing in diameter with each branching. *The smallest branched artery is called an* **arteriole** *and is the vessel that moves blood into the capillaries.* The smaller arteries and arterioles are less elastic than the larger ones and retain much of their diameter as the pressure of the blood rises and falls with each heartbeat. This effect is what causes the *pulse,* or regular, recurrent expansion and contraction of an artery in response to the contraction of the heart. The pulse can be easily detected in the superficial arteries, such as those in the wrist and neck.

Blood flow through the capillaries is in large part determined by the arterioles. The flow may be either increased or decreased in response to neural stimuli or local chemical influences. The arterioles may dilate to increase blood flow to an area or, conversely, may constrict to bypass or limit blood flow.

Capillaries.   Capillaries are the smallest blood vessels in the body, with extremely thin walls and a diameter only large enough for cells to pass through in single file. They are directly responsible for serving the metabolic needs of the tissues. Blood flows slowly through the intricate, lattice-like network of the capillaries. This allows adequate time for the exchange of substances between the plasma and the tissues.

The role of the capillaries depends on the tissues in which they are located. For example, renal capillaries send waste products into tubules where urine is formed, while pulmonary capillaries facilitate the exchange of oxygen and carbon dioxide in the alveoli of the lungs. Capillaries of the muscles exchange carbon dioxide and metabolic by-products for oxygen and nutrients, while capillaries of the intestines absorb nutrients from broken-down food sources. The capillaries connect the arterial system with the "return" mechanism, or venous system.

Veins.   The venous system is responsible for carrying deoxygenated blood from the capillary beds toward the heart. In contrast to the arterial system, the venous vessels increase in diameter and their walls become thicker as they leave the capillary beds en route to the heart. **Venules** *are the smallest and thinnest of these vessels and are found immediately after the capillary beds where the capillaries unite.* Venules continue to become larger and converge to form veins that eventually return the blood into the right atria of the heart.

Even though their walls are thinner than those of arteries, veins possess large lumens to accomodate blood returning to the heart at the same rate at which it was pumped. Valves, formed by a folded interior lining, are present within the veins to help prevent the backflow of blood against the force of gravity. Approximately 65% of the body's blood supply is within the veins at any given time.

Physiology

Blood pressure *is the pressure exerted by the blood on the walls of a blood vessel and the chambers of the heart*. It is created by the contraction of the ventricles. Maintaining adequate blood pressure is essential, and is in fact one of the "vital signs" of life. Systemic pressure is highest in the aorta, closest to the ventricle, and decreases as the blood travels farther from the heart. Pressure continues to decrease in the vast surface area of the capillaries, allowing necessary filtration and exchanges to occur. As blood leaves the capillaries and enters the venous system, pressure decreases even further, approaching zero as blood enters the right atrium.

Pressure is regulated by several factors. In general, if the heart rate and force increase, blood pressure also increases. If the venous return of blood increases, as is seen in exercise, the heart responds by pumping more forcefully. Other factors, such as nervous stimulation and renal function, will also affect the blood pressure.

Blood pressure is most commonly measured with the use of a sphygmomanometer and is measured in millimeters of mercury (mm Hg). *Two readings are obtained: the* **systolic pressure,** *which represents the blood pressure at its highest (when the ventricle is contracting), and the* **diastolic pressure,** *which represents the time when the ventricle is most relaxed.* The systolic pressure is always the higher of the two readings. The diastolic pressure is maintained in the arteries due to their elastic attributes. Normal brachial artery blood pressure is around 120/80 (systolic/diastolic) mm Hg.

Blood pressure and pulse rate are two useful tools in evaluating the performance of the circulatory system.

BLOOD

Long before today's medicine and current clinical laboratory testing, blood was known to be the source of life—for when it is drained from the body, so is life itself. Clinicians analyze this tissue more than any other in a quest for the explanation of illness and disease.

Composition

In the body, the blood is in constant motion and the blood cells are evenly dispersed throughout the plasma. There are three major blood cell types, the erythrocytes that transport oxygen to the tissues; the leukocytes that are involved in the body's defense mechanisms; and the platelets that are involved in the clotting of blood. The plasma is a clear, straw-colored liquid composed of a highly complex mixture of 90% water and over 100 dissolved organic and inorganic substances. These constituents include a number of different proteins, electrolyte ions, nutrients, byproducts of cellular metabolism, and respiratory gases. Plasma composition varies continuously as cellular metabolism takes place. The different systems of the body (e.g., liver and kidney) constantly remove or add substances to the plasma in order to maintain the homeostatic relationship necessary for our survival. The composition and function of blood are described in more detail in Chapter 11.

RESPIRATORY OR PULMONARY SYSTEM

The joyous laughter of a child, the vocalization of an inspiring speech, and the ability to sing a favorite song aloud are all functions of the respiratory system. The most important function, however, is the fulfillment of the body's need for oxygen. In order for the cells of the body to carry on their metabolic activities under aerobic conditions, a continual supply of oxygen as well as an efficient means of removing carbon dioxide and waste products of the cells' activities is required. As discussed previously, this is accomplished with the assistance of the cardiovascular system.

Respiration involves several integrated processes:

- The movement of air into and out of the lungs
- The exchange of oxygen and carbon dioxide between the air in the lungs and the blood
- The transport of oxygen and carbon dioxide by the blood
- The exchange of oxygen and carbon dioxide between the blood and the tissues
- The utilization of oxygen in cellular metabolism

This section of the chapter investigates the anatomy and physiology of this system and demonstrates its relationship with the cardiovascular system as well as other systems of the body.

ANATOMY

The respiratory system can be divided into the *upper respiratory tract* (nose, nasal cavities, sinuses, pharynx, and larynx) and the *lower respiratory tract* (trachea, bronchi, and lungs) (Fig. 6–8). Also associated with the respiratory system are the pleural membranes and the respiratory muscles that form the chest cavity: the intercostal muscles and the diaphragm (Fig. 6–9).

Upper Respiratory Tract

Air enters the respiratory system through the *external nares* (nostrils) of the nose and then passes through to a portion of the nasal cavities termed the *vestibule*. This area is lined with hairs that trap large particles of dust in the air. The two nasal cavities are within the skull and are separated by the nasal septum. The lining of the nasal cavities possesses a moist, ciliated, mucosal surface that prevents dust and bacteria from entering the respiratory tract. This lining also serves to warm, moisten, and humidify the air as it passes through on its way to the lungs. The nasal cavities link the external nose to a muscular passage, the *pharynx*, common to routes followed by both air and food. The pharynx branches into two paths: the esophagus, through which food passes, and the *trachea*, through which air passes. At the entrance to the trachea lies the *larynx,* or voice box. The larynx not only possesses the vocal cords that allow us to speak, but also provides for the passage of air from the pharynx into the lower respiratory tract. Cilia found along the interior linings of these passages (except for the vocal cords) continuously sweep upward and serve as a protective device for the lower respiratory tract.

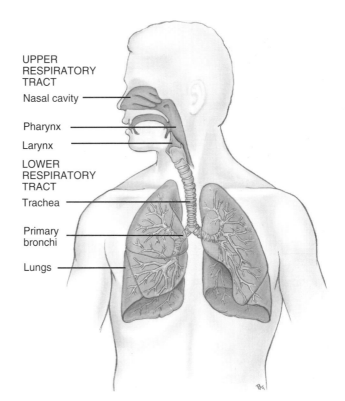

FIGURE 6-8
The anatomy of the respiratory system.
(From Applegate, E.J.: The Anatomy and Physiology Learning System. Philadelphia, W.B. Saunders, 1995, with permission.)

UPPER RESPIRATORY TRACT
Nasal cavity
Pharynx
Larynx
LOWER RESPIRATORY TRACT
Trachea
Primary bronchi
Lungs

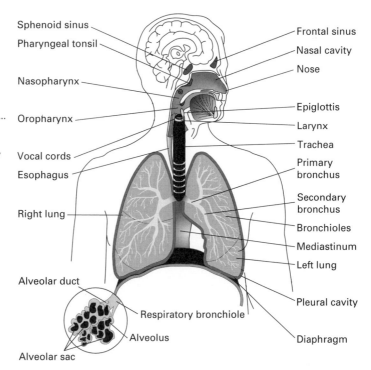

FIGURE 6-9
The location of the respiratory system.
(From Gould, B.: Pathophysiology for the Health-Related Professions. Philadelphia, W. B. Saunders, 1997, with permission.)

Sphenoid sinus
Pharyngeal tonsil
Nasopharynx
Oropharynx
Vocal cords
Esophagus
Right lung
Alveolar duct
Respiratory bronchiole
Alveolus
Alveolar sac
Frontal sinus
Nasal cavity
Nose
Epiglottis
Larynx
Trachea
Primary bronchus
Secondary bronchus
Bronchioles
Mediastinum
Left lung
Pleural cavity
Diaphragm

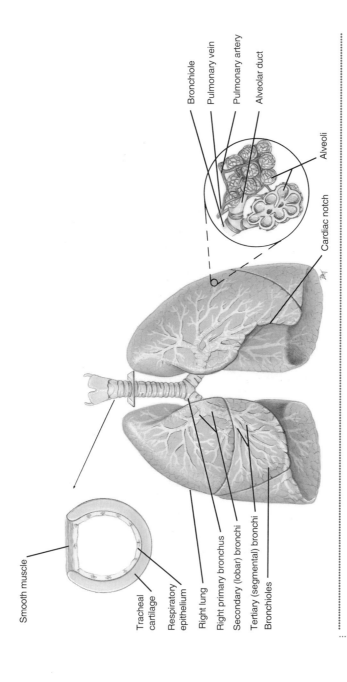

Smooth muscle

Tracheal
cartilage

Respiratory
epithelium

Right lung

Right primary bronchus

Secondary (lobar) bronchi

Tertiary (segmental) bronchi

Bronchioles

Bronchiole

Pulmonary vein

Pulmonary artery

Alveolar duct

Alveoli

Cardiac notch

FIGURE 6-10

Alveolar structure. The exchange of oxygen and carbon dioxide takes place within the capillary beds of the alveoli. (From Applegate, E.J.: The Anatomy and Physiology Learning System. Philadelphia, W. B. Saunders, 1995, with permission.)

Lower Respiratory Tract

The *trachea*, or windpipe, is about 4 to 5 inches long. It extends from the larynx and then branches into the left and right primary *bronchi*. These primary bronchi are the air passages that enter the *lungs*. The lungs are located within the thoracic cavity and are separated by the mediastinum and protected by the ribs. Each lung is divided into lobes: the right lung has three lobes and the left lung has two. The lungs are covered by a double-layered pleural membrane. Within the lungs, the bronchi continue to branch into secondary bronchi and then into smaller tubes called *bronchioles* that service each lobe of the lung. This branching resembles an inverted tree and is often called *the bronchial tree*. The bronchioles terminate in the lungs as small air sacs, known as alveoli. *The **alveoli** are very thin-walled sacs surrounded by numerous capillaries where the exchange of gases takes place* (Fig. 6–10).

PHYSIOLOGY
Mechanics of Breathing

Breathing is a natural phenomenon that occurs without thought on our part. We can hold our breath for a short period of time, but will eventually be forced to breathe.

The *respiratory control centers* are responsible for stimulating the muscles of the respiratory system, the diaphragm and the intercostal muscles. They are regulated by the concentration of carbon dioxide in the bloodstream. *Neurons within the medulla oblongata and pons of the brain control inhalation (inspiration) and expiration, collectively known as* **respiration**.

When the muscles of inspiration contract, the volume of the chest increases and the lungs expand. The pressure within the lungs decreases and air rushes in. As these same muscles relax, the volume of the chest decreases, the lungs are compressed, and air is expelled.

Coughing and sneezing are two inherent protective reflexes within the system. These reflexes serve to remove foreign matter or irritants from the respiratory tract.

Gas Exchange in the Lungs

There are two sites of gas exchange within the body: the alveoli of the lungs and the tissues of the body. The exchange of oxygen and carbon dioxide in the lungs is known as *external respiration* while the exchange between the tissues and the blood is known as *internal respiration*.

The air we inhale contains approximately 21% oxygen and 0.04% carbon dioxide. The concentration of each gas is expressed in a value called *partial pressure*. **Partial pressure (measured in millimeters of mercury) is the pressure that a particular gas exerts within a mixture of gases or in a liquid.** This pressure is directly related to the concentration of the gas and to the total pressure of the mixture. This partial pressure allows for the exchange of oxygen and carbon dioxide throughout the body. Each will diffuse from an area of greater concentration to an area of lesser concentration. For example, freshly inhaled air in the alveoli has a high partial pressure of oxygen and a low partial pressure of carbon dioxide. Conversely, blood in the capillaries of the alveoli that has returned from the tissue of the body has a high partial pressure of carbon dioxide and a low partial pressure of oxygen. As a result, gases diffuse across the capillaries, oxygenate the blood, and release carbon dioxide into the alveoli. The carbon dioxide is then expelled from the body through exhalation. Similarly, gaseous exchange occurs when oxygenated blood is transported to the tissues of the body. Cells utilize oxygen in the process of aerobic metabolism and produce carbon dioxide as a waste product. As arterial (oxygen-rich) blood reaches the capillaries of the tissues, oxygen is given up by the erythrocytes and carbon dioxide is picked up and transported via the cardiovascular system back to the lungs.

Control of Respiration

As with the heart, the inspiratory muscles of the respiratory system contract rhythmically, but the origins of the contractions are quite different. While cardiac muscle is self-stimulating, the muscles of the respiratory tract are composed of skeletal muscle and require neural stimulation for contraction. Breathing is regulated in two ways: the nervous mechanism associated with the respiratory control centers in the brain, and chemical influences such as hypoxia.

   Nervous regulation *refers to the neural communication between the respiratory control centers in the brain and the lungs.* Neural impulses from the inspiration center in the brain cause the respiratory muscles to contract and the chest to expand. Receptors in the lungs detect the stretching and in turn send impulses to the respiratory control centers to depress inspiration, preventing overinflation. The expiration center becomes more active as the inspiration center is depressed, and the respiratory muscles relax. The relaxation brings about exhalation. The respiratory centers work together in an effort to produce a normal rhythm of breathing. Disruption of the nervous regulation of breathing during sleep can result in apnea, the temporary absence of spontaneous breathing. Impulses from various sources can also modify the normal patterns of breathing. For example, voluntary adjustments of respiration occur during singing or swimming under water. The normal respiratory rate is between 12 and 20 breaths/min.

   Chemical regulation *refers to the effect that blood pH and blood levels of oxygen and carbon dioxide (blood gases) have on respiration.* The body is very sensitive to changes in the chemical makeup of the blood, especially changes in pH and gas levels. Excess levels of carbon dioxide in the blood directly affect and lower its pH. Chemoreceptors detect this change and send impulses to the respiratory centers. These impulses cause an increase in respiratory rate, thereby eliminating excess carbon dioxide. A decreased level of oxygen in the tissues (*hypoxia*) will also activate the chemoreceptors and increase respiratory rate and volume in order to compensate for this less-than-optimal condition.

Respiration and the Acid-Base Balance

The body exists within a very strict blood pH range. Changes in this balance must be corrected in order for life to continue. An inappropriate pH may be respiratory or metabolic in origin, or both. **Respiratory acidosis** *is a state in which inefficient respiration allows for an excess buildup of carbon dioxide and, in turn, a low pH.* This is most commonly associated with a sudden inability of the respiratory system to meet the body's demands, as in the case of a collapsed lung (*pneumothorax*). This may also occur in severe pulmonary disease. **Respiratory alkalosis** *occurs when respirations are increased and the exhalation of carbon dioxide is so fast that less carbonic acid (a source of hydrogen ions) is formed and the pH increases.* Hyperventilation may bring about this phenomenon. The respiratory system offers the most rapid and most effective means to remedy pH imbalances.

An acid-base imbalance is considered metabolic if it originates from a source other than a change in the respiratory rate. For example, *metabolic acidosis* can occur as the result of hydrogen ion (acid) buildup in the tissues in such conditions as strenuous exercise, certain complications of diabetes mellitus, and kidney disease. The respiratory system attempts to compensate for this imbalance by increasing the rate of respiration. This occurs in order to eliminate carbon dioxide and prevent the formation of carbonic acid. *Metabolic alkalosis* is not a common occurrence, but may be caused by an excessive loss of acids or by an increase in blood alkali. Loss of hydrochloric acid from persistent vomiting, as well as overuse of medications such as antacids, may bring about metabolic alkalosis. The respiratory system attempts to compensate for this condition by decreasing respirations in order to retain carbon dioxide.

CONDITIONS OF CLINICAL SIGNIFICANCE ASSOCIATED WITH THE CARDIOPULMONARY SYSTEM

There are too many diseases and conditions of the cardiopulmonary system to furnish a comprehensive list in this text. However, an attempt is made to provide an abbreviated survey of some of the more commonly encountered problems. The disease states presented could be categorized in many different ways, but have been arranged here as "noninfectious" or "infectious" for the sake of this presentation.

HEART AND VESSELS
Noninfectious Conditions

High blood pressure, also known as *hypertension*, affects many people and is generally defined as a resting arterial systolic pressure of greater than 140 mm Hg, a diastolic pressure of greater than 90 mm Hg, or both. Hypertension may result from several entities, such as increased volume due to excessive sodium intake or retention, kidney disease, or certain tumors. Hypertension usually produces no symptoms, but the long-term consequences can be very serious. High blood pressure has the most effect on the arteries and subsequently the heart by causing them to work harder, and may result in myocardial infarction, heart failure, stroke, and/or kidney damage.

As people age, a large number of them undergo degenerative changes in the walls of their vessels known as *atherosclerosis*. These changes are characterized by the deposition of *plaques* consisting of lipid materials, connective tissue, and abnormal smooth muscle cells. The slower blood flow through these regions also promotes the formation of *thrombi* (clots). Plaques may become larger, narrowing the lumen of the vessel, and thereby affecting the organs and tissues that are serviced by it. Early indications of this phenomenon may be manifested in a condition known as *angina pectoris*. In this condition, blood flow to a portion of the heart is temporarily restricted, resulting in chest discomfort. Once the vessel dilates, the symptoms cease and no permanent damage results. *Conversely, a prolonged deprivation of blood flow to a portion of the cardiac muscle leads to tissue death, also known as a* **myocardial infarction** *or heart attack.*

Similarly, a *stroke* is caused by decreased blood flow to a portion of the brain, resulting in tissue death. This damage may be the result of an occluded vessel or hemorrhage from a vessel.

Atherosclerotic plaques may become calcified, giving rise to *arteriosclerosis*, commonly known as "hardening of the arteries." This condition severely limits the elasticity of the vessels and, as a result, the vessels cannot respond to the pressure changes exerted by the heart.

Aneurysms *are localized dilations of an artery due to weakness in the artery wall.* This weakening may be due to atherosclerotic disease, congenital defects, or trauma. Aneurysms are often symptom free and pose the greatest danger to life if they rupture. They are also a common site for thrombus formation.

Congestive heart failure occurs when there is inadequate blood flow through the kidneys, resulting in fluid retention and subsequent increase in blood volume. This in turn places the heart under considerable stress as it attempts to compensate for the increased volume. Pressure builds within the vessels due to the heart's inability to pump adequately. This leads to distention of the heart and vessels, *edema* (the abnormal accumulation of fluid in the subcutaneous tissues), and possible tissue impairment.

Circulatory shock *is a condition in which the body tissues fail to receive adequate blood supplies due to reduced cardiac output.* Thus, lack of oxygen to the tissues impairs their function and may cause tissue damage; in severe cases, it may cause the death of the patient.

Varicose veins *are veins that are enlarged, extended, and tortuous.* They often develop in the superficial leg veins of persons with a congenital or inherited weakness of the walls and valves of the vessels. This condition may be present in persons who stand for long periods of time. The weakened vessels are unable to efficiently return blood to the heart, and the blood tends to pool in the veins of the legs. This may cause discomfort and cramping in the legs.

Phlebitis *is an inflammation of a vein and can result from a number of conditions, such as obesity, poor circulation, advancing age, and infection.* The inflammation of the vein may lead to thrombus formation and a condition called *thrombophlebitis.* The clots may occlude the vessel or may break loose and travel through the bloodstream as an *embolus* and obstruct a vessel in another portion of the body (*embolism*).

Infectious Conditions

Rheumatic heart disease results from an infection of group A *Streptococcus*, although the organism is no longer present when the disease manifests itself. Rheumatic fever is classified as an autoimmune disease with an affinity for heart tissue.

Bacterial endocarditis *is a condition in which the interior lining of the heart becomes inflamed due to the presence of bacteria.* This bacteria is usually a strain of *Streptococcus* that enters the bloodstream and forms vegetations within the heart.

UPPER RESPIRATORY SYSTEM
Noninfectious Conditions

Hay fever, also called **allergic rhinitis,** *is an allergic disease.* Patients exhibit a sensitivity to certain foreign proteins, such as the pollen of ragweed, and exposure to these proteins elicits an immune response.

Infectious Conditions

Everyone has had experience with the *common cold*. A cold is caused by a variety of viruses and is an acute inflammation of the mucous membranes of the upper respiratory tract. There is no known cure for the common cold and, because of the various etiologic agents and their mutations, our body does not provide adequate immunity. **Influenza,** *or the flu, is a similar viral illness caused by the influenza viruses.* The severity of influenza can range from very mild to life threatening.

Tonsillitis *is defined as an inflammation of the tonsils, which are patches of lymph tissue at the rear of the throat.* The tonsils are important in defending against infections, but at times become infected themselves. They may be red and swollen and will narrow the opening to the throat. Untreated streptococcal tonsillitis may lead to rheumatic heart disease.

LOWER RESPIRATORY SYSTEM

Noninfectious Conditions

Asthma is usually triggered by an allergic reaction that affects the smooth muscle and glands of the bronchioles. The muscles of the bronchioles constrict and may close completely. Mucous secretion is also increased during an attack, so that already constricted passageways become even more congested by the mucus. Severity of the illness ranges from mild to life threatening, with wheezing and *dyspnea* (shortness of breath or difficulty breathing) as symptoms of this condition.

Emphysema *is a degenerative, chronic lung obstruction in which the alveoli lose their elasticity.* As the alveoli break down, larger air cavities are created that are not efficient in gas exchange. The most common (and most avoidable) cause of emphysema is cigarette smoking.

Cystic fibrosis *is a hereditary disease that affects the glands of the body that secrete mucus, sweat, and digestive enzymes.* The abnormality causes excessively viscous mucous secretion that obstructs the airways. The sweat glands are also affected, and the patient tends to lose large amounts of salt as a result. This abnormal secretion of salt is the basis for the "sweat test" used to confirm cystic fibrosis.

Pneumothorax *is the presence of air in the pleural space that causes the collapse of the lung.* The area between the pleural membranes normally contains only serous fluid and is maintained at slightly below atmospheric pressure. If, by trauma or weakened alveoli, air at atmospheric pressure enters the pleural cavity, the suddenly higher pressure outside the lung will cause the lung to collapse.

Two terms related to the respiratory system that are not disease conditions in and of themselves, but are manifestations of respiratory distress, are hypoxia and cyanosis. **Hypoxia** *is any state in which there is insufficient oxygen available to the tissue.* For example, transient cerebral hypoxia can result in a brief loss of consciousness, known as *syncope*. **Cyanosis** *refers to a bluish discoloration of the skin and mucous membranes as a result of hypoxia.*

Infectious Conditions

Laryngitis *is an inflammation of the mucosal epithelium of the vocal cords occurring as an acute disorder caused by a cold, exposure to irritating fumes, or sudden temperature changes.*

Pneumonia *is an acute inflammation of the lungs that causes a fibrous exudate to be produced within the alveoli.* The alveoli and bronchioles become plugged with the exudate, and gas exchange is inhibited. Most cases of pneumonia are caused by a variety of viruses and bacteria.

Bronchitis *is an acute or chronic inflammation of the bronchial tree caused by either infection or inhalation of irritants.* **Pleurisy** *is an inflammation of the pleural membranes that surround the lungs.* It is characterized by dyspnea and pain during breathing.

Tuberculosis *is an infection caused by the microorganism Mycobacterium tuberculosis.* The tubercular bacillus most often enters the body by inhalation and may infect the lungs as well as other portions of the body. The lungs react to the organism by forming tubercles (small nodules) around them. If the organisms are not successfully contained, they can cause extensive damage to the lungs. The presence of the fibrous masses may also interfere with gas exchange.

LABORATORY TESTING ASSOCIATED WITH THE CARDIOPULMONARY SYSTEM

Literally hundreds of laboratory tests require blood (cells, plasma, or serum) as the specimen of choice. Diseases such as diabetes, hepatitis, and renal failure can be detected by testing the blood. The following list of tests covers those areas directly associated with the cardiopulmonary system and its function, and is in no way complete.

Blood gases   Analysis performed on arterial blood to determine its pH, as well as the concentration (partial pressure) of oxygen and carbon dioxide.

Cardiac enzymes   Analysis of plasma to detect elevated levels of the enzymes creatine kinase (CK), lactate dehydrogenase (LDH), and aspartate transaminase to aid in the diagnosis of possible cardiac injury. Isoenzymes of LDH and CK are routinely used as specific indicators of myocardial injury.

Chemistry profile   Analysis of a variety of substances that are found within the blood of normal, healthy individuals. Disease states may be indicated if a patient's test values fall outside established normal ranges. For example, previously unknown diabetic patients can be diagnosed by testing their blood glucose. Renal failure may be predicted by measuring blood urea nitrogen and creatinine. General health profiles usually include testing for electrolytes, glucose, and renal and liver function.

CBC with differential   The determination of the number of formed elements in a cubic millimeter of whole blood. This includes erythrocytes, leukocytes, and platelets. Also included are determinations of the hemoglobin content and the hematocrit. The differential is an examination and enumeration of the distribution of leukocytes expressed in percentages. Erythrocyte morphology is also examined. Many suspected disease states may be diagnosed with use of this simple test.

Lipid profile and cardiac risk   Determination of the levels of the various free fatty acid substances in the blood, such as cholesterol and triglycerides. Patients with high levels of these substances are more likely to develop cardiovascular disease over time.

Microbial cultures Techniques used to isolate and identify microorganisms that may be responsible for disease. Blood cultures are routinely done as a means of diagnosing septicemia and endocarditis.

CHAPTER SUMMARY

As we have seen, the very source of life is contained within the cardiopulmonary system. It is by this remarkable network that oxygen and nutrients are delivered to each cell in the body and the by-products of metabolism are efficiently discarded. Without the coordinated efforts of the components of this system, the maintenance of life would be impossible.

Review Questions

1. Name the three major types of blood vessels and describe their functions briefly.

2. List five functions of the respiratory system and describe where these functions take place.

3. List three infectious and three noninfectious conditions associated with the cardiopulmonary and respiratory systems. Briefly discuss each condition.

BIBLIOGRAPHY

Martini, F.H.: Anatomy and Physiology, 3rd ed. Englewood Cliffs, NJ, Prentice-Hall, 1995.

Seely, R.R., Stevens, T.D., and Tate, P.: Anatomy and Physiology, 3rd ed. St. Louis, C.V. Mosby, 1995.

Tortora, G.J., and Grabowski, S.R.: Principles of Anatomy and Physiology, 8th ed. New York, HarperCollins, 1996.

The Urinary System

INTRODUCTION

ANATOMY OF THE URINARY SYSTEM

Gross Anatomy
The Kidney
  Internal structure of the kidney
  Microscopic anatomy of the kidney
  Blood supply to the nephron

FUNCTIONS OF THE URINARY SYSTEM

Formation of Urine
  Glomerular ultrafiltration
  Tubular reabsorption
  Tubular secretion
  Summary
Composition of Urine

ABNORMAL CONDITIONS THAT AFFECT THE KIDNEY

Renal Conditions
  Acute poststreptococcal glomerulonephritis

Chronic glomerulonephritis
  Nephrotic syndrome
  Urinary tract infections
  Arteriolar nephrosclerosis
  Diabetes mellitus
Postrenal Conditions
  Renal calculi
Acute and Chronic Renal Failure
  Acute renal failure
  Chronic renal failure

LABORATORY TESTS FOR ASSESSING RENAL FUNCTION

Routine Urinalysis
  History
  Definition
  Macroscopic examination of physical characteristics
  Macroscopic examination of constituents by chemical tests
  Microscopic examination of the urine
  Automation in urinalysis

Chemistry Tests That Assess Renal Function
    Serum creatinine
    Creatinine clearance
    Urea nitrogen

OTHER DIAGNOSTIC TESTS FOR ASSESSING RENAL FUNCTION
Radiologic Studies
    Intravenous pyelography
    Ultrasonography
    Computed tomography

Nuclear Medicine Studies
Cytologic and Histologic Studies
Cystoscopy
Proton Nuclear Magnetic Resonance Urinalysis

CHAPTER SUMMARY

REVIEW QUESTIONS

Objectives

1. List and describe the primary structures of the urinary system and explain the function of each.

2. Describe the parts of the nephron and their function.

3. Explain how blood circulates through the nephron.

4. Explain how urine is formed, including the major substances that are secreted and those that are reabsorbed throughout the nephron.

5. Identify the primary hormones that affect kidney function.

6. Discuss the normal composition of urine.

7. Describe the following disease states: acute and chronic glomerulonephritis, nephrotic syndrome, urinary tract infection, arteriolar nephrosclerosis, diabetes mellitus, and acute and chronic renal failure.

8. Define and briefly discuss the clinical significance of the following observations/tests performed during the macroscopic examination of urine: color, clarity, specific gravity, pH, protein, glucose, ketones, bilirubin, blood, nitrite, leukocyte esterase, urobilinogen, and ascorbic acid.

9. Briefly discuss the significance of microscopic structures that are commonly found in urine, such as various cells, casts, crystals, and organisms.

10. Describe the importance of serum creatinine, creatinine clearance, and blood urea nitrogen in assessing renal function.

11. Identify other diagnostic tests that are used to assess renal function.

KEY TERMS

kidney
ureter
bladder
urethra
nephron
glomerulus
proximal convoluted
    tubule
loop of Henle
distal convoluted tubule
afferent arteriole
efferent arteriole
peritubular capillaries
vasa recta
glomerular filtration
    rate

tubular reabsorption
osmosis
renin-angiotensin-al-
    dosterone system
renin
angiotensin II
aldosterone
antidiuretic hormone
tubular secretion
glomerulonephritis
cystitis
pyelonephritis
arteriolar nephro-
    sclerosis
diabetic nephropathy
postrenal

renal calculi
routine urinalysis
color
clarity
specific gravity
refractometry
dipsticks
proteinuria
glucosuria
ketonuria
hematuria
hemoglobinemia
bilirubinuria
urobilinogen
nitrite test
leukocyte esterase

pyuria
false-negative
bacteriuria
crystals
casts
creatinine
creatinine clearance
urea
intravenous pyelog-
    raphy
ultrasonography
computed tomography
cytologic examination
renal biopsy
cystoscopy

Introduction

The urinary system includes all organs involved in the production of urine and its subsequent elimination from the body. The urinary system is the major excretory system of the body, and therefore plays an essential role in maintaining *homeostasis*. The primary structures of the urinary system are two kidneys, two ureters, a bladder, and a urethra. This chapter describes the basic anatomy and physiology of the urinary system, common abnormal conditions of the kidney, and laboratory tests associated with kidney function. Laboratory analysis of urine (*urinalysis*) is a noninvasive, cost-effective procedure that provides important data to aid physicians in diagnosing a variety of abnormal conditions.

ANATOMY OF THE URINARY SYSTEM

GROSS ANATOMY

The **kidneys** *are paired bean-shaped organs located on the posterior abdominal wall, just above the waistline and between the level of the 12th thoracic and the third lumbar vertebrae* (Fig. 7–1). The left kidney is slightly larger than the right kidney. The right kidney is usually located a little lower than the left kidney, probably due to the position of the liver above the right kidney. The average kidney is 4 to 5 inches long and weighs approximately 150 g (5.25 oz). Each kidney is surrounded by a heavy cushion of fat that serves to hold the kidney in place and provide protection. An adrenal gland sits on top of each kidney.

Each kidney is connected to a **ureter,** *a slender muscular tube that squirts urine by peristaltic action into the* **bladder,** *a single muscular sac located on the floor of the pelvic cavity.* The bladder has the capacity to store up to approximately 400 ml of urine. *Urine is eliminated from the body through the* **urethra,** *a muscular tube that opens to the outside of the body* (Fig. 7–2). In men, the urethra also serves to discharge seminal fluid. The scientific term for the process of urine elimination from the body is *micturition.* When approximately 150 ml of urine accumulates in the bladder, a reflex is initiated causing a sensation of the "urge" to urinate.

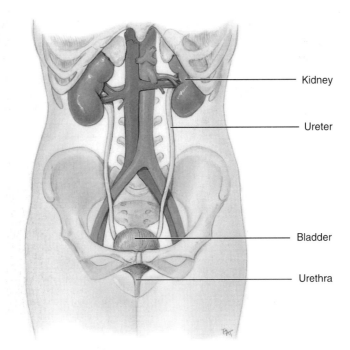

FIGURE 7–1
Location of the kidneys in the body.
(From Applegate, E.J.: The Anatomy and Physiology Learning System. Philadelphia, W.B. Saunders, 1995, with permission.)

Kidney

Ureter

Bladder

Urethra

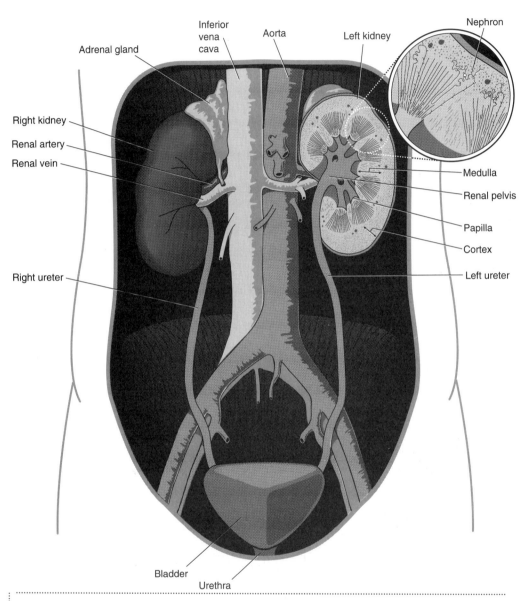

FIGURE 7-2

A schematic representation of the urinary tract, showing the relationship of the kidneys to the nephrons and the vascular system.

(From Brunzel, N.: Fundamentals of Urine and Body Fluid Analysis. Philadelphia, W.B. Saunders, 1994, with permission.)

THE KIDNEY

Internal Structure of the Kidney

The kidney is made up of an outer portion, the *cortex*, and an inner portion, the *medulla* (see Fig. 7–3). The cortex contains the *glomeruli*, which are the filtering system of the kidney. The medulla, in contrast, consists of numerous *pyramids* of renal tissue. A few channels, called the *papillae*, open at the tip of each pyramid. Each papilla juts inward toward a

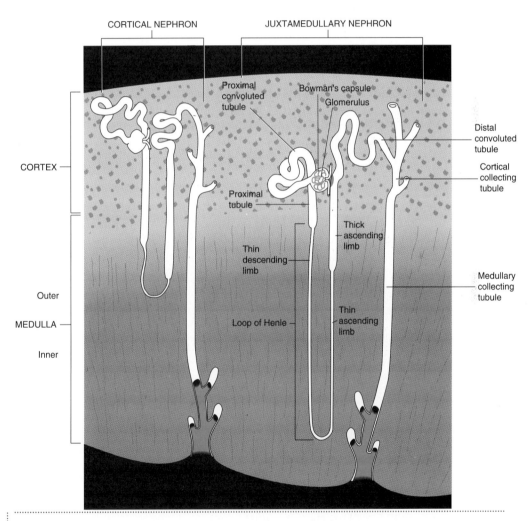

FIGURE 7-3

A schematic diagram showing the relationship of the nephron and its components to the renal cortex and the medulla.
(From Brunzel, N.: Fundamentals of Urine and Body Fluid Analysis. Philadelphia, W.B. Saunders, 1994, with permission.)

calyx. The calyces or channels join together and empty the urine received from the cortex into the *renal pelvis*, which subsequently empties the urine into the corresponding ureter.

Microscopic Anatomy of the Kidney

The **nephron** *is the functional unit of the kidney and is essentially a tiny funnel with a complex stem.* There are approximately 1.2 million nephrons per kidney. Every nephron consists of five distinct parts, each of which has a unique function in the formation of urine. The five components of the nephron are listed in Table 7–1. The cells in each of the five areas of the nephron have different microscopic structures. The structure is related to a specific function of either selectively reabsorbing or secreting various constituents from the blood. The section on urine formation discusses these functions in more detail. The following text briefly describes each of these parts.

Glomerulus.   *The* **glomerulus** *is the filtering system of the kidney and is located in the cortex.* It consists of a tuft of capillaries surrounded by a membrane known as *Bowman's capsule*. The space between the two walls of the capsule connects with the lumen (space) of the first tubule, the proximal convoluted tubule.

Proximal Convulated Tubule.   *The* **proximal convoluted tubule** *(PCT) is the small, coiled tube that is closest to the glomerulus.* The PCT travels through the cortex, toward the medulla.

Loop of Henle.   *The PCT straightens out and becomes thinner as it enters the medulla and is now called the* **loop of Henle.** There is a thin descending limb; a sharp, hairpin turn (loop); and a thin and thick ascending limb. The thick ascending limb is actually the straight portion of the distal convoluted tubule. In Figure 7–3, note the differences in length between the loop of Henle in the medulla and the cortex. The significance of this difference is discussed shortly.

Distal Convoluted Tubule.   *As the loop of Henle ascends, thickens, and heads back into the cortex, it becomes the* **distal convoluted tubule** (DCT). As its name suggests, this tubule is distal to the glomerulus and a portion of it is also convoluted. Several DCTs converge at one collecting tubule.

Table 7–1 ■ **Major Components of the Nephron**
Glomerulus
Proximal convoluted tubule (PCT)
Loop of Henle
Distal convoluted tubule (DCT)
Collecting tubule

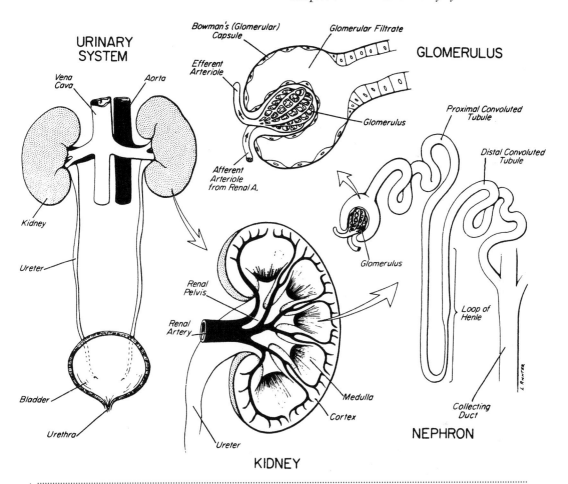

FIGURE 7-4

The urinary system.
(From Linne, J.J., and Ringsrud, K.M.: Basic Techniques in Clinical Laboratory Science. St. Louis, C.V. Mosby, 1992, with permission.)

Collecting Tubule.   Once the urine enters the collecting tubule, it passes through several ducts and empties into the calyces of the renal pyramids. The urine then drains into the renal pelvis and into the ureters. The urine collects in the bladder and remains there until it is excreted via the urethra. Figure 7–4 summarizes the entire urinary system and the major parts of the kidney.

Blood Supply to the Nephron

The kidney is a highly vascularized organ with a blood flow rate of approximately 1,200 ml/min through the glomerulus. Blood flow through the kidney begins with the *renal artery*, which supplies blood to the kidney from the abdominal aorta. *The **afferent** (entering)* **arteriole** *receives blood from the renal artery and branches to form the capillary network* *of the glomerulus. As the capillary network exits the glomerulus, it becomes the* **efferent** *(leaving)* **arteriole.** This arteriole branches into yet another capillary network called the **peritubular capillaries,** which encompass the outer cortical tubules. In the medulla, the peritubular capillaries divide into a series of long, U-shaped vessels called the **vasa recta,** which closely parallel the loop of Henle. The close proximity of the peritubular capillaries and the vasa recta to the tubules allows for efficient exchange of substances throughout the nephron. The peritubular capillaries and vasa recta eventually converge into the *renal vein.* Blood is carried away from the kidney and back to the heart through the renal vein (Fig. 7–5). Blood flow through the kidney is summarized in Figure 7–6.

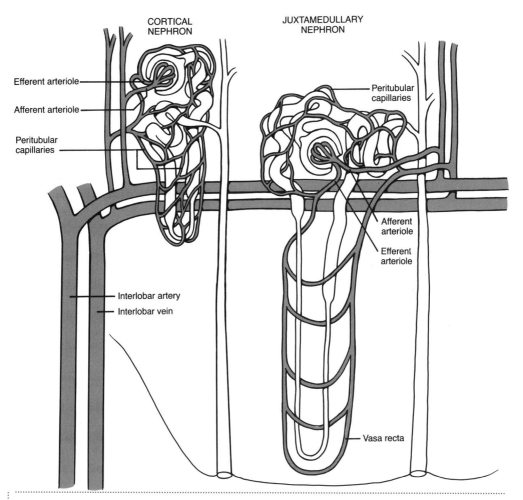

FIGURE 7-5

The vascular circulation of the nephron in the renal cortex and medulla.
(From Brunzel, N.: Fundamentals of Urine and Body Fluid Analysis. Philadelphia, W.B. Saunders, 1994, with permission.)

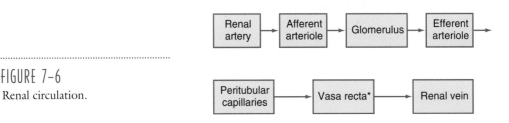

FIGURE 7-6

Renal circulation.

*only found in juxta-medullary nephrons

FUNCTIONS OF THE URINARY SYSTEM

The urinary system is the major excretory system of the body. Although there are other excretory systems in the body, such as the skin, lungs, and digestive system, the kidney is the most important because of its role in maintaining homeostasis. The major functions of the kidney are

- Regulate excretion and retention of various substances during the process of urine formation
- Maintain the delicate fluid (i.e., water), electrolyte (i.e., sodium, chloride), and acid-base balance of the blood
- Remove toxins, drug metabolites, and nitrogenous waste products such as urea from the body
- Produce substances such as erythropoietin and prostaglandins that are involved in other metabolic activities.

The focus of this section is on urine formation and the fluid, electrolyte, and acid-base balances in the body.

FORMATION OF URINE

There are three basic processes that occur within the nephron that result in the formation of urine—glomerular ultrafiltration, tubular reabsorption, and tubular secretion. At this rate of filtration, the final urine volume is 600 to 1,800 ml/24 hr.

Glomerular Ultrafiltration

The function of the glomerulus is to passively filter plasma from the afferent arteriole. The normal **glomerular filtration rate** (GFR) of the kidneys is approximately 125 ml of filtered plasma/min (180,000 ml filtered plasma/24 hr). Substances are filtered through the glomerulus or retained in plasma based on their size, molecular weight, and charge. The majority of solutes (substances dissolved in solution) that come in contact with the glomerulus are of low molecular weight and pass through the glomerulus into Bowman's capsule. Nearly all proteins and cells, such as erythrocytes and leukocytes, are unable to pass through the glomerulus because of their size or high molecular weight. Therefore, the specific gravity of the filtrate is essentially the same as cell and protein-free plasma. This filtered plasma is called the *glomerular filtrate.*

The mechanisms for reabsorption and for secretion are complex and highly variable according to the substance involved and its location within the tubules. The existence of various mechanisms allows for selective adjustments in one or more substances in order to "fine tune" urine composition, acidity, volume, or osmolality based upon the current needs of the body. In fact, only 1% of original glomerular filtrate is excreted as urine.

Tubular Reabsorption

Tubular reabsorption *occurs when substances filtered by the glomerulus into the tubular lumen are returned to blood in peritubular capillaries.*

A significant amount of reabsorption occurs in the PCT. Essentially 100% of the glucose, amino acids, and potassium (K^+) and about 70% of water, sodium (Na^+), and chloride (Cl^-) that are present in the glomerular filtrate are reabsorbed in the PCT. Sodium is actively reabsorbed while water is passively reabsorbed through a process called osmosis. **Osmosis** *is the movement of water across a membrane from a solution of low osmolality to an area of high osmolality.* Substances such as phosphate, urea, and calcium (Ca^{2+}) are partially reabsorbed here. The glomerular filtrate is reduced to about one third of its original volume after passing through the PCT, but the osmotic pressure is unchanged. This is because water and salts have been reabsorbed together.

There is, however, a limit on the amount of tubular reabsorption of an analyte. This is referred to as the *renal plasma threshold* and varies depending on the substance. For example, glucose has a plasma renal threshold value of approximately 180 mg/dl. This means that, once the glucose concentration in the blood exceeds 180 mg/dl, glucose in urine is not reabsorbed by the PCT. The excess glucose remains in the glomerular filtrate and is eliminated from the body through the urine. This excess glucose can be described as "spilling over" into the urine and can be detected by a urinalysis.

Reabsorption also occurs in the loop of Henle and involves the vasa recta. The descending loop of Henle is permeable to water but not to solutes. This results in a more concentrated fluid as water moves from the lumen of the descending loop of Henle into the capillaries of the vasa recta. As the remaining fluid passes into the ascending limb of the loop of Henle, it becomes more dilute as sodium and chloride ions are actively reabsorbed. Water loss is prevented because the ascending loop of Henle is impermeable to water. As the fluid leaves the loop of Henle, it is slightly *hypo-osmotic.* This means that more sodium and chloride leave the tubule than does water when compared to the plasma.

The final concentration of the urine through sodium and water reabsorption takes place in the DCT and collecting tubule. These important processes are under the control of hormones and enzymes, several of which are discussed here.

The **renin-angiotensin-aldosterone system** *plays an important role in fluid and electrolyte balance and in maintaining blood pressure by regulating sodium reabsorption in the DCT* (Fig. 7–7). The enzyme **renin** is produced by the *juxtaglomerular apparatus,* which

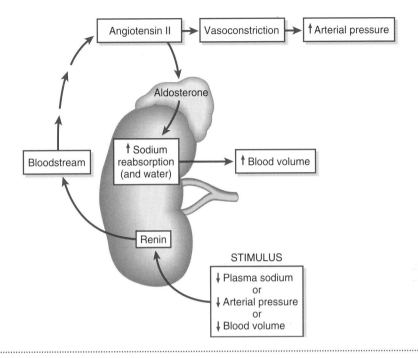

FIGURE 7-7

Renin-angiotensin-aldosterone system. The kidney releases renin into the bloodstream in response to a fall in blood pressure or blood volume, or a decrease in plasma sodium level. This initiates production of angiotensin II, which causes vasoconstriction and the production of aldosterone by the adrenal glands. Aldosterone, in turn, promotes increased sodium reabsorption and water retention (by osmosis). This results in an increase in blood volume.

is located in the nephron near the point where the afferent and efferent arterioles exit Bowman's capsule. Renin is released into the bloodstream in response to sodium depletion, decreased arterial pressure, or decreased blood volume. Once released, renin produces **angiotensin II,** a powerful vasoconstrictor that increases the blood pressure and stimulates the production of aldosterone. **Aldosterone** *is a mineralocorticoid produced by the adrenal glands in response to changes in blood volume.* Aldosterone accelerates the reabsorption of sodium in exchange for the excretion of potassium in the DCT. Following sodium reabsorption, water is reabsorbed by osmosis.

The hormone that is involved in controlling water reabsorption in the DCT and the collecting tubule is *vasopressin,* or **antidiuretic hormone** *(ADH).* ADH is produced by the hypothalamus and stored in the posterior pituitary gland. When there is a decrease in plasma volume or in arterial pressure, ADH is released. This makes the DCT and collecting tubule permeable to water reabsorption. The result is a decrease in the final urine volume. Conversely, when the plasma volume or blood pressure is increased, ADH is not released and the tubules are impermeable to water reabsorption (Fig. 7–8).

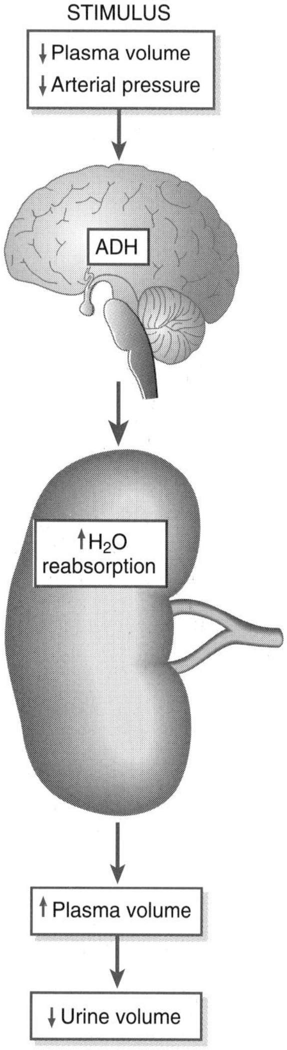

STIMULUS

↓ Plasma volume
↓ Arterial pressure

ADH

↑H₂O reabsorption

↑ Plasma volume

↓ Urine volume

FIGURE 7-8

Regulation of fluid balance. In response to a decrease in plasma volume or arterial pressure, antidiuretic hormone (ADH) is released from the posterior pituitary gland. Once released, ADH causes water retention by the distal convoluted tubule (DCT) and the collecting tubule within the kidney. This results in an increase in plasma volume and, thus, a decrease in urine volume.

Tubular Secretion

In **tubular secretion** *(excretion), substances move from the peritubular capillaries into the lumen of the tubule for elimination in the urine.* For the most part, tubular secretion is an active process involving the removal of waste products or substances from the blood. Tubular secretion also helps maintain the acid-base balance of the blood through the secretion of hydrogen ($H+$) ions.

Tubular secretion takes place throughout the nephron except for the loop of Henle. In the PCT, hydrogen ions are secreted in exchange for sodium ions. Other substances that are secreted here include ammonia, phosphate, and drugs such as penicillin. In the DCT and the collecting tubule, potassium, hydrogen, and ammonia are secreted.

Table 7–2 ■ Major Activities within the Nephron

Part of Nephron	Reabsorption	Secretion
Glomerulus*	—	—
Proximal convoluted tubule	Water, sodium, chloride, amino acids, glucose, urea, potassium	Hydrogen, ammonia, penicillin
Loop of Henle	Water (descending only), sodium and chloride (ascending only), urea (throughout loop)	None
Distal convoluted tubule	Sodium,† water,‡ chloride	Potassium, ammonia hydrogen
Collecting tubule	Sodium,† chloride, water,‡ urea	Potassium, ammonia, hydrogen

* Ultrafiltration is unique to the glomerulus.
† Controlled by renin-angiotensin-aldosterone system.
‡ Controlled by antidiuretic hormone (ADH).

Summary

Table 7–2 lists the major substances that are reabsorbed or secreted throughout the nephron. Water is reabsorbed throughout the tubules except for the ascending limb of the loop of Henle. The majority of the solutes are reabsorbed through the PCT. Secretion of hydrogen, potassium, and ammonia is similar all along the nephron with the exception of the loop of Henle. Tubular secretion occurs primarily in the DCT and collecting tubule.

COMPOSITION OF URINE

In a normal, healthy individual, the end result of tubular reabsorption and secretion is the excretion of urine composed of approximately 94% water and 6% dissolved substances. The major organic components of urine include the nitrogenous wastes, urea (primary end product of protein metabolism), creatinine, and uric acid. The major inorganic solutes in urine are sodium, chloride, potassium, calcium, and ammonia. It is the kidney's ability to adjust the excretion of water and the various solutes to meet the body's needs that makes the kidney the principal regulator of body fluids.

ABNORMAL CONDITIONS THAT AFFECT THE KIDNEY

There are several abnormal conditions that can affect kidney function. Table 7–3 outlines the prerenal, renal, and postrenal causes of kidney dysfunction. In this section, only renal and postrenal causes are presented.

Table 7–3 ■ Causes of Kidney Dysfunction

Prerenal

Hemorrhage

Shock

Dehydration

Cardiac failure

Renal

Acute poststreptococcal glomerulonephritis

Chronic glomerulonephritis

Nephrotic syndrome

Pyelonephritis

Arteriolar nephrosclerosis

Diabetic nephropathy

Postrenal

Renal calculi

Tumor that compresses bladder, ureter, or urethra opening

Enlarged prostate gland

RENAL CONDITIONS

Renal causes of kidney problems are those that occur within the kidney itself and may affect the GFR, the various tubular activities, and/or the renal blood vessels. Conditions that initially affect the GFR include different types of glomerulonephritis and nephrotic syndrome. Pyelonephritis, in contrast, is an example of a urinary tract infection than can affect tubular activities. Arteriolar nephrosclerosis is a condition that affects the renal blood vessels. Finally, diabetes mellitus is a metabolic disease that can affect the kidney in several ways.

Acute Poststreptococcal Glomerulonephritis

Acute poststreptococcal glomerulonephritis gets its name because it occurs shortly after a group A beta-hemolytic streptococcus infection such as strep throat. Glomerulonephritis is characterized by hematuria (blood in the urine) and proteinuria (protein in the urine). Edema, hypertension, fever, nausea, and renal insufficiency may also occur in varying degrees. Other abnormal laboratory tests include a decreased creatinine clearance, an increased blood urea nitrogen (BUN)–to–creatinine ratio, and an elevated antistreptolysin O (ASO) titer. This form of glomerulonephritis is often self-limiting in children and is usually not serious in adults.

Chronic Glomerulonephritis

Chronic glomerulonephritis usually develops in patients who have previously had some other form of glomerulonephritis. This disease develops slowly and silently, often taking several years to progress. It is characterized by a gradual loss of renal function. Common clinical findings include proteinuria, hypertension, edema, and azotemia (increased BUN and creatinine). The patient must often be maintained on renal dialysis or must undergo renal transplantation.

Nephrotic Syndrome

Nephrotic syndrome is caused by lesions that develop in the glomerular membrane. These lesions increase the permeability of the membrane and allow large molecules that normally do not pass through the membrane to "leak" into the urine. The classic findings in nephrotic syndrome are *hyperlipidemia* (increased lipids in blood), *hypoproteinemia* (decreased protein in blood), *lipiduria* (lipids in urine), proteinuria, and edema. Causes of nephrotic syndrome include glomerulonephritis, diabetes mellitus, and systemic lupus erythematosus.

Urinary Tract Infections

An estimated 5.2 million physician office visits annually are due to urinary tract infections (UTIs). A UTI can involve only the lower portion of the urinary tract (bladder, urethra, or both) or may extend to the upper portion of the tract (kidneys, ureters, or both). **Cystitis** *is the term that refers to inflammation of the bladder, while* **pyelonephritis** *refers to inflammation within the kidney itself.*

UTIs are caused by bacterial organisms that infect an otherwise sterile urinary tract. The most common agent is *Escherichia coli*, which is a normal stool flora. The bacteria ascend from the urethra to the bladder or on into the kidney. Incidence and risk factors for UTIs vary with age and gender. In adults, women are 30 times more likely to develop UTIs than men. This predisposition is due to several factors, including the shorter urethra in females and the "milking" of bacteria up the urethra during sexual intercourse. UTIs can usually be successfully treated with appropriate antibiotic therapy. However, repeated or chronic infections can damage renal tissue and subsequently decrease renal function.

Cystitis has more recently been referred to as uncomplicated UTI and is the most common of all clinical forms of urinary tract infections. This form is often observed in otherwise healthy women and comprises approximately 70% of UTIs in women. *Dysuria* (painful urination) and urine frequency are the most common symptoms. Other findings may include increased urge to urinate, hematuria, low back pain, suprapubic pain, and mild fever. Routine urinalysis reveals bacteria in urine (bacteriuria) and increased numbers of leukocytes in the urine (pyuria).

The most common type of upper UTI is *acute pyelonephritis*, which occurs when bacteria move from the lower urinary tract to the kidneys. Predisposing conditions include pregnancy, catheterization, reflux, and urinary obstruction. Signs and symptoms of an upper UTI are similar to those observed with a lower UTI but often also include fever, chills, and flank or back pain. Routine urinalysis shows bacteriuria, leukocyturia, and the presence of casts (not seen in lower UTIs). Patients can also have a UTI without having any symptoms.

Arteriolar Nephrosclerosis

Hypertension, or high blood pressure, can cause serious, irreversible kidney damage. Hypertension can affect the blood flow to the kidney but can also be caused by abnormalities *within* the renal blood vessels themselves. **Arteriolar nephrosclerosis** *is the thickening of the lining of the renal arterioles to such a degree that the arteriolar blood pressure increases because the lumen is decreased.* Impairment of renal function occurs because of the destruction (*necrosis*) of the blood vessels due to the increased blood pressure and thickening of the arteriolar walls. If the high blood pressure cannot be controlled by medication or other means, the development of chronic renal failure is inevitable.

Diabetes Mellitus

Several systemic diseases can also result in renal disease. One of the most well-known examples is *diabetes mellitus.* Diabetes is caused by ineffective glucose utilization due to either decreased pancreatic insulin production or the production of dysfunctional insulin. Diabetes mellitus affects carbohydrate, fat, and protein metabolism. Classic findings in patients with undiagnosed/uncontrolled diabetes mellitus are *hyperglycemia* (increased glucose in the blood), glucosuria (glucose in the urine), ketonuria (increased ketones in urine), *polydipsia* (increased thirst), and *polyuria* (increased urine production). *Renal disease caused by diabetes is referred to as* **diabetic nephropathy.**

POSTRENAL CONDITIONS

Postrenal *means that the cause of renal dysfunction occurs beyond the kidney but somewhere within the remainder of the urinary system.* Postrenal factors include renal calculi (stones) or tumors that may constrict the ureters, urethra, or bladder opening. In men, an enlarged prostate gland that partially blocks the urethra can cause renal dysfunction.

Renal Calculi

Although only about 0.1% of the population develop renal calculi, it is important to understand how and why calculi form, and to identify the composition of renal calculi. For the purposes of this chapter, a brief overview of these concepts is presented.

Renal calculi, *also known as "kidney stones," are solid aggregates of chemicals that form within the urinary tract (renal calyces, pelvis, ureters, or bladder).* When the urine becomes supersaturated with chemical components and the pH is optimal, crystals precipitate and renal calculi form. Calculi often form as a result of some type of metabolic or endocrine disturbance, such as gout, cystinuria, and hyperparathyroidism. Stone formation can be enhanced by bacterial infections or conditions in which the urinary pH is fixed.

Most calculi are actually mixtures of several chemical components, including a mineral salt. Calcium is the most common element and is found in approximately 75% of all calculi. The composition of renal calculi can be determined in a specialized laboratory. Identification of the type of stone aids in the prevention and treatment of renal calculi.

ACUTE AND CHRONIC RENAL FAILURE

Acute Renal Failure

Acute renal failure (ARF) is discussed separately because it is a condition that can have prerenal, renal, or postrenal causes. ARF is caused by abnormally functioning nephrons. Clinically, the patient will present with a decreased GFR, azotemia, and *oliguria* (urine output less than 400 ml).

Prerenal ARF may result from a decrease in the renal blood flow due to decreased cardiac output (i.e., congestive heart failure), burns, or surgery. Urinalysis results are not helpful in this situation. Instead, measuring urine electrolytes, such as sodium, is helpful. In response to the decreased blood flow to the kidney, the kidney reabsorbs more water and sodium in an attempt to restore blood volume. Therefore, the urine sodium will be low. In addition, the BUN-to-creatinine ratio will be increased in prerenal ARF.

The most common *renal* cause of ARF is damage within the kidney itself. The majority of patients present with renal tubular destruction, resulting in the loss of water and electrolytes (sodium and potassium). In contrast to prerenal ARF, renal ARF shows an increased urinary sodium concentration.

Postrenal causes of ARF are obstructions in urinary flow because of neoplasms or deposits of crystals from drugs or solutes. In postrenal ARF, the obstruction increases hydrostatic pressure within the tubules and disrupts normal glomerular filtration pressures. Tubular damage and subsequent loss of renal function can occur.

Chronic Renal Failure

Chronic renal failure (CRF) is an extremely serious condition owing to the progressive and irreversible loss of renal function. As with chronic glomerulonephritis, CRF occurs slowly and silently. Numerous diseases can result in CRF, including glomerulonephritis, systemic lupus erythematosus, hypertension, and chronic pyelonephritis.

Clinical findings associated with CRF include azotemia, acid-base imbalance, and water and electrolyte imbalance. Anemia, hypertension, nausea, and vomiting can also be present. Urinalysis findings include a fixed specific gravity of 1.010, proteinuria, hematuria, and the presence of several types of casts, especially broad and waxy casts. With CRF, the GFR continuously decreases over time, and the condition eventually is referred to as "end-stage renal disease." At this point, the patient must undergo renal dialysis or renal transplantation in order to survive.

LABORATORY TESTS FOR ASSESSING RENAL FUNCTION

Laboratory tests for renal function encompass several disciplines within clinical laboratory science. Areas include clinical chemistry, urinalysis, microbiology, and virology. This section focuses on urinalysis and clinical chemistry tests that are commonly used to assess renal function. Because of its multiple functions, the kidney plays an important role in several regulatory mechanisms in the body. Therefore, the detection of abnormal constituents in the urine can be extremely helpful in the diagnosis and monitoring of disease, whether renal or nonrenal (systemic). Examination of urine also provides an assessment of the body's general health status.

ROUTINE URINALYSIS

History

The study of urine began over 2,000 years ago because of the basic belief that changes in the appearance of urine were associated with disease (Table 7–4). In ancient times, urine was poured on the ground and then observed as to whether or not it attracted insects. If insects were attracted, the urine was called "honey urine." This phenomenon was usually observed with urine from people with boils. It is now known that this "honey urine" probably

Table 7–4 ■ Historical Overview of the Development of Urinalysis

Time in History	Discovery/Event
Ancient times (>400 B.C.)	"Honey" urine attracted insects
400 B.C.	Hippocrates observed color and odor changes in urine related to fever
1000 A.D.	Ismail of Jurjani made seven observations while studying urine
1500–1600s	"Pisse prophets" made numerous predictions about health and future just by visual observation of urine
1674	Boerhaave correlated specific gravity with dehydration
1827	Bright developed a method for detecting protein in renal disease by using heat and acid
1911	Benedict developed a test for sugar that used an alkaline copper reduction method
early 1900s	Addis developed method for quantitation of urine sediment (Addis count)
1940s	Compton developed CLINITEST for determining reducing sugars in urine
1956	Both Lilly and Ames companies developed a urine dip-and-read test for glucose

contained glucose, which attracted the insects. Even today, untreated diabetics often develop boils.

Since this early practice of urinalysis, a variety of procedures, including qualitative chemical test strip procedures, microscopy, and microbiologic techniques, have become available to aid in the diagnosis of renal disease.

In the 20th century, the laborious "wet" chemistry tests were eventually replaced by "dry" chemistry spot tests. As a result, urinalysis gradually became a practical laboratory procedure. In 1956, the modern era of urine test strips emerged. Two companies, Lilly and Ames, developed a urine dip-and-read test for glucose that was more specific and sensitive than any previously developed test. Its introduction was called "a revolution in lab diagnostics." Eventually, several manufacturers developed a number of different urine test strips, some of which measure as many as 10 different parameters.

Definition

A **routine urinalysis,** better known as a UA, normally consists of both a macroscopic and a microscopic examination of urine. A macroscopic examination includes physical observations and chemical testing of urine. These tests are performed first. Then the microscopic examination is performed. This procedure involves identifying cellular components, organisms, casts, and crystals in the urine. Table 7–5 lists the individual tests and observations commonly performed in a routine urinalysis.

Table 7–5 ■ **Components of a Routine Urinalysis**

Macroscopic Examination		*Microscopic Examination*
Physical Observations	*Chemical Tests*	
Color	Specific gravity*	Leukocytes
Clarity	pH	Erythrocytes
(Odor)	Protein	Epithelial cells
(Volume)	Glucose	Bacteria
	Ketones	Crystals
	Blood	Casts
	Bilirubin	Yeast
	Urobilinogen	Parasites
	Nitrite	
	Leukocyte esterase	
	Ascorbic acid	

* Also a physical test.

Most routine urinalysis testing is done on a freshly voided random urine specimen. If the specimen cannot be tested within 2 hours of collection, it should be refrigerated until testing is performed. This is because urine stored at room temperature for more than 2 hours undergoes changes that can alter the physical, chemical, and microscopic test results.

Macroscopic Examination of Physical Characteristics

The physical findings portion of a urinalysis is routinely performed prior to the chemical portion. Several physical characteristics that are routinely observed include the color, clarity, and specific gravity of the urine. The volume of urine is also noted on timed urine collections. Urine odors characteristic of certain diseases are also recorded when present.

The **color** of urine is determined by visually inspecting the urine sample in a clear container using adequate lighting. There are endogenous pigments that contribute to the color of urine. *Urochrome*, a yellow pigment, contributes the most color to urine. The color of urine is primarily influenced by the amount of water present in the urine; that is, the more water present in the specimen, the lighter the color of urine. Normal colors of urine range from colorless (very dilute) to yellow to amber or dark yellow (very concentrated). The presence of an abnormal urine color may be attributed to physical activity, medication, diet, disease, or therapy. Therefore, an abnormal color does not necessarily mean a pathologic condition exists. For example, increased physical activity can cause temporary hematuria, giving a pink-red color to the urine. Pyridium is a medication that is frequently prescribed to patients with UTIs and may give the urine an orange-red color. Patients with hepatitis produce urine that is dark yellow or orange-yellow, indicating the abnormal presence of bilirubin. Likewise, a blue to green urine color can be observed in patients with a UTI caused by a *Pseudomonas* (bacteria) infection. Table 7–6 lists frequently observed colors of urine and their possible causes.

Table 7–6 ■ Common Colors of Urine and Their Causes

Color of Urine	Possible Causes
Dark yellow to yellow-brown	Bilirubin
Pink to red	Blood (hemoglobin), beets, various dyes and other foods
Dark reddish brown	Porphyrins
Green to greenish brown	Biliverdin
Blue to green	*Pseudomonas* infection
Orange	Pyridium (aminopyrine drugs), bilirubin
Dark brown–black	Melanin

The **clarity,** or appearance, of urine is determined by visually inspecting a well-mixed sample of urine in a clear container. A normal urine specimen usually appears clear. The fact that a specimen is clear, however, does not mean it is entirely normal—clinically significant microscopic elements or chemical constituents may be present. A urine specimen that is not clear in appearance is described as *cloudy* or *turbid.* Just as various urine colors can be pathologic or nonpathologic, cloudy urines may or may not be clinically significant. Some pathologic conditions that cause urine to become cloudy include the presence of pathologic crystals, increased numbers of leukocytes and bacteria as seen with a UTI, and the presence of erythrocytes. Nonpathologic conditions that result in cloudy urine include a small number of epithelial cells, trace amounts of mucus or spermatozoa, or precipitation of crystals in a refrigerated urine specimen.

The **specific gravity** of urine reflects the relative degree of concentrating and diluting abilities of the kidney. The specific gravity varies greatly because it is so dependent on the state of hydration. The specific gravity of a random specimen can range from 1.001 to 1.035. However, the majority of random urine specimens have a specific gravity between 1.015 and 1.025. A specific gravity of more than 1.023 on a random urine specimen indicates normal renal concentrating ability. Chronic glomerulonephritis and conditions involving renal tubular dysfunction show a loss of concentrating ability. Urine from patients with these conditions has a decreased specific gravity. A "fixed" specific gravity of 1.010, which is equivalent to the specific gravity of the glomerular ultrafiltrate, is indicative of severe renal damage. Conversely, high specific gravities are seen with excessive loss of water, as in chronic sweating, diarrhea, or vomiting. The specific gravity of urine is determined by comparing the density (mass) of urine with that of water. The most common laboratory method for measuring specific gravity is **refractometry**.

Urine volume is considered a physical test but is not performed routinely. It is important in assessing renal damage or when a specific urinary constituent is measured quantitatively. This necessitates a timed urine collection. A 24-hour urine collection is the most frequently ordered timed collection. After the urine is collected for the specified time, the urine volume is measured and used to calculate the concentration of the urinary analyte of interest. In renal disease, the urinary output decreases as the degree of renal damage increases.

The *odor* of urine is not routinely reported except when abnormal. Fresh urine from a healthy individual has a characteristic odor due to the presence of volatile acids. Upon standing, urine develops a strong ammonia odor because bacteria present in the urine decompose urea to ammonia. A fruity urine odor is characteristic of diabetes mellitus, while a foul-smelling urine can be caused by a UTI. Two metabolic disorders that produce urine with characteristic odors are *maple syrup urine disease* (maple syrup odor) and *phenylketonuria* (PKU) (musty or mousy odor). The accumulation of increased amounts of amino acids or their metabolites produce the unique odors in both of these conditions.

Macroscopic Examination of Constituents by Chemical Tests

Several manufacturers have developed chemically impregnated reagent test strips (**dipsticks**) that are used for the rapid determination of urine constituents. Thus, urine specimens can be screened for a number of analytes in a matter of minutes. Each pad on the strip contains the necessary reagents to detect a specific chemical constituent. The reagent strip is dipped into a well-mixed urine specimen, and specific substances in the urine react with the reagents on the strip to produce a color change. The color produced on each pad is compared with the color chart that is provided (see Color Figure 6). The intensity of color change reflects the concentration of the substance being measured. Qualitative or semi-quantitative results are obtained depending on the particular substance being measured.

Commercial reagent test strips are available in several combinations of the following constituents: specific gravity, pH, protein, glucose, ketones, bilirubin, blood, nitrite, leuko-cyte esterase, urobilinogen, and ascorbic acid (vitamin C). In addition, other reagent strips and chemical tablets are available for specialized testing. A summary of these 11 analytes and their major clinical significance is found in Table 7–7.

The *pH* of urine is a measurement of its hydrogen ion concentration. It plays an important role in the acid-base balance of the body. Urine with a pH greater than 7.0 is known as *alkaline urine*, while a pH less than 7.0 denotes *acidic urine*. The pH range of urine is about 5 to 8, with a healthy individual having a slightly acidic urine of 6. High alkalinity is often associated with UTIs, high fruit/vegetable diets, and urine that has not been properly preserved. Individuals on high-protein diets and those with diabetes mellitus have very acidic urine.

Table 7–7 ■ Clinical Significance of Positive Chemical Tests in Urine

Measured Analyte	Major Clinical Significance
pH	Alkaline Acidic: diabetes mellitus
Protein	Renal disease
Glucose	Uncontrolled diabetes mellitus
Ketones	Anorexia, prolonged vomiting or fasting, uncontrolled diabetes mellitus
Blood	Renal disease, trauma, or neoplasms
Bilirubin	Hepatic disease (i.e., hepatitis, biliary obstruction)
Urobilinogen	Increased in hemolytic anemia, malaria, hepatitis, cirrhosis; decreased in neoplasms and cholelithiasis
Nitrite	UTI
Leukocyte esterase	UTI
Ascorbic acid	Can interfere with interpretation of other chemical tests such as blood, glucose
Specific gravity	Increased in chronic sweating, diarrhea, or vomiting; decreased in renal tubular dysfunction and "fixed" with severe renal damage

A small amount of low-molecular-weight *protein* is normally found in urine. Because of its low concentration, it is not usually detected by the reagent strip. Larger molecular weight proteins are usually unable to pass through a healthy glomerulus. Therefore, when increased urine protein (**proteinuria**) is detected, it means that damage to the glomerulus or disruption of the tubular reabsorption processes has occurred. In fact, proteinuria is considered to be one of the earliest indicators of renal disease. Transient forms of proteinuria that are not clinically significant may occur in pregnancy, stress, and increased physical activity. Nonrenal diseases such as multiple myeloma and leukemia may also cause proteinuria.

Glucose is a sugar (carbohydrate) that is an important source of body energy. It is completely reabsorbed in the PCT unless the plasma renal threshold is surpassed. *When the renal threshold is exceeded, glucose begins to appear in the urine* (**glucosuria**). Diabetes mellitus, a disorder of glucose metabolism, is the disease most frequently associated with glucosuria. Other sugars can appear in the urine and are detected by different screening methods.

Ketones are intermediary products of fat metabolism that appear in blood. **Ketonuria, the presence of ketones in urine, is usually observed when there is an inadequate amount of carbohydrate in the diet and fatty acids are metabolized.** Conditions such as anorexia, prolonged vomiting, and fasting often result in ketonuria. It is also present when there is a defect in carbohydrate metabolism or absorption (diabetes mellitus).

The clinical significance of *blood* in the urine is dependent on the patient's history and clinical presentation. When blood appears as intact erythrocytes, referred to as **hematuria,** the urine may appear pink, red, or brown in color. When blood is present as free hemoglobin (**hemoglobinuria),** the color of the urine may not be affected at all. The presence of blood in the urine in either form is detected by the urine reagent strip and is usually due to bleeding somewhere in the urinary tract caused by renal disorders, infectious disease, trauma, or neoplasms. A common nonpathologic condition in women that causes a positive result for blood on the dipstick is menstruation. Vigorous exercise can also cause a transient hematuria. Blood detected by the dipstick is routinely confirmed and correlated with the microscopic examination.

Bilirubin detected in the urine is indicative of some sort of hepatic (liver) disease, either a hepatocellular disease or hepatic biliary obstruction. Bilirubin is formed when hemoglobin is catabolized in the reticuloendothelial cells of the bone marrow and spleen. Bilirubin is carried to the liver and then to the intestinal tract, where it is further metabolized. Conjugated bilirubin, a water-soluble form of bilirubin, can be excreted by the kidneys. In healthy individuals, trace amounts of this bilirubin are excreted. This trace amount is not detected by the reagent strip. An increased amount of bilirubin in the urine (**bilirubinuria**) is caused by a concomitant increase in bilirubin in the bloodstream *(hyperbilirubinemia)*.

Urobilinogen is formed from the breakdown of bilirubin by bacteria in the intestinal tract. The majority of urobilinogen is excreted in the feces. It is estimated that as much as 50% of the urobilinogen formed in the intestines is reabsorbed into the hepatic portal circulation and re-excreted by the liver. However, a small amount is also excreted in urine. The concentration of urobilinogen in a normal, random urine specimen is 0.1 to 1.0 Ehrlich units/dl. Therefore, the result is usually reported as "normal" instead of "negative." An increase in urinary urobilinogen occurs in any condition that causes an increase in the production of bilirubin. Such conditions include hemolytic anemias and malaria, where there is excessive destruction of erythrocytes. An increased urinary urobilinogen is also found with any disease that prevents the liver from removing reabsorbed urobilinogen from the portal circulation. Hepatitis and cirrhosis are hepatic diseases that affect the reabsorption of urobilinogen in this manner. In contrast, a decreased urinary urobilinogen occurs when normal amounts of bilirubin are not excreted into the intestinal tract. This situation usually involves some type of bile duct obstruction. Neoplasms and cholelithiasis (gallstones) cause bile duct obstruction. Together, the urinary bilirubin and urobilinogen results can be used to help establish a differential diagnosis. Table 7–8 shows the correlation between these two parameters in making a diagnosis.

Two tests, the nitrite and the leukocyte esterase tests, are used to screen for possible UTI. A probable diagnosis can be made sooner, and the urine can be cultured for confirmation and identification of the bacterial agent and the antimicrobial susceptibility patterns. The **nitrite test** is based upon the principle that the majority of the microorganisms that cause UTIs contain reductase enzymes that reduce nitrate to nitrite. The reagent strip measures the nitrite concentration. However, a negative nitrite test does not always mean that significant numbers of bacteria are not present. Correlation between the dipstick result and the microscopic examination should always be done.

Leukocyte esterase *(LE) is an enzyme that is present in certain types of leukocytes, which are found in increased numbers in UTIs. The presence of leukocytes (pus cells) is referred to as* **pyuria.** A urinary tract infection is the most likely diagnosis if both bacteriuria and pyuria are present. These results should also be correlated with the microscopic examination findings and, as stated previously, confirmed with a microbiologic culture.

Ascorbic acid (vitamin C) can be detected by the dipstick method, but is not a commonly ordered test. Ascorbic acid is a water-soluble vitamin, and any excess vitamin ingested is excreted in the urine. It is a strong reducing agent, and can interfere with several of the other chemical tests on the dipstick. This interference can result in "false-negative" test results for a number of analytes. *A* **"false-negative"** *result is one that erroneously reports the absence of an analyte that is actually present.* The most common interference caused by ascorbic acid is observed when there is a negative result on a blood dipstick test but the microscopic exam reveals the presence of erythrocytes. Consequently, detecting the presence of vitamin C in urine can be extremely helpful in the interpretation of the results of other dipstick tests.

Table 7–8 ■ **Differential Diagnosis Using Urinary Bilirubin and Urobilinogen Results**

Type of Disease	*Urine Bilirubin*	*Urine Urobilinogen*
Prehepatic (i.e., hemolytic anemia)	Negative	Increased
Hepatic (i.e., cirrhosis)	Positive or negative	Increased
Posthepatic (i.e., biliary obstruction)	Positive	Decreased or absent

Summary. Table 7–9 lists the reference (expected) ranges for some of the physical and chemical tests performed on a random, routine urine specimen from a healthy individual. Factors such as the amount of physical activity and recent diet (including amount of fluid intake) affect the composition of an individual's urine. Therefore, establishing normal reference ranges for many of the other urinary components is difficult. To minimize variability and ensure accuracy, 24-hour urine collections are often obtained. Urinary constituents that are collected in this manner include sodium, chloride, urea, and creatinine.

Microscopic Examination of the Urine

The microscopic examination of urine consists of centrifuging an aliquot of urine, pouring off the supernatant, and examining the remaining urine sediment under the microscope. Casts, cells, and crystals are the formed elements commonly observed in the sediment. In addition, the microscopic examination serves as a confirmatory test for some of the results obtained by the macroscopic examination. In fact, the macroscopic and microscopic examination results are routinely compared with each other to ensure they correlate before reporting out the final urinalysis results. The following paragraphs briefly discuss examples of the more common formed elements found in urine. Color Figures 7 through 16 show several of these formed elements.

Table 7–9 ■ Reference Ranges for Macroscopic Tests

Test	Reference Range
Color	Light yellow to amber
Clarity	Clear
Specific gravity	1.001–1.035 (random urine)
pH	5–9*
Protein	Negative
Glucose	Negative
Ketones	Negative
Blood	Negative
Bilirubin	Negative
Urobilinogen	0.2–1.0 Ehrlich units/ml
Nitrite	Negative
Leukocyte esterase	Negative

* Both the normal and abnormal urinary pH range is 5 to 9.

Large numbers of *leukocytes* present in the urine sediment usually indicate the presence of a UTI. If the LE test is positive on the dipstick, leukocytes should also be seen on the microscopic exam. An exception to this occurs when the urine has been allowed to stand at room temperature too long, causing the leukocytes to disintegrate.

The presence of more than about three *erythrocytes* in the urine sediment is indicative of an abnormal condition. Kidney trauma due to passage of kidney stones, neoplasms, pyelonephritis, glomerulonephritis, and cystitis can all cause blood in the urine. Nonpathologic conditions causing hematuria include menstruation in females and strenuous exercise. The presence of erythrocytes in the urine microscopically should correspond with a positive blood result on the dipstick. However, a correlation will not exist if the erythrocytes *lyse* (dissolve) before the urine is examined microscopically. This can occur if the urine is very dilute or has an alkaline pH.

There are several types of *epithelial cells* that appear in urine. *Squamous* epithelial cells appear frequently in normal urine because they are sloughed off the walls of the external genitalia and the urethra, especially in females. *Transitional* epithelial cells originate in the upper urethra and renal pelvis, and *renal tubular* epithelial cells come directly from the tubules, hence their name. Transitional epithelial cells are present in significant amounts in bladder disease. Renal tubular epithelial cells are present in conditions associated with acute tubular damage, such as viral infections, poisons, or salicylate intoxication.

Bacteria in urine (**bacteriuria**) is most often associated with a UTI. Their presence microscopically should almost always correlate with a positive nitrite or LE test, or both, and a positive microbiologic culture. They appear as tiny, motile, and often rod-shaped organisms that can easily number more than 40 organisms/high-power field. A note of caution— bacteria can also be present in a urine specimen that has been allowed to sit at room temperature for more than 2 hours. The presence of bacteria in the absence of leukocytes is more indicative of contamination than of a UTI.

Urine can contain a number of different types of **crystals** that may or may not be clinically significant. Crystals are formed from the precipitation of solutes in the urine. They frequently form during refrigeration storage of the urine and are not clinically significant. Crystals are identified by their microscopic appearance and by noting the pH of the urine in which they appear. Nonpathologic crystals include the *amorphous urates* (acid urine) and *amorphous phosphates* (alkaline urine). Calcium oxalate (often acid or neutral urine) and triple phosphate (often alkaline or neutral urine) can be observed in nonpathologic and pathologic conditions. Other abnormal crystals in acidic urines include uric acid, cystine, cholesterol, and tyrosine.

Yeasts often appear as "budding" structures and are present in women with vaginal yeast infections (candidiasis). Yeast infections also occur in diabetic patients.

Casts *are unique types of formed elements that form in the DCT or collecting tubules.* Four conditions/components enhance cast formation: an acid environment, the presence of a special protein called Tamm-Horsfall, a high salt concentration, and a reduction of urine flow (stasis). The various types of casts differ in their composition. Eventually, the casts will detach from the tubular epithelium and be excreted in the urine. In general, detection of casts in the urine suggests renal disease with tubular involvement.

Hyaline casts have a colorless matrix and are the most predominant form of cast found in urine. Their presence in high numbers is usually due to nonpathologic conditions such as fever, stress, or vigorous exercise, but they may also be seen in renal disease. The names given to the other types of casts are derived from the chemical or formed element that is contained within a cast's matrix. *Erythrocyte* casts are present in acute glomerulonephritis and renal infarction. *Leukocyte* casts are also observed in pyelonephritis and nephrotic syndrome. *Broad* casts get their name from being several times wider than other casts. This type of cast is also known as a "renal failure" cast because it is seen in individuals with chronic renal failure. *Fatty* casts are observed in nephrotic syndrome and toxic renal poisoning.

Urine sediment findings are reported in qualitative or semiquantitative terms. The term used for each finding is dependent on the element observed and the reporting methods of the laboratory that is performing the test. Expected values are difficult to establish because of the numerous factors that contribute to the composition of the final urine. However, in most cases, the presence of one or two erythrocytes, leukocytes, or both per high-power field and a few epithelial cells is not abnormal. Adult women normally shed more squamous epithelial cells. An occasional hyaline cast can also be considered a normal finding.

In summary, it takes a great deal of practice to accurately identify the numerous formed elements that can be present in a urine specimen. Furthermore, one must be able to distinguish significant formed elements from artifacts and contaminants.

Automation in Urinalysis

The urine reagent test strips can also be read by a semiautomated or automated instrument. In fact, one manufacturer has even developed a system that can perform the entire urinalysis, including a "slideless" microscopic examination of the urine. Automation has several advantages over manual (visual) methods, including increased efficiency, standardization, and improved accuracy and precision.

CHEMISTRY TESTS THAT ASSESS RENAL FUNCTION

Serum Creatinine

The measurement of serum creatinine is a good indicator of renal function. **Creatinine** is a waste product formed when creatine phosphate, a high-energy compound stored in muscle, is broken down when the body needs energy. Creatinine is filtered by the glomerulus but is not reabsorbed by the tubules and, hence, is excreted. Creatinine is excreted at a fairly constant rate. Extrinsic factors such as diet, gender, age, and exercise do not affect the amount of creatinine that is excreted. Consequently, an increase in serum creatinine means an impairment of renal function. The causes of impairment are either a reduction of the GFR or an obstruction that interferes with urinary excretion. Healthy nephrons are unique in that they can compensate for unhealthy ones until about half of the nephrons have lost their ability to function. Unfortunately, as a result, elevated serum creatinine levels are normally not observed until about 50% of normal kidney function is lost.

Prerenal causes of an elevated serum creatinine level include congestive heart failure, excessive sweating, shock, prolonged vomiting or diarrhea, and diabetes insipidus. *Renal* causes involve damage to the glomeruli, tubules, or renal blood vessels. *Postrenal* causes of increased serum creatinine include neoplasms, renal calculi (blocking ureters), and prostatic hypertrophy.

Creatinine Clearance

The creatinine clearance test is considered to be the most sensitive chemical method available for assessing renal function. **Creatinine clearance** actually estimates the GFR. Creatinine clearance is calculated based on the serum and urine creatinine measurements. For this test, the volume of the 24-hour urine is measured and the concentration of creatinine in a 24-hour urine sample and in a single serum sample are determined.

Decreased creatinine clearance indicates a decreased GFR. As with the serum creatinine, prerenal, renal, or postrenal factors can be involved in decreasing the creatinine clearance. Decreased creatinine clearance with a normal serum creatinine level most likely suggests a problem with specimen collection or method of analysis.

Urea Nitrogen

In addition to creatinine, urea is found in increased concentration with renal function impairment. **Urea** is a nitrogenous substance that is a product of protein catabolism. It is solely excreted by the kidney. Urea is filtered by the glomerulus but, unlike creatinine, some urea is reabsorbed by the tubules. With a normal GFR and normal renal function, approximately 40% of the filtered urea is reabsorbed by the tubules.

In earlier times, clinical chemists measured nitrogen-containing substances by converting the nitrogen into ammonia, which was trapped and measured. Hence, *blood urea nitrogen* (BUN) was the name used to designate the measurement of urea. This name is still used today.

Elevated levels of BUN can be caused by the same prerenal, renal, and postrenal factors as seen with creatinine. In fact, the creatinine and BUN concentrations usually parallel each other in renal impairment. Unlike creatinine, however, extrinsic factors such as hormones or diet can affect the urea concentration in blood. For example, a high-protein diet will cause an elevated BUN, as will the hypersecretion or injection of adrenal steroids. Both of these factors increase protein catabolism. Therefore, an elevated BUN does not always indicate renal impairment.

OTHER DIAGNOSTIC TESTS FOR ASSESSING RENAL FUNCTION

Several other diagnostic tests can aid in the assessment of renal function. Radiologic studies are the most common tests that are performed outside the clinical laboratory. Some studies require the use of radioisotopes while other studies employ cytologic or histologic methods. Proton nuclear magnetic resonance spectroscopy is one of the most recently developed methods used to study urine.

RADIOLOGIC STUDIES

Intravenous Pyelography

Intravenous pyelography *(IVP) involves the injection of radiographic contrast media into blood so that the urinary tract can be visualized.* Several radiographs are then taken as the contrast media pass through the urinary system. IVP can be helpful in detecting renal calculi, cysts, tumors, or scarring in the kidney. It can also reveal changes in the kidney due to renal failure or other renal disorders.

Ultrasonography

Ultrasonography (ultrasound) *is a noninvasive radiologic technique that uses high-frequency sound to produce images of sections of the urinary tract.* It is an extremely useful imaging system that can detect masses or stones within the urinary system. It can even detect small tumors or blood clots within the renal veins or vena cava that cannot be seen on IVP.

Computed Tomography

Computed tomography (CT) is the most sensitive method available for diagnosing and staging renal carcinoma. It is also the most expensive radiographic imaging procedure available. **CT** *utilizes computer processing to generate an image (CT scan) of the tissue density in a transverse plane of the patient's body.* Radiographic contrast media are injected or barium sulfate is ingested prior to the CT scan.

NUCLEAR MEDICINE STUDIES

Similarly, radioisotopic methods have been utilized for more than 40 years to evaluate renal function. Radioisotopic methods do not require urine or blood samples, which is an advantage over the creatinine clearance test and other traditional methods. However, radioisotopic methods require more sophisticated equipment (gamma counter and computer) and highly trained personnel.

CYTOLOGIC AND HISTOLOGIC STUDIES

Cytologic examination *of urine involves special centrifugation and staining procedures for cell identification and enumeration.* This allows cells found in the urine to be studied in more detail than routine urinalysis. *Cytodiagnostic urinalysis,* a modification of the routine cytologic examination of urine, is often used to monitor renal or pancreatic transplant rejection or to detect opportunistic infections such as cytomegalovirus. Finally, cytodiagnostic urinalysis can be performed to aid in the diagnosis of renal disease.

Renal biopsy *is an invasive diagnostic procedure used to examine renal tissue.* Renal biopsy is usually not performed unless the diagnosis cannot be made using routine clinical and laboratory findings. Histologic examination of a biopsy sample can help assess the severity and nature of the pathologic processes that are present. It can also aid the physician in choosing the appropriate treatment as well as in monitoring renal transplant management.

CYSTOSCOPY

Cystoscopy *is the visual examination of the urethra and bladder using a specialized probe that is inserted into the urethra.* This technique is often utilized to diagnose bladder tumors (neoplasms). The procedure can also aid in the removal of kidney stones (renal calculi).

PROTON NUCLEAR MAGNETIC RESONANCE URINALYSIS

One of the most recently developed procedures for analysis of urine is proton nuclear magnetic resonance (NMR) urinalysis. The major advantage that this technique has over other detection techniques is that NMR has the ability to "see" every proton in a urine sample, whether it is expected or not. Although this technique is gaining more acceptance in the medical community, there are some disadvantages to it. One disadvantage is that no "commercially" prepared kits are available yet. Another disadvantage is the cost of the instrument. Nevertheless, investigators see NMR urinalysis finding its way into the hospital. Diagnostic applications using NMR that have been studied so far include screening for drugs (*toxicology*) and for congenital metabolic diseases. NMR methods have also been developed for use as chemical markers for renal tubular injury or dysfunction.

CHAPTER SUMMARY

The importance of examining urine to detect disease is reflected by the fact that urine has been studied in a variety of ways for thousands of years. Urine tests have evolved from examining physical properties such as color and clarity to determining many chemical constituents by automated methods. It is probably the easiest specimen to collect from the body since collection is noninvasive and, normally, specimen production happens quite naturally as a reflex.

The urinary system has one of the most important functions in the body: to maintain homeostasis. The urinary system consists of several complex parts, each working with the others to retain and excrete various substances that are filtered from the blood. As you have discovered from reading this chapter, urine is much more than simply a waste product composed mainly of water. Regardless of the direction of health care, examination of urine will continue to play an important role. Routine urinalysis is an inexpensive, quick, and easy way to assist physicians in making definitive diagnoses.

Review Questions

1. The correct order for the flow of urine through the nephron is
   a. Bowman's capsule, proximal convoluted tubule, loop of Henle, distal convoluted tubule, collecting duct
   b. Bowman's capsule, distal convoluted tubule, proximal convoluted tubule, loop of Henle, collecting duct
   c. Bowman's capsule, distal convoluted tubule, loop of Henle, proximal convoluted tubule, collecting duct
   d. Collecting duct, proximal convoluted tubule, loop of Henle, distal convoluted tubule, Bowman's capsule

2. All of the following are functions of the nephron *except*
   a. secretion

    b. ultrafiltration

    c. reabsorption

    d. reduction

3. The structure that conducts urine from the kidney to the bladder is the

    a. urethra

    b. ureter

    c. renal pelvis

    d. papillae

    e. minor calyx

4. The enzyme produced by the juxtaglomerular apparatus that regulates blood pressure through its action on angiotensinogen is

    a. aldosterone

    b. vasopressin

    c. renin

    d. antidiuretic hormone

    e. adrenalin

5. The primary constituent of urine is

    a. sodium

    b. urea

    c. chloride

    d. water

    e. creatinine

6. Chronic renal failure is characterized by all of the following *except*

    a. bacteriuria

    b. azotemia

    c. "fixed" specific gravity of 1.010

    d. broad casts

    e. acid-base imbalance

7. A strong ammonia odor in urine is caused by

    a. the breakdown of urea by bacteria

    b. the excretion of ammonia

    c. the presence of glucose in the urine

    d. the lysis of erythrocytes

    e. the presence of large amounts of leukocytes

8. The test that is considered to be the most sensitive indicator of renal function is
    a. blood urea nitrogen (BUN)
    b. ultrasonography
    c. cholesterol
    d. creatinine clearance
    e. renal biopsy

BIBLIOGRAPHY

Allen, K.A.: Cytodiagnostic urinalysis: Effective in detecting transplant rejection. Adv Med Lab Professionals *7*:8, 1995.

Brunzel, N: Fundamentals of Urine and Body Fluid Analysis. Philadelphia, W.B. Saunders, 1994, pp. 71, 97, 281, 292.

Comer, J.P.: Semiquantitative specific test paper for glucose in urine. Anal. Chem. *28*: 1748, 1956.

Free, A.H., Adams, E.C., Kercher, M.L., Free, H.M., and Cook, M: Simple specific test for urine glucose. Clin. Chem. *3*:163, 1957.

Free, H.M.: Modern Urine Chemistry, 7th ed., Elkhart, IN, Miles, Inc., Diagnostics Division, 1991, pp. 10, 61.

Henry, J.B., Nelson, D.A., Tomar, R.H., et al.: Clinical Diagnosis and Management by Laboratory Methods, 18th ed. Philadelphia, W.B. Saunders, 1991, pp. 396–397, 415.

Hooton, T.M., and Stamm, W.E.: Management of acute uncomplicated urinary tract infection in adults. Med. Clin. North Am. *75*:339, 1991.

Kaplan, A., Jack, R., Opheim, K.E., Toivola, B., and Lyon, A.W.: Clinical Chemistry: Interpretation and Techniques, 4th ed. Baltimore, Williams & Wilkins, 1995, pp. 156, 174, 177, 182.

Krieger, T.N.: Urinary tract infections in women: Causes, classification, and differential diagnosis. Urology *35*:(suppl.):S4, 1990.

National Committee for Clinical Laboratory Standards: Routine Urinalysis and Collection, Transportation, and Preservation of Urine Specimens: Tentative Guidelines. Villanova, PA, 1992, 23 (26) GP 16-T, p. 8.

Noe, D.A., and Rock, R.C.: Laboratory Medicine: The Selection and Interpretation of Clinical Laboratory Studies. Baltimore, Williams & Wilkins, 1994, p. 426.

Powers, R.D.: New directions in the diagnosis and therapy of urinary tract infections. Am. J. Obstet. Gynecol. *164*:1387, 1991.

Sherbotie, J.R., and Cornfeld, D.: Management of urinary tract infections in children. Med. Clin. North. Am. *75*:327, 1991.

Taplin, G., Meredith, O., Kade, H., et al.: The radioisotope renogram: An external test for individual kidney function and upper urinary tract patency. J. Lab. Clin. Med. *48*:886, 1956.

Videen, J.S., and Ross, B.D.: Proton nuclear magnetic resonance urinalysis: Coming of age. Kidney Int. Suppl. *47*:S122, 1994.

Voswinckel, P.: A marvel of colors and ingredients: The story of urine test strips. Kidney Int. Suppl. *47*:S3, 1994.

The Digestive System

INTRODUCTION

ANATOMY OF THE DIGESTIVE TRACT
Major Organs
  Mouth and oral cavity
  Esophagus
  Stomach
  Small intestine
  Large intestine
Accessory Organs
  Liver
  Gallbladder
  Pancreas

CONDITIONS ASSOCIATED WITH THE DIGESTIVE SYSTEM
**Mouth, Oral Cavity, and
  Esophagus**

Stomach and Peritoneal Cavity
Diarrheal Illnesses
Other Conditions

LABORATORY EVALUATION OF THE DIGESTIVE TRACT
Stool Analysis
Serum Gastrin Analysis
Gastric Analysis
Fecal Fat Analysis
Pancreatic Tests

CHAPTER SUMMARY

REVIEW QUESTIONS

Objectives

1. Name and locate the organs that comprise the digestive system.

2. Trace the pathway of food through the digestive system.

3. Describe the functions of each organ in the digestive process.

4. Name and locate the following accessory organs of digestion and describe their functions in the digestive process: liver, pancreas, and gallbladder.

5. List the diseases that may be diagnosed by stool examination.

6. Give the purpose of gastric analysis.

7. List the laboratory tests used to evaluate diarrheal illnesses and give the significance of abnormal results.

8. Explain the significance of increased levels of serum amylase.

9. Discuss the clinical applications of fecal fat analysis.

10. Explain how serum gastrin analysis is used in the diagnosis of Zollinger-Ellison syndrome and pernicious anemia.

11. Describe the following conditions and correlate the laboratory test findings with each condition: hepatitis, pancreatitis, steatorrhea, stomatitis, gastritis, diverticulitis, peritonitis, diarrhea, achlorhydria, jaundice, appendicitis, Crohn's disease, colitis, and cholecystitis.

KEY TERMS

digestive system	stomach	hematemesis	hepatitis
mouth	pepsinogen	diarrhea	pancreatitis
deglutition	small intestine	achlorhydria	gastrin
esophagus	crypts of Lieberkuhn	cholecystitis	
peristalsis	emulsification	colitis	
gastroesophageal	gastritis	Crohn's disease	
sphincter	ulcer	diverticulitis	

Introduction

The human body requires food to survive. Food provides sources for growth and energy, for sustaining cellular components and structures, and for maintaining bodily functions and processes. Basic nutrients derived from food include water, vitamins, inorganic salts, carbohydrates, proteins, and fats. Most of these nutrients, however, are not readily available for the body to utilize because they are too large to simply pass through the cellular membranes of tissues and cells, and the process of digestion must first take place. Nutrients must be extracted from food before they become available for cellular use. The digestive system is primarily responsible for this process.

The digestive system includes the mouth and oral cavity, esophagus, and small and large intestines. Accessory organs located outside the digestive tract secrete enzymes and digestive juices that aid in the digestive process. The salivary glands, pancreas, liver, gallbladder, and bile ducts are the accessory organs. Food is ingested through the mouth, where it is initially broken down into smaller pieces. As food travels through the digestive tract, digestive juices and enzymes secreted by glands and accessory organs further prepare the partially digested food material for absorption by converting complex food molecules to a simpler state. These nutrients, in their simplest form, are absorbed across the intestinal wall into the bloodstream and are carried to the cells and tissues of the body. Metabolic waste products and unused materials are propelled to the end of the digestive tract and eliminated from the body. Therefore, the major functions of the digestive system include preparation of food for cellular consumption, absorption of nutrients, and, finally, excretion of undigested materials.

This chapter describes the anatomy and functions of the digestive tract. By tracing food as it travels through the system, this chapter discusses the processes that occur at each site. This chapter also presents the clinical conditions and laboratory tests related to the digestive system.

ANATOMY OF THE DIGESTIVE TRACT

The **digestive tract,** *or alimentary canal, is a long, continuous tube that begins at the mouth and ends at the anus* (Fig. 8–1). This tract is approximately 9 m (30 ft) long and runs through the ventral body cavity. It consists of the mouth and esophagus, stomach, small intestine, and large intestine. Accessory organs that are necessary in achieving the functions of the digestive system include the liver, gallbladder, and pancreas.

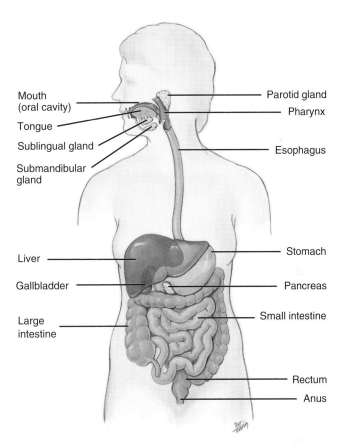

FIGURE 8-1
The digestive tract.
(From Applegate, E.J.: The
Anatomy and Physiology
Learning System. Philadelphia,
W.B. Saunders, 1995, with
permission.)

Labels in figure:
Mouth (oral cavity)
Tongue
Sublingual gland
Submandibular gland
Parotid gland
Pharynx
Esophagus
Liver
Gallbladder
Large intestine
Stomach
Pancreas
Small intestine
Rectum
Anus

MAJOR ORGANS
Mouth and Oral Cavity

The Mouth. Food is ingested through the mouth. *The **mouth,** formed by the cheeks, hard and soft palates, and tongue, is also referred to as the oral or buccal cavity.* The mouth is armed with teeth that cut and grind food into smaller pieces, a process called *mastication.* Cheeks are the muscular structures that form the lateral walls of the mouth. They are covered on the outside by skin and lined with stratified squamous epithelial cells on the inside, and end anteriorly in the superior and inferior lips. The lips, which are fleshy folds covered on the outside by skin and on the inside by mucous membrane, surround the opening of the mouth. During mastication, or chewing, the cheeks and lips serve to keep the food between the upper and lower teeth. The hard palate, lined by mucous membrane, is the anterior portion of the roof of the mouth, while the soft palate frames the posterior portion of the roof of the mouth. A finger-like muscular structure, called the *uvula*, hangs from the middle of the lower portion of the soft palate.

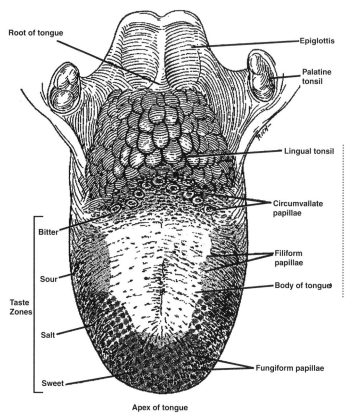

Root of tongue

Epiglottis

Palatine tonsil

Lingual tonsil

Circumvallate papillae

Bitter

Filiform papillae

Sour

Body of tongue

Taste Zones

Salt

Fungiform papillae

Sweet

Apex of tongue

FIGURE 8-2

The tongue, showing the regions of tastes.
(Modified from Fehrenbach, M.S. and Herring, S.W.: Illustrated Anatomy of the Head and Neck. Philadelphia, W.B. Saunders, 1996, with permission.)

The Tongue. The tongue, composed of skeletal muscle and mucous membrane, covers the floor of the oral cavity. The primary function of the tongue is to maneuver food for chewing and swallowing. The upper surface and sides of the tongue are covered with papillae, in which taste buds are located. Taste zones of the tongue are shown in Figure 8–2.

The Teeth. The teeth, or *dentes*, break down food, mix it with saliva, and reduce the food into a soft, malleable mass that is easily swallowed. The teeth, therefore, aid in the mechanical digestion of food. The tooth has three principal parts: the *crown*, which is the portion that shows above the gum level; the *root*, which anchors the tooth in the socket and is made up of one to three projections; and the *cervix*, a constricted junction between the crown and the root. The parts and structures of a typical tooth are shown in Figure 8–3.

Teeth are made up primarily of three components:

■ The *dentin*, which forms the main bulk of the tooth and gives the tooth its basic shape and rigidity. The dentin, a bone-like material, encloses a cavity. The enlarged portion of this cavity is called the *pulp cavity* and the narrow extension that ends up at the root of the tooth is called the *root canal*. The pulp cavity, which lies in the crown, contains the pulp, a soft connective tissue containing blood vessels, nerves, and lymphatics. At the base of the root canal is

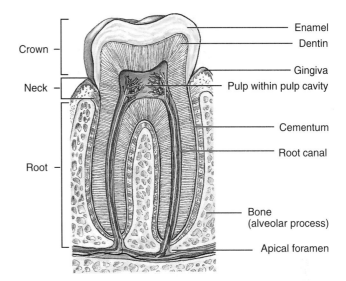

FIGURE 8-3
The tooth.
(From Applegate, E.J.: The Anatomy and Physiology Learning System. Philadelphia, W.B. Saunders, 1995, with permission.)

an opening called the *apical foramen*, where blood vessels that bring nourishment, lymphatics for protection, and nerves to provide sensation enter.

■ The *enamel*, which is the hardest structure in the body and forms the calcified outer covering. It protects the tooth from wear of chewing and serves as a deterrent against acids that may readily dissolve the dentin.

■ The *cementum*, which covers the dentin of the root. The cementum is also bone-like material that connects the root to the periodontal ligament.

Everyone has two *dentitions*, or sets of teeth. The first set—called *deciduous* or *baby* or *milk teeth*—appears at about 6 months of age. These teeth continue to appear in pairs monthly until all 40 (20 pairs) are present. Generally, between 6 and 12 years of age, all deciduous teeth are lost and replaced by the *permanent dentition.*

The dentitions, both deciduous and permanent, consist of incisors, canines or cuspids, and molars. The chisel-shaped incisors are designed for cutting the food and are located closest to the center, while the canines, located next to the incisors, are used for tearing and shredding food. Next to the canines are the first and second molars, which are used for crushing and grinding food.

Permanent dentition resembles the deciduous dentition with a few exceptions. Deciduous molars are replaced with premolars or bicuspids that have two cusps and one root. Upper first bicuspids are used for crushing and grinding. Permanent molars appear behind the bicuspids as the jaw grows to accommodate them. The first set of molars appear at age 6 years, the second molars at 12, and the third molars (or wisdom teeth) after the age of 18 years. The human jaw often does not have enough room to accommodate the third molars and they may become embedded (impacted) in the alveolar bone. Because of the pain and pressure impacted wisdom teeth may cause, they are oftenly surgically removed. Occasionally, in some individuals, third molars may be dwarfed in size or may not develop at all.

Food Digestion in the Mouth.   Buccal glands located in the mucous membrane lining of the mouth continuously produce a fluid (*saliva*) that keeps the mucous membranes of the mouth moist. When food enters the mouth, the secretion of saliva is increased to help in lubricating, dissolving, and breaking down the food. Saliva is made up of primarily water and a certain amount of solutes, such as chlorides, bicarbonates, and phosphates. It also contains other substances such as mucin, albumin, bacteriolytic enzyme (lysozyme), and digestive enzyme (salivary amylase). The major portion of the saliva is secreted by three pairs of salivary glands, the parotid, submandibular, and sublingual, which are situated outside the mouth. The salivary glands drain their contents into ducts that empty into the oral cavity. The parotid glands, found under and in front of the ears, secrete the enzyme salivary amylase. Amylase starts the digestion of carbohydrates. The submandibular glands are located posteriorly beneath the base of the tongue, while the sublingual glands are anterior to the submandibular. The submandibular glands secrete a small amount of enzyme in addition to mucus. The sublingual glands contain primarily mucus-producing cells, hence they secrete a thick fluid made up of mucus with a very small amount of enzyme.

When food has been reduced to smaller particles or transformed into a mass, or *bolus*, the tongue directs the mass to the back of the mouth. The mass is swallowed by upward and backward movements of the tongue against the palate. *Swallowing, or* **deglutition,** *transports food from the mouth to the stomach.* The partially digested food is funneled to the stomach by way of the esophagus.

Esophagus

The **esophagus**, a long muscular tube that measures approximately 23 to 25 cm (10 in), is located behind the trachea. It produces a wave-like muscular contraction called *peristalsis.* With peristaltic movement, food is directed to and enters the stomach through a sphincter, an opening with a thick, ring-like muscle around it. The sphincter at the inferior part of the esophagus is known as the lower esophageal or **gastroesophageal sphincter**. During swallowing, the sphincter relaxes, which helps movement of the bolus from the esophagus to the stomach. It takes approximately 4 to 8 seconds for solids or semisolids, and about 1 second for soft foods and liquids, to pass from the mouth to the stomach. No further digestion or absorption takes place in the esophagus, but the esophagus does secrete mucus that eases the transport of partially digested food to the stomach.

Stomach

The superior part of the stomach is a continuation of the esophagus while the inferior portion connects with the duodenum, the superior part of the small intestine. *The* **stomach,** *is a J-shaped pouch located directly underneath the diaphragm, occupying the epigastric, umbilical, and left hypochondriac regions* (Fig. 8–4). The size of the stomach varies with each individual, and the stomach can expand to accommodate an enormous amount of food. The stomach is divided into three areas: the fundus, the body, and the pylorus (see Fig. 8–4). The rounded portion of the stomach is the *fundus*, the large central portion is the *body*, and the narrow, inferior portion is the *pylorus*. The stomach wall is lined with temporary folds, called *rugae*, which allow for distention and expansion. When the stomach fills and distends, the rugae smooth out and disappear. The inner wall of the stomach is equipped with a layer of columnar epithelium containing gastric glands that secrete gastric or digestive juices. Gas-

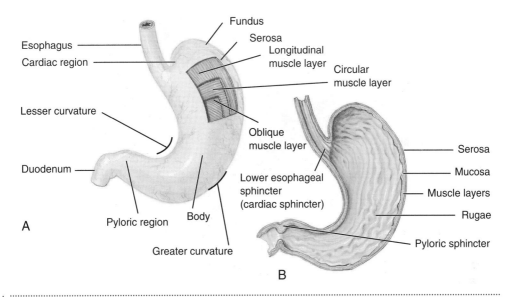

FIGURE 8-4

The stomach.
(From Applegate, E.J.: The Anatomy and Physiology Learning System. Philadelphia, W.B. Saunders, 1995, with permission.)

tric juices include secretions such as the gastric enzymes pepsinogen and lipase, hydrochloric acid, mucus, and intrinsic factor, a substance necessary for the absorption of vitamin B_{12}.

Food Digestion in the Stomach.   The stomach is responsible for storing ingested food and further digestion of the particles into a more refined state. As food enters the stomach, peristalsis, muscular contraction, and digestive juices further digest the food. Digestive juices include pepsinogen, hydrochloric acid, and mucin. **Pepsinogen** *is an inactive form of pepsin, the principal gastric enzyme responsible for digesting proteins.* Pepsin is activated when pepsinogen comes in contact with hydrochloric acid. Mucus prevents pepsin from digesting the stomach cells, which are made up of proteins. Another gastric enzyme, *gastric lipase*, is responsible for breaking down butterfat in milk. *Hydrochloric acid*, in addition to activating pepsinogen, breaks down connective tissues and cell membranes.

The stomach wall is not permeable to most materials to be absorbed into the bloodstream; however, it allows absorption of some water and salts, certain drugs, and alcohol. Otherwise, absorption only takes place in the small intestine. After 2 to 6 hours of digestion, food passes through the pyloric sphincter into the small intestine. Further digestion occurs in the small intestine.

Small Intestine

The **small intestine** *is a long, coiled tube occupying the central and lower portion of the abdominal cavity that begins at the pyloric sphincter and ends at the opening of the large intestine.* It measures approximately 6 m (20 ft) in length and 2.5 cm (1 in) in diameter. There

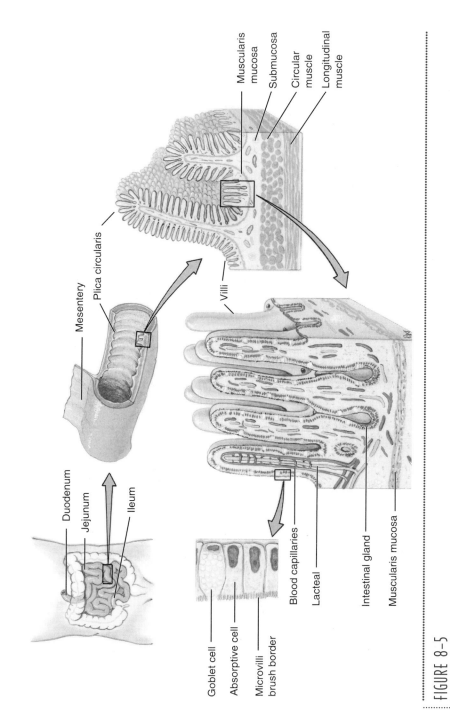

Duodenum

Jejunum

Ileum

Mesentery

Plica circularis

Villi

Muscularis
mucosa

Submucosa

Circular
muscle

Longitudinal
muscle

Goblet cell

Absorptive cell

Microvilli
brush border

Blood capillaries

Lacteal

Intestinal gland

Muscularis mucosa

FIGURE 8–5

The small intestine.
(From Applegate, E.J.: The Anatomy and Physiology Learning System. Philadelphia, W.B. Saunders, 1995, with permission.)

are three regions in the small intestine (Fig. 8–5): the duodenum, the jejunum, and the ileum. The *duodenum* connects the stomach and the small intestine. The broadest of the three segments, the duodenum originates from the pyloric valve of the stomach and stretches out 25 cm (10 in) until it meets the jejunum. The *jejunum* is about 2.5 m (8 ft) long and extends to the final region of the small intestine, the ileum. The *ileum* measures approximately 3.6 m (12 ft) and connects with the large intestine at what is called the *ileocecal region.*

Food Digestion in the Small Intestine. Because final digestion takes place in the small intestine, the walls of the small intestine are equipped with intestinal glands—the **crypts of Lieberkuhn**—that secrete additional enzymes. The submucosa of the duodenum also secretes an alkaline mucus produced by Brunner's glands, to protect the walls of the small intestine from the actions of the digestive enzymes and neutralize the acid in incompletely digested food. To complete the digestive process, digestion of carbohydrates, lipids, and proteins requires secretions from the accessory organs (the pancreas, liver, and gallbladder). Bile, produced by the liver and temporarily stored in the gallbladder, emulsifies large fat droplets. It is released from the gallbladder through the common bile duct. Pancreatic and intestinal juices further digest carbohydrates, proteins, and fats.

Digestion of Carbohydrates. Salivary amylase secreted in the mouth initiates the digestion of complex polysaccharides into dextrin, which contains numerous monosaccharide units. An enzyme found in pancreatic juice, *pancreatic amylase*, breaks dextrin down into the disaccharide maltose. Maltose is further degraded by an intestinal enzyme, maltase, into two molecules of glucose. Other disaccharides (sucrose and lactose) are acted upon by other enzymes (sucrase and lactase, respectively). Sucrase splits sucrose into a molecule of glucose and a molecule of fructose, while lactase digests lactose into one molecule of glucose and one molecule of galactose.

Digestion of Proteins. Most of the protein digestion begins in the stomach by the action of pepsin. Proteins are broken into short chains of amino acids called peptones and proteoses. In the small intestine, proteins are further digested by pancreatic juice, which contains the enzyme trypsin. Trypsin continues the breakdown of peptones and proteoses into simple amino acids, and also digests any intact proteins.

Digestion of Lipids. Bile initiates lipid digestion. It starts with the emulsification of fats, which are the most abundant lipids in the diet. **Emulsification** *is the breaking down of fat globules into droplets, which become accessible to the fat-splitting enzyme pancreatic lipase.* Lipase is found in pancreatic juice and hydrolyzes fat molecules to produce fatty acids, glycerol, and glycerides, the end products of lipid digestion.

Absorption of Nutrients from the Small Intestine. Absorption of nutrients is also accomplished in the small intestine. The walls of the small intestine are particularly equipped for this function. Columnar epithelial cells line the mucosa and epithelial covering. Some of the epithelial cells have been converted into goblet cells, capable of secreting additional mucus. The remaining cells contain finger-like projections called *microvilli* that promote absorption by increasing the surface area of the plasma membrane. Nutrients are then able to diffuse through the epithelial cells, pass through the capillary walls, and enter the bloodstream. Absorption of water, vitamins, minerals, and electrolytes take places in the small intestine. Digestive products from carbohydrates, proteins, and lipids are further processed by the liver before they are eventually transported to the cells of the body.

As food is pushed down the small intestine by means of peristalsis, the composition of the food materials is drastically changed so that most of the remains are water and undigested materials. After the nutrients are absorbed through the walls of the small intestine, waste products and undigestable materials are moved by peristalsis into the large intestine.

Large Intestine

There are three regions in the large intestine (Fig. 8–6): a short tube, the cecum, that connects the large intestine with the small intestine; a long central region, the colon; and the terminal end, or rectum. The large intestine, which measures approximately 6.25 cm (2.5 in) in width and 1.8 m (6 ft) in length, is, in general, wider and shorter than the small intestine. A fold of mucus membrane, called the *ileocecal valve*, guards the opening from the ileum into the large intestine and allows materials from the small intestine to pass into the large intestine. Just below the ileocecal valve is the *cecum*, which measures about 6 cm (2 to 3 in) long. Attached to the cecum is a coiled, tube-like structure called the *vermiform appendix*. The cecum opens into a long tube called the *colon*. The colon is divided into four regions: *ascending, transverse, descending*, and *sigmoid* (see Fig. 8–6). The colon is colonized by indigenous bacteria that help break down waste products. Water, salts, and vitamins produced by colon organisms are absorbed into the bloodstream through the walls of the large intestine. When all the usable materials are absorbed, waste products are stored in the rectum and later passed out (by elimination or defecation) through the anus.

The last 20 cm (7 to 8 in) of the digestive tract is the *rectum*, which lies anterior to the sacrum and coccyx. The terminal end, about 2 to 3 cm of the rectum, is the anal canal. The anal canal is lined with mucous membranes arranged in longitudinal folds called anal columns that hold a network of blood vessels. The anal canal has an exterior opening called the *anus*, which is guarded by an internal sphincter of smooth muscle and an external sphincter of skeletal muscle. The anus is normally closed, except during the elimination of waste or feces.

Digestion and Elimination in the Large Intestine.   The mucosa of the large intestine contains primarily columnar epithelium with goblet cells that secrete mucus. Mucus helps lubricate colon contents as they move through the colon. Digestion and absorption are just about finished when intestinal materials reach the large intestine. The digested food, now turned into a liquid substance called *chyme*, moves into the ileocecal valve and accumulates in the ascending colon. The chyme is prepared for elimination by the action of bacteria in the large intestine. As absorption occurs, chyme eventually turns into a solid or semisolid matter known as *feces*, or fecal material. Feces is made up of water, inorganic salts, bacteria, bacterial by-products, undegraded parts of food, and epithelial cells that line the digestive tract.

Indigenous colon flora ferment any remaining undigested carbohydrates, reduce proteins to amino acids, and break down amino acids into simpler forms such as indole, skatole, hydrogen sulfide, and fatty acids. Colon flora also help in the absorption of vitamins such as K and B. Skatole and indole contribute to the odor of feces as these substances are deposited in the feces. Massive and strong peristaltic movements force colon contents into the sigmoid and rectum.

Defecation, *or elimination, is the process of emptying of the rectum of fecal material, or feces*. Fecal matter is pushed into the rectum, which results in the distention of the rectal

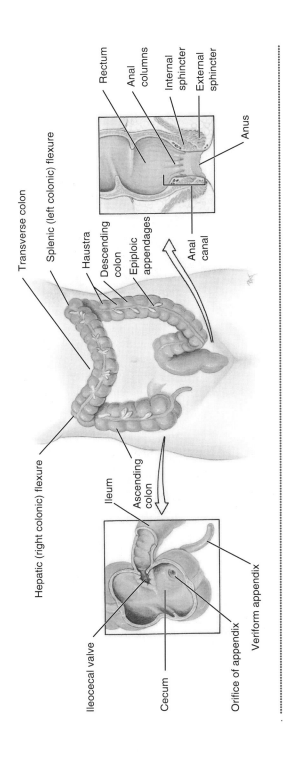

FIGURE 8-6

The large intestine.
(From Applegate, E.J.: The Anatomy and Physiology Learning System. Philadelphia, W.B. Saunders, 1995, with permission.)

walls. Pressure-sensitive receptors are stimulated, initiating the feeling of wanting to defecate. The longitudinal rectal muscles contract, which shortens the rectum, creating pressure inside and forcing the sphincter to open and expel the feces through the anus.

ACCESSORY ORGANS

Chemical digestion of food, which occurs in the small intestine, is dependent not only on the secretions produced by the small intestine but also on the participation of three significant accessory organs: the liver, pancreas, and gallbladder.

Liver

The liver, located under the diaphragm, takes up most of the right hypochondrium and part of the epigastrium of the abdomen. The liver weighs approximately 1.4 kg (4 lb) in an average adult and is divided into two principal lobes—the right lobe and the left lobe—separated by a ligament called the falciform ligament. The right lobe is the main lobe and with it are associated two smaller lobes, the inferior quadrate lobe and the posterior caudate lobe. Numerous units called *lobules* make up the lobes of the liver. Each lobule consists of cords of hepatic cells that are arranged in a radial pattern around a central vein. Blood passes through spaces between the cords. These spaces, called *sinusoids*, are lined with endothelial cells as well as phagocytic cells termed *Kupffer cells*.

Hepatic cells manufacture a yellowish-brownish or olive green liquid called *bile*. Bile is made up of water, bile salts, bile acids, lipids and two pigments called *biliverdin* and *bilirubin*. Bile is partly a product of excretion; when erythrocytes die out, iron, globin, and bilirubin are released. Bile helps in the digestion and absorption of fats by emulsifying them. Bilirubin is broken down in the intestines, and its by-product, urobilinogen, is responsible for the color of feces.

Bile is secreted into bile capillaries or canaliculi that empty into small ducts that eventually become larger ducts, the left and right hepatic ducts. As these larger ducts leave the liver, they combine as the *common hepatic duct*, which further joins the cystic duct from the gallbladder. These two ducts combined make up the *common bile duct* that drains into the duodenum at the *ampulla of Vater*. The flow of bile into the small intestine is monitored by the *sphincter of Oddi*, which is a valve in the common bile duct. The sphincter closes when the small intestine is empty and the bile backflows into the gallbladder, where it is stored and becomes concentrated. Concentrated bile in the gallbladder has the potential to be saturated with cholesterol, which may later form crystals that make up gallstones.

The liver performs several essential functions, so essential that the human body cannot survive without the liver. The liver is responsible for

- Manufacturing heparin, an anticoagulant, and other plasma proteins such as albumin. It also produces prothrombin and fibrinogen.
- The phagocytosis of erythrocytes and leukocytes and bacteria by Kupffer cells.
- Clearing toxic compounds produced by the body. The liver produces enzymes that either break down the toxins or change them into less hazardous substances.
- Collecting recently absorbed nutrients and converting excess monosaccha-

rides into glycogen or fat, both of which can be stored. Depending on the body's needs, the liver can later transform glycogen, fat, or protein into glucose. It also stores vitamins such as A, D, E, and K and minerals such as copper and iron.

■ Manufacturing bile, necessary for the emulsification and absorption of fat in the small intestine.

Gallbladder

Along the underside of the liver is a small sac, the gallbladder. Bile, which is manufactured in the liver, is temporarily stored in the gallbladder. The inner walls of the gallbladder are made up of mucous membranes arranged in rugae much like those found in the stomach. The gallbladder is able to expand to about the size and shape of a pear when filled up with bile. Bile is channeled into the cystic duct and then the intestine as needed when the wall of the gallbladder contracts.

Pancreas

The pancreas is an accessory gland located posterior to the greater curvature of the stomach (see Fig. 8–1). This oblong-shaped gland measures approximately 12.5 cm (5 in) long and 2.5 cm (1 in) thick and is divided into three parts: a head, body, and tail. The pancreas consists of small clusters of glandular epithelial cells that include the *islets of Langerhans*, the endocrine portion of the pancreas, and the ascini, the exocrine portion of the gland. The islets of Langerhans secrete glucagon and insulin, hormones that regulate the blood glucose level. Acini consist of cells that release a mixture of digestive enzymes, water, salts, and sodium bicarbonate, referred to as pancreatic juice. Pancreatic juice assists in the digestion of food in the small intestine, particularly carbohydrates and fat. Pancreatic enzymes include *pancreatic amylase*, which breaks down dextrin, and pancreatic lipase, responsible for hydrolysis of fat molecules. From the pancreas, pancreatic juice is channeled through the pancreatic duct, a large main tube that connects with the common bile duct from the liver and gallbladder and terminates in the duodenum by way of the ampulla of Vater.

CONDITIONS ASSOCIATED WITH THE DIGESTIVE SYSTEM

There are numerous pathologic conditions that are associated with the digestive system. Diseases may be caused by a wide variety of infectious agents, such as viruses, bacteria, and parasites. Other conditions may occur as a result of complications from conditions occurring in other organ systems. This section discusses the clinical conditions most commonly encountered.

MOUTH, ORAL CAVITY, AND ESOPHAGUS

Oral candidiasis, or *thrush*, caused by the yeast *Candida albicans*, is a common affliction experienced by individuals who are immunosuppressed. Immunosuppression caused by prolonged antibiotic therapy, chemotherapy, or human immunodeficiency virus (HIV) infection predisposes patients to oral fungal infections such as thrush. Other infections in the mouth and nearby structures include *pyorrhea*, an inflammation of the periodontal ligament and adjacent gums, and *periodontitis*, a disease of the structures surrounding the tooth that results in the bone and the gum shrinking away from the tooth.

Dental caries, or tooth decay, the decomposition of the tooth enamel down to the pulp, is usually caused by poor dental hygiene. Dental caries begin when bacteria feed on the carbohydrates settled on the tooth. Fermentation of the carbohydrates result in acids that demineralize the enamel. *Lactobacillus acidophilus* and *Streptococcus mutans* are bacterial species commonly associated with dental caries. When this condition remains untreated, more serious events such as bacterial invasion of the pulp may take place. This condition may also progress into subsequent necrosis (death) of the pulp and abscess formation. Root canal therapy is the recommended treatment.

The most serious pathologic condition of the salivary glands is a viral inflammatory disease, *parotitis*, or mumps. *Stomatitis* is a nonspecific inflammation of the mouth that can be caused by a variety of agents, including bacteria such as streptococci, viruses (*Herpes virus*), or vitamin deficiency (vitamin B_{12} deficiency, or scurvy).

The most serious disorder of the esophagus is a malignant tumor, which usually occurs in men older than 50 years of age. *Dysphagia*, or difficulty in swallowing, is the most common complaint as the tumor invades the muscular tube.

STOMACH AND PERITONEAL CAVITY

Gastritis, *an inflammation of the stomach mucous membrane, is a common disease that elicits redness, swelling, and inflammatory cell infiltration.* There are two types of gastritis: type A, which is associated with a blood dyscrasia called *pernicious anemia*, and type B, which is now attributed to a bacterial organism called *Helicobacter pylori*. In type A gastritis, erythrocytes do not mature normally due to vitamin B_{12} deficiency which is a result of the lack of intrinsic factor secretion by the stomach. Type B gastritis has been strongly associated with the spiral-shaped bacillus *H. pylori*. This newly recognized pathogen seems to survive the low pH of the stomach and cause a chronic but continuous inflammation of the gastric mucosa. Patients with *H. pylori* infection may be symptomatic or asymptomatic. When present, symptoms include nausea, vomiting, heartburn, anorexia, and epigastric pain. *H. pylori* has also been associated with peptic ulcer disease and, more recently, a serious consequence of this chronic inflammatory process, gastric carcinoma.

Ulcers *are crater-like lesions that develop in a membrane.* In general, an ulcer that occurs in any portion of the gastrointestinal tract is referred to as a *peptic ulcer.* An ulcer that occurs in the stomach is called a *gastric ulcer* because of the peptic acid or gastric juice present in this area. Ulcers that occur in the duodenum are called *duodenal ulcers*. These ulcers have long been referred to as the "executive stress" syndrome, the etiology of which has been associated with increased production of acid stimulated by stress.

Bleeding is the most serious occurrence in acute gastritis and ulcers. If the bleeding is minor, it may remain undetected in the gastric contents. It may be detected, however, when vomiting occurs in acute inflammation. *Vomiting of blood is called* **hematemesis.** In gastric ulcer, the vomitus may appear like "coffee grounds" because of the action of the gastric juice on the blood. If the blood is passed in the stool, the stool may appear blackish in color (tarry stools) and the condition is known as *melena*.

Appendicitis, an inflammation of the vermiform appendix, may occur as a result of fecal obstruction of the lumen. Inflammation, the presence of a foreign body, and carcinoma of the cecum are other predisposing factors. Infection may result from the obstruction and may further cause edema, gangrene, ischema, and ultimately perforation. Symptoms of acute appendicitis begin with pain in the umbilical region of the abdomen, anorexia, nausea, and vomiting. The pain later shifts to the lower right quadrant and becomes more severe and intense as infection develops. If early appendectomy is performed in a suspected case, the risk of rupture and subsequent peritonitis may be avoided.

Peritonitis, an acute inflammation of the thin layer of serous membrane that lines the abdominal cavity, may occur as a result of a ruptured appendix. Spillage of septic material from perforated or ruptured walls of organs that contain bacteria may cause bacterial contamination of the cavity and lead to inflammation. An example is the release of normal colonic bacterial flora in the large intestine. If, for one reason or another, these organisms traverse the intestinal mucosal wall and gain entrance to the peritoneal cavity, infection of the surrounding vital organs may follow. Peritonitis has been known to be fatal.

DIARRHEAL ILLNESSES

Diarrhea, *a very common condition, is an abnormal increase in stool liquidity and frequency.* This condition, usually accompanied by urgency, abdominal pain, and discomfort, may be a result of interference in transport of water and electrolytes through the intestinal wall. There are a number of pathophysiologic mechanisms of diarrhea as well as numerous causes, both infectious and noninfectious. For example, when laxatives such as citrate of magnesia, a hypertonic solute, are taken, *osmotic diarrhea* occurs. Another form of diarrhea called *secretory diarrhea* is a result of the malfunction of the secretory cells lining the small intestine. This manifestation may be caused by enterotoxins produced by bacterial species such as *Vibrio cholerae* and enterotoxin-producing *Escherichia coli.* Neoplasms, cathartics such as castor oil, and various drugs cause increased secretion of electrolytes and water into the intestinal lumen. Lumen-dwelling parasites such as *Giardia lamblia* may result in impaired absorption that may be the cause of the diarrheal illness. Heavy infection with *G. lamblia* may eventually result in a *malabsorption syndrome,* usually evidenced by *steatorrhea,* the presence of gas and fat in the stool. Finally, altered motility, either hypomotility or hypermotility, in the small intestine may be a cause of diarrhea.

OTHER CONDITIONS

Achlorhydria *is the condition in which the stomach does not secrete hydrochloric acid or secretes too little of it.*

Cholecystitis *is inflammation of the gallbladder.* In 85 to 95% of cases, the presence of calculi or gallstones (cholelithiasis) is the primary cause. Bacteria seem to be the cause in approximately 50 to 70% of acute cholecystitis cases in which a combination of facultative and obligate anaerobic organisms have been cultured.

Colitis *is the acute inflammation of the bowel.* Protozoans such as *Entamoeba histolytica* may cause amebic colitis and ulcers. Acute inflammation in the walls of the large intestine may lead to what is known as *amebic dysentery.* In dysentery, the patient experiences profuse diarrhea in which the liquid, watery stool contains pus, blood, and mucus. Antibiotic-associated colitis may occur in patients who receive prolonged antibiotic or chemotherapy. A common colon flora, *Clostridium difficile*, survives the broad-spectrum antibiotic while the rest of the colon flora are eliminated. This provides *C. difficile* the opportunity to thrive and cause an acute inflammatory process in the intestinal mucosa.

Crohn's disease was first described by Crohn in 1932. **Crohn's disease** *is an inflammatory bowel disorder the etiology of which remains unknown.* A form of enteritis, Crohn's disease is characterized by the presence of inflammation of the gastrointestinal tract in any location from the mouth to the anus. Other symptoms include diarrhea, abdominal pain and mass, rectal bleeding, malabsorption with weight loss, and occasionally fever. Inflammatory bowel disorders (IBDs) such as Crohn's disease are difficult to assess, and differential diagnosis of Crohn's disease from other forms of IBD, such as ulcerative colitis, may only be made by exclusion.

Diverticulitis *is inflammation of the diverticula.* Diverticula are small pouches that form in the lining and wall of the large intestines when the muscles weaken. Muscle spasms, abdominal cramps, and pain are the usual symptoms, probably due to the inflammation caused by the bacteria and other irritants settled in these pouches. When numerous diverticula are present, the condition is referred to as *diverticulosis*. Complications of diverticulitis include peritonitis, pelvic abscesses, obstruction, and bleeding.

Hepatitis *is inflammation of the liver.* There are a multitude of causes for hepatitis. A complete discussion of this disease is found in Chapter 9. Hepatitis is often accompanied by *jaundice*, a yellow coloration of the skin, whites of the eyes, and other body fluids caused by the increased production of bilirubin.

Pancreatitis *is inflammation of the pancreas.* Symptoms include pain in the upper abdomen, rigid and tender abdomen, and shock. Typically the pain subsides when the patient assumes a fetal position, with the knees drawn up and the body folded. Chronic pancreatitis is often seen in alcohol abusers and in individuals with biliary tract disease.

LABORATORY EVALUATION OF THE DIGESTIVE TRACT

STOOL ANALYSIS

Feces, or stool, consists of residues of food that have not been absorbed and products of material excreted from the blood. Colon flora also make up more than 10% of the bulk of the feces. Stool analysis reveals information pertaining to the activities of the digestive tract and the disorders that may involve it.

The normal color and form of the stool vary from yellow to brown and soft to formed, respectively. Gross or macroscopic examination of the stool sample will show numerous conditions such as bleeding, diarrheal events such as dysentery, and the presence of the adult forms of some parasites. Bleeding in the upper or lower gastrointestinal tract may be detected by the presence of blood in the stool. This blood may appear bright red, which indicates that bleeding is occurring in the lower part of the intestinal tract. Dark or tarry stool indicates that the erythrocytes have come in contact with gastric juices; therefore, the bleeding must be occurring in the upper level of the digestive tract. If the bleeding is only slight, the presence of blood may not be detected visually. Test for hidden blood, or *occult blood*, may then be performed. Chemical compounds such as benzidine, orthotoulidine, and gum guiac may be used to detect the occult blood.

The blood may be accompanied by mucus and pus, especially in cases of acute dysentery and ulcerative colitis. Mucus is a slimy-looking material that comes from the cellular lining of the mucous membrane of the large intestine. When inflammation is present, mucus is produced along with inflammatory cells such as polymorphonuclear cells (PMNs). In cases of diarrheal illnesses, PMNs, detected microscopically, are indicative of an infectious process rather than a toxin.

Microscopic examination of stool samples will reveal the presence of parasitic ova and protozoans. Some of the most common protozoans are *Giardia lamblia* and *Entamoeba histolytica* (see Color Figures 17 and 18). *Cryptosporidium parvum* (Color Figure 19), commonly recovered from immunosuppressed patients such as those with acquired immunodeficiency syndrome (AIDS), has been associated recently with outbreaks in day care centers. Helminth eggs, such as *Ascaris lumbricoides* (see Color Figure 20), *Trichuris trichuria*, and hookworm (see Color Figures 21 and 22), are also common findings.

Diarrheic illnesses may also be due to a wide variety of bacterial and nonbacterial agents. It is extremely costly and time-consuming for the laboratory to detect all possible causes. Therefore, patient history of travel and food taken prior to onset of illness is critical information. Bacterial culture to recover enteric pathogens such as *Salmonella* (see Color Figure 23), *Shigella*, *Campylobacter*, and *Vibrio* species is necessary, particularly in patients experiencing fever and severe or prolonged symptoms. Infections caused by these bacterial species can be life threatening, and therapy should be initiated as soon as possible. Further work-up has not been necessary in other cases, such as suspected food poisoning or in patients without profuse diarrhea and danger of dehydration.

Examination of stool for PMNs may help differentiate diarrheal events caused by an invasive bacterial agent, in which PMNs are present, from those caused by toxin-elaborating species, in which PMNs are absent. For example, detection of food poisoning caused by toxin-producing *Staphylococcus aureus*, *Clostridium perfringens*, and *Bacillus cereus* is usually done by history of food taken and onset of symptoms, and only rarely by culturing for the organisms. In cases of invasion by organisms such as *Salmonella* or *Shigella*, numerous PMNs are found.

Diagnosis of inflammatory bowel disorders such as Crohn's disease and ulcerative colitis has remained an exclusionary one. A single test or examination has not been determined. Diagnostic evaluation includes a detailed history and physical examination in conjunction with radiologic, endoscopic, and histologic evaluations.

SERUM GASTRIN ANALYSIS

Serum gastrin analysis is used to detect hypergastrinemia in the diagnosis of Zollinger-Ellison syndrome and in pernicious anemia. **Gastrin** *is a hormone manufactured by the G cells in the gastric antrum and released when the vagus nerve is stimulated by senses such as smell, taste, and other reflexes.* When gastrin is released into the bloodstream, it induces the release of hydrochloric acid and stimulates secretion of pepsin and intrinsic factor from the stomach. Gastrin release is controlled by a negative feedback mechanism in which extremely acid pH (1.0) suppresses gastrin production.

Increased levels of serum gastrin are found in *Zollinger-Ellison syndrome*, a condition characterized by extensive ulceration in the gastrointestinal tract. Elevated levels of gastric acid and development of gastrinomas are usually found in the pancreas. Patients with peptic ulcers usually have normal gastrin levels, while those with gastric ulcers may show slightly elevated levels.

Patients with pernicious anemia also show marked elevations in serum gastrin concentrations. In pernicious anemia, however, patients are unable to secrete gastric hydrochloric acid, and intragastric infusion of hydrochloric acid will reduce the gastrin level.

GASTRIC ANALYSIS

In conjunction with gastrin levels, gastric analysis is performed to determine gastric acid secretion, which varies in different disease states. Gastric analysis is performed on gastric contents, collected by nasal or tubal aspiration. Volume, pH, and titratable acidity are measured. Lack of acidity in pernicious anemia and in some cases of stomach carcinoma is detected by this laboratory test. This test will also detect hypersecretion, a characteristic of Zollinger-Ellison syndrome. In gastric peptic ulcers, gastric analysis shows normal volume and acid secretion.

FECAL FAT ANALYSIS

Malabsorption syndrome may be determined by fecal fat analysis. Steatorrhea, an excessive amount of fats in the stool, characterized by foul-smelling, foamy feces, is associated with malabsorption syndrome, celiac disease, and any situation in which fats are not completely absorbed by the small intestine.

PANCREATIC TESTS

Amylase is a serum enzyme useful in detecting acute pancreatitis. Within a few hours of onset of the disease, serum amylase levels tend to show a dramatic increase. Other conditions in which serum amylase is frequently increased include parotitis, cholecystitis, hepatitis, and cirrhosis. Serum *lipase* is another test that may be used to diagnose pancreatic diseases. Serum lipase tends to increase in about 50% of patients with acute pancreatitis and remains elevated up to 14 days after the serum amylase level has returned to normal. It is recommended that the serum lipase level be determined whenever an amylase assay is performed, since the amylase may have already returned to normal at the time of testing.

CHAPTER SUMMARY

By processes such as ingestion of food into the body, digestion, absorption of essential nutrients, and elimination of waste products, the digestive system plays a major role in sustaining life. It mainly prepares sources of nutrients for cells and tissues for consumption. Gastrointestinal illnesses can be diagnosed by a wide variety of laboratory tests to aid the clinician in making a diagnosis and developing a therapeutic regimen for the patient.

Review Questions

1. Define the following terms.

diarrhea	nausea
febrile	jaundice
hepatomegaly	hepatitis
pancreatitis	

2. Match the enzyme responsible for digesting each of the following substances.

starch	*a.*	trypsin
lipids	*b.*	amylase
proteins	*c.*	bile
	d.	lipase

3. The involuntary wave-like contraction of the gastrointestinal tube that propels food through the digestive system is known as
   a. deglutition
   b. mastication
   c. peristalsis
   d. anastomosis
   e. cirrhosis

4. Absorption of nutrients during digestion occurs primarily in the
   a. stomach
   b. small intestine
   c. liver
   d. large intestine

5. Ima Jinks came to the emergency room due to severe back pains, nausea, and vomiting. The physician explained to her that she has an inflammation of the gallbladder. This condition is referred to as
   a. acute hepatitis
   b. stomatitis
   c. cholecystitis
   d. ascites
   e. colitis

BIBLIOGRAPHY

Hruska, J.: Gastrointestinal and intra-abdominal infections. *In* Reese, R., and Douglas, R.G., Jr. (eds.): A Practical Approach to Infectious Diseases, 2nd ed. Boston, Little, Brown, and Co., 1986, p. 285.

Kazmierczak, S.: Gastrointestinal and pancreatic function. *In* Anderson, S., and Cockayne, S. (eds.): Clinical Chemistry: Concepts and Applications. Philadelphia, W.B. Saunders, 1993, p. 570.

Sheldon, H.: Boyd's Introduction to the Study of Disease, 3rd ed. Philadelphia, Lea & Febiger, 1992.

Tortora, G., and Anagnostakos, N.: Principles of Anatomy and Physiology, 3rd ed. New York, Harper & Row, 1981, p 595.

Wallach, J.: Interpretation of Diagnostic Tests. Boston, Little, Brown and Co., 1986.

The Hepatic System

INTRODUCTION

ANATOMY
The Liver
The Gallbladder

FUNCTIONS OF THE LIVER
Bilirubin Metabolism
Production of Bile
**Synthesis and Metabolism of
    Proteins**
**Synthesis and Metabolism of
    Coagulation Factors and
    Vitamins**
Regulation of Glucose
Synthesis of Lipids

LIVER DISEASES
Jaundice
    Congenital conditions
        producing jaundice
    Neonatal jaundice
Hepatitis
    Prophylaxis
Cirrhosis
Metabolic Damage
Cancer

DISEASES/CONDITIONS OF THE
GALLBLADDER

LABORATORY TESTS
Liver Function Tests
    Bilirubin
    Enzyme assays
    Ammonia
Adjunct Tests
    Urine bilirubin and
        urobilinogen
    Prothrombin time
    Autoantibodies
Tests for Hepatitis

PARASITES THAT INFECT THE
LIVER

CHAPTER SUMMARY

REVIEW QUESTIONS

1. *Describe the size and location of the liver.*

2. *List and describe four major functions of the liver.*

3. *Explain the function of the gallbladder, its relationship to the liver, and its role in digestion of fats.*

4. *Explain the significance of jaundice in a patient and differentiate between prehepatic, hepatic, and posthepatic jaundice.*

5. *List three enzymes that, when elevated, are indicators of liver damage.*

6. *Explain the etiology and significance of gallstones.*

7. *List the major viral agents that cause hepatitis and explain the route of infection, relative severity and complications, and preventive measures.*

8. *Define the following terms and explain how they regulate glucose metabolism in the body: glycogenesis, glyconeogenesis, and glycogenolysis.*

KEY TERMS

liver	glycogenesis	Dubin-Johnson syndrome	gamma-glutamyl transpeptidase
lobule	glycogenolysis	Gilbert's disease	protein electrophoresis
Kupffer cells	glyconeogenesis	hepatitis	alkaline phosphatase
ampulla of Vater	jaundice	cirrhosis	alpha-fetoprotein
sphincter of Oddi	prehepatic jaundice	cholecystitis	ceruloplasmin
gallbladder	hepatic jaundice	cholestasis	alpha$_1$-antitrypsin
bilirubin	posthepatic jaundice	cholelithiasis	*Entamoeba histolytica*
bile	Crigler-Najjar syndrome	unconjugated bilirubin	*Echinococcus granulosus*
biliverdin	kernicterus	conjugated bilirubin	
albumin		aminotransferases	
glucose			

Introduction

The liver is one of the most complex organs in the body. It plays a role in many body functions and processes related to providing energy. Some of the primary processes include (1) fat metabolism, (2) glucose regulation and storage, (3) bilirubin metabolism and bile production, and (4) the synthesis of vitamins, proteins, and substances necessary for blood clotting. It also plays a role in phagocytosis and the detoxification of alcohol, drugs, and poisons. From about 6 weeks of fetal life until around 3 to 4 months of gestation, it serves as a major organ of hematopoiesis until the bone marrow takes over the majority of blood cell production. After birth, the liver ceases production of blood cells completely. However, in adults whose bone marrow function has become impaired, the liver may again resume erythropoietic activity. As with a number of other organs in the body, much of the liver tissue can be destroyed before its functions are significantly impaired. The liver also has the ability to regenerate tissue. The structural and functional complexity of this organ make it vital to life.

This chapter describes the anatomy and functions of the liver and an accessory organ, the gallbladder. It also discusses bilirubin metabolism, bile production, and synthesis of coagulation factors. Liver and gallbladder diseases are also described.

ANATOMY

THE LIVER

The **liver** *is a large triangular-shaped organ located in the upper right quadrant of the abdomen just under the diaphragm* (Fig. 9–1). It weighs about 1.5 kg (3 to 4 lb) and has two major lobes. The smaller or left lobe lies toward the centerline of the abdomen; the larger or right lobe is divided into three smaller lobes. A strong ligament (the falciform ligament) joins the two lobes and also serves to attach the liver to the diaphragm and underlying abdominal wall. Most of the liver is protected by the rib cage, but in hepatomegaly the edges of the liver may extend below the margin of the ribs. On the underside of the right lobe is the gallbladder (Fig. 9–2).

The **lobule** *is the functional unit of the liver* (Fig. 9–3). Each lobe is separated into lobules that contain arrangements of liver cells (*hepatocytes*), blood vessels, and bile ducts. The lobule is composed of a stack of hepatocytes that radiate from a central vein that brings blood to the cells. At the sides of adjacent lobules, in interconnective tissue, are branches of the portal vein, hepatic artery, and bile duct. Groups of hepatic cells are separated from each other by *sinusoids*. Blood from the portal vein empties into the sinusoids and supplies the cells with nutrients, while blood from the hepatic artery also empties into the sinusoid to

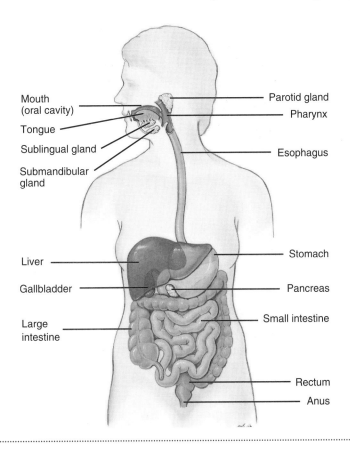

Mouth
(oral cavity)

Tongue

Sublingual gland

Submandibular
gland

Parotid gland

Pharynx

Esophagus

Liver

Gallbladder

Large
intestine

Stomach

Pancreas

Small intestine

Rectum

Anus

FIGURE 9–1

Location of the liver.
(From Applegate, E.J.: The Anatomy and Physiology Learning System. Philadelphia, W.B.
Saunders, 1995, with permission.)

supply oxygen to the cells. *Phagocytic cells, known as* **Kupffer cells,** *line the sinusoids and function to remove bacteria, damage erythrocytes, and other substances from the portal blood as it enters the lobule.* The filtered blood from sinusoids goes to the central vein of the lobule to be returned to the lungs and heart by the hepatic veins (Fig. 9–4).

There is a unique dual blood supply to the liver. The hepatic artery carries oxygenated blood from the aorta to the liver. The artery branches into many small arterioles, giving the liver an abundant blood supply. The second source of blood, the portal vein, carries nutrient-rich blood from the intestinal tract and spleen to the liver. The liver uses some of these nutrients to synthesize energy and stores others, such as glucose and proteins, for future energy needs. The hepatic vein returns blood to the heart.

The liver produces bile, a combination of water, cholesterol, bilirubin pigments, inorganic salts, and bile acid salts. Bile canals (canaliculi) within the lobule accept bile secretions from the hepatocytes. These small canals converge to form larger and larger ducts until they merge into the common hepatic duct. This duct combines with the common bile duct and

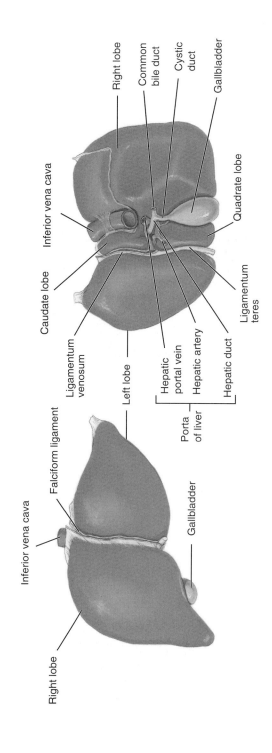

FIGURE 9-2

Gross anatomy of the liver.
(From Applegate, E.J.: The Anatomy and Physiology Learning System. Philadelphia, W.B. Saunders, 1995, with permission.)

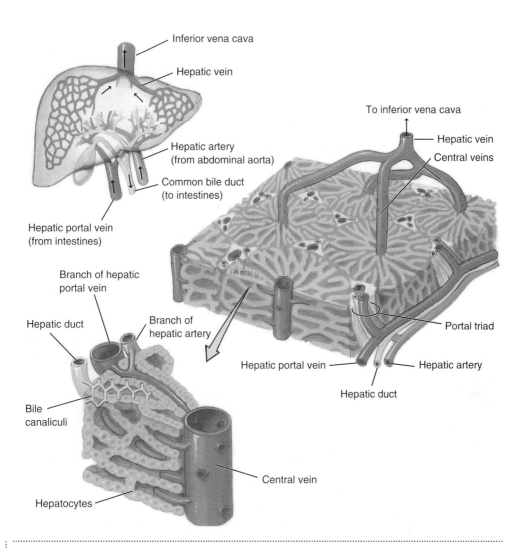

FIGURE 9-3

Microscopic structure of the hepatic lobule.

(From Applegate, E.J.: The Anatomy and Physiology Learning System. Philadelphia, W.B. Saunders, 1995, with permission.)

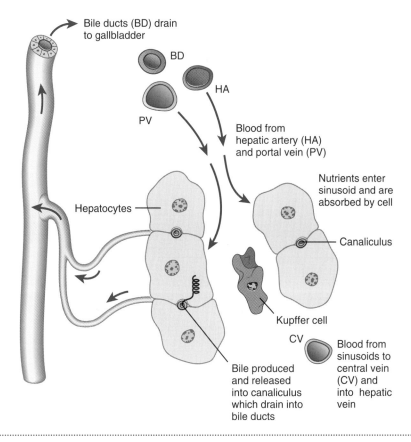

Bile ducts (BD) drain
to gallbladder

BD

HA

PV

Blood from
hepatic artery (HA)
and portal vein (PV)

Nutrients enter
sinusoid and are
absorbed by cell

Hepatocytes

Canaliculus

Kupffer cell

CV

Blood from
sinusoids to
central vein
(CV) and
into hepatic
vein

Bile produced
and released
into canaliculus
which drain into
bile ducts

FIGURE 9-4

Flow of blood and bile within the hepatic cells.

drains into the intestine at the **ampulla of Vater**. The flow of bile is controlled by a valve, the **sphincter of Oddi,** in the common bile duct. When the small intestine is full, the valve opens; when the small intestine is empty, the valve closes and causes bile to remain in the gallbladder. Bile is released from the gallbladder into the duodenum in response to the stimulus caused by dietary fats.

THE GALLBLADDER

The **gallbladder** *is a small, sac-like organ that can store up to about 50 ml of bile. Its major function is to concentrate and store bile produced in the liver.* The mucous membrane lining the gallbladder can expand to allow storage of bile or contract to empty bile. The gallbladder is connected to the liver by the cystic duct and accepts drainage of bile from the liver. The cystic duct joins with the hepatic duct to form the common bile duct, which empties into the duodenum. The hormone *cholyecystokinin* controls the emptying of the gallbladder.

FUNCTIONS OF THE LIVER

The primary functions of the liver encompass a variety of metabolic activities, including

- Catabolism of bilirubin production and excretion of bile
- Synthesis and metabolism of proteins, including albumin, fibrinogen, and prothrombin
- Regulation, metabolism, and storage of blood glucose
- Detoxification of drugs
- Metabolism of nitrogenous waste
- Storage of vitamins and iron
- Synthesis of lipids
- Phagocytosis of old erythrocytes, bacteria, and other foreign particles

Most of these functions are interrelated. Impairment of one or more activities affects not only other liver functions but also the function of other organs.

BILIRUBIN METABOLISM

The most important activity associated with the liver is the metabolism of bilirubin. **Bilirubin** *is a by-product of the destruction of senescent (old) erythrocytes. Hemoglobin from erythrocytes is converted to bilirubin in the spleen and bound to albumin in the blood.* This form of bilirubin, which is not water soluble, is transported to the liver, where it is then linked with glucuronic acid by the enzyme *glucuronyltransferase.* This linking process makes bilirubin water soluble and allows it to be excreted. Bilirubin is sent through the biliary system and is passed into the intestine, where most of it is converted to urobilinogen by intestinal bacteria and then excreted in the feces. A small portion (10%) is recycled through the liver or excreted in the urine (Fig. 9–5).

Under normal conditions, the liver is able to process released hemoglobin when erythrocyte destruction occurs at a relatively constant level. When there is an excessive breakdown of erythrocytes, however, the elevated bilirubin level cannot be processed by the liver. Bilirubin will therefore appear in the plasma—leading to a yellow discoloration of skin, mucous membranes, sclera (white of eye), and body fluids in the patient, a condition called *jaundice.* Jaundice occurs when there is an elevated level of circulating bilirubin. Jaundice may also occur when the liver cells are nonfunctional and cannot process even the normal load of bilirubin.

PRODUCTION OF BILE

Another function associated with the liver is the production of bile, which helps digest fats in the intestine. **Bile,** *a yellow-brown fluid, is composed of water, bile salts, bile acids, and bile*

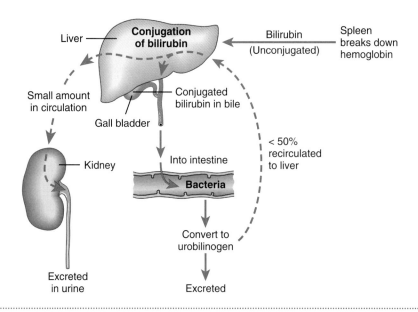

FIGURE 9-5

Metabolism of bilirubin.

pigments (bilirubin and **biliverdin**). Bile acids are synthesized from cholesterol by the cells lining the canaliculi and ductules. The bile acids help to break down fats in the intestine so that these lipids can be digested. The liver produces approximately 500 to 1,000 ml of bile daily. The gallbladder decreases this amount through concentration and stores approximately 50 ml. Bile is released from the gallbladder into the digestive tract through the bile duct. The hormone cholyecystokinin is produced in response to fat ingestion and stimulates gallbladder contraction to release bile.

SYNTHESIS AND METABOLISM OF PROTEINS

The liver is responsible for regulating the interchange of stored and circulating proteins. Proteins present in food are converted into amino acids in the intestine and transported to the liver via the portal vein. The liver stores these amino acids from the blood and releases them as proteins when protein sources are not present in the diet. In time of starvation, the liver may convert these amino acids into an energy source by the process of *glyconeogenesis.* In this process, the amino acids are converted to glucose, a ready source of energy.

Another metabolic function of the liver is the manufacture of a number of substances, such as albumin, fibrinogen, and alpha- and beta-globulins. **Albumin,** *a key plasma protein, is synthesized exclusively in the liver.* This substance serves to maintain osmotic pressure and to bind hormones, drugs, anions, and fatty acids for transport throughout the body. Production of normal amounts of albumin is used as an index or marker of liver function. Albumin production will be decreased when the liver is damaged; the lower the amount of albumin, the more severe the underlying disease.

SYNTHESIS AND METABOLISM OF COAGULATION FACTORS AND VITAMINS

The liver also synthesizes the following proteins, which are necessary for the proper clotting of blood (*coagulation*). For example:

- ◼ Prothrombin (factor II)
- ◼ Fibrinogen (factor I)
- ◼ Proconvertin (factor VII)
- ◼ Stuart factor (factor X)

Damage to the liver results in the decreased production of these factors and an increase in the time it takes for the blood to clot. Tests such as the prothrombin time indirectly measure levels of coagulation proteins. The longer it takes for plasma to clot, the less coagulation proteins that are present.

The liver also stores vitamin B_{12}, which is necessary for proper blood cell production. In addition, fat-soluble vitamins such as vitamins A, D, and E and folic acid are stored in the liver.

Although specific lymphocytes in the blood produce the majority of immunoglobulins (antibodies), some are made in the liver. The liver also produces increased amounts of specific proteins called *acute-phase reactants*. Acute-phase reactants are proteins produced in increased amounts by the liver when tissue injury, inflammation, or both occur in the body. Reactants such as C-reactive protein, haptoglobin, $alpha_1$-antitrypsin, and ceruloplasmin serve to mediate processes important to host defense.

REGULATION OF GLUCOSE

Glucose *is a major product of carbohydrate metabolism.* It is vital in supplying energy to the brain, heart, and other tissues in the body. The role of the liver in glucose metabolism is one of buffering or leveling out the amount of glucose in the blood—storing it when blood levels are high, releasing it when blood levels are low. Glucose derived from food digested in the intestine is transported to the liver via the portal vein. After a meal, the level of glucose in the portal vein is twice the normal level. A certain amount of glucose is immediately oxidized into energy for the rest of body while approximately two thirds is removed by the hepatocytes and stored as *glycogen* (a polymer of glucose). When the glucose level in the blood decreases, the stored glycogen will be converted back into glucose. The terms glycogenesis, glycogenolysis, and glyconeogenesis describe liver functions as they relate to glucose metabolism.

Glycogenesis *describes the conversion of glucose to glycogen for storage. In* **glycogenolysis,** *the stored glycogen is broken down into glucose and then re-enters the blood. The term* **glyconeogenesis** *describes what happens when both glucose and stored glycogen are unavailable as sources of energy. In glyconeogenesis, liver glucose is manufactured from sources other than glycogen.* For example, during starvation, tissue protein is broken down and converted to glucose in order to provide energy to the body.

SYNTHESIS OF LIPIDS

Cholesterol and phospholipids are synthesized in the liver. These substances are important constituents of cell membranes, and the cholesterol molecule is the precursor for a number of important hormones, including estrogen.

LIVER DISEASES

As you have seen in the previous sections, the liver has a wide variety of functions and therefore is susceptible to many diseases of either infectious or noninfectious origin. Infectious agents include hepatitis viruses, Epstein-Barr virus (the cause of infectious mononucleosis), and cytomegalovirus. Noninfectious causes of inhibited or disrupted normal liver function include autoimmune antibodies, neoplasms, biliary obstruction, and toxic agents.

Diseases that affect the liver can be broadly classified into acute and chronic conditions. The acute condition most often seen is viral hepatitis, while common chronic liver diseases include chronic hepatitis and cirrhosis. Hepatocellular carcinoma often follows chronic hepatitis or cirrhosis. Most other liver cancer is the result of metastases from the primary site, such as the breast, colon, or lung. Other chronic conditions include biliary atresia, which is seen in newborns as a result of an inflammatory process that destroys the bile ducts.

JAUNDICE

Jaundice *is not a disease but rather is a general symptom that reflects liver damage from an underlying condition.* It is characterized by a yellow discoloration of skin, mucous membranes, the sclera of the eye, and body fluids such as plasma or urine due to an increased level of bilirubin. Although jaundice is most often linked to viral hepatitis, there are other causes for increased bilirubin in the circulation. In general, jaundice can be classified by the underlying site or cause of the jaundice: prehepatic, hepatic, and posthepatic jaundice.

Prehepatic jaundice *is generally due to causes other than damage to the liver tissue.* In this type of jaundice, too much bilirubin is produced, and the liver is unable to process it. A typical cause of prehepatic jaundice is hemolytic anemia, in which large numbers of erythrocytes are rapidly destroyed. This massive breakdown exceeds the liver's ability to process the bilirubin that is produced from the hemolyzed erythrocytes. The excess bilirubin therefore accumulates in the plasma.

Hepatic jaundice *reflects damage in the liver itself.* The classic example is viral hepatitis, which affects the hepatocytes. Chemicals, drugs, and other substances can also cause liver damage. Bilirubin levels in the blood are usually elevated in these cases.

The term **posthepatic jaundice** *is used to describe conditions in which the liver is functioning normally but the bilirubin is not being released into the intestine through the bile duct.* The most common reason for posthepatic jaundice is the presence of gallstones blocking the bile duct and preventing bile from entering the intestinal tract. The conjugated bilirubin backs up into the circulation. The glomerulus then filters it from the blood into the urine. Because there is no bile being released into the intestinal tract due to the blockage, there is no urobilinogen produced. The patient's stool in these cases has a characteristic light color. In addition, since there is no urobilinogen being produced in the intestinal tract, none is re-circulated and excreted through the kidney. Hence, urine urobilinogen levels are decreased.

Congenital Conditions Producing Jaundice

Jaundice may also appear as a result of a congenital condition in which there are defects in the enzymes necessary to process bilirubin in the liver. The symptoms, severity, and process affected will depend on the specific enzyme deficiency. **Crigler-Najjar syndrome** *is a rare autosomal recessive condition in which there is a deficiency in glucuronyltransferase and therefore bilirubin is not conjugated.* Bilirubin rises to up to 20 times normal during the first 48 hours of life. Infants develop **kernicterus** and nervous system disorders, and die in early infancy. **Dubin-Johnson syndrome** is characterized by a chronic nonhemolytic jaundice due to inability to excrete bilirubin. **Gilbert's disease** is characterized by hyperbilirubinemia due to the liver's inability to pick up and process bilirubin that is presented to hepatocytes.

Neonatal Jaundice

Newborns may present with jaundice shortly after birth that may be due to normal physiologic jaundice of the newborn or a more serious condition, *hemolytic disease of the newborn* (HDN). Normal physiologic jaundice occurs in newborns because the liver is one of the last organs to become fully functional. Up until birth, the mother's liver takes care of the removal of bilirubin from fetal circulation. After birth, it takes several days for the newborn's liver to begin working; in premature infants, this process often takes even longer. Therefore, the fetal erythrocytes that are being normally destroyed produce bilirubin that is not conjugated by the liver. Hence, the level of unconjugated bilirubin increases and the infant appears jaundiced. The risk involved in this situation is that this type of bilirubin can settle in brain cells and cause mental retardation. In most cases, placing the infant under ultraviolet (UV) lights will help destroy the bilirubin until the infant's liver is functional.

In HDN, in contrast, there is an increased destruction of the infant's erythrocytes due to the presence of maternal antibody against a specific antigen on the baby's erythrocytes. After birth, the destruction continues at a higher rate than normal. Although there is a certain amount of enzyme present, it is insufficient to process the increased bilirubin and jaundice occurs. As a means of therapy, the infant may be placed under UV lights or, in very severe cases, may require an exchange transfusion, depending on the amount and type of antibody present and the severity of the erythrocyte destruction. This exchange transfusion involves removing part of the infant's blood and replacing it with the donor's fresh blood. This process will remove antibody-coated erythrocytes and replace them with erythrocytes that will not be prematurely destroyed.

HEPATITIS

Hepatitis *is a general term that refers to inflammation of the liver.* There are many viruses as well as parasitic, bacterial, and chemical agents that may cause this condition. Most commonly, however, hepatitis is caused by five different recognized hepatotropic viruses:

- ■ Hepatitis A virus (HAV)
- ■ Hepatitis B virus (HBV)
- ■ Hepatitis C virus (HCV)

   ■ Hepatitis D virus (HDV)
   ■ Hepatitis E virus (HEV)

These viruses vary in their routes of transmission as well as in their ability to cause acute and chronic disease (Table 9–1). HAV and HEV are transmitted by fecal-oral contamination; HBV, HCV, and HDV are transmitted via parenteral (blood/body fluids) means. HDV requires a part of the HBV in order to replicate; therefore, it is only seen in patients who also have HBV. HAV, HBV, and HCV are the most common viruses in the United States. HDV is most commonly seen in the Middle East, southern Europe, and parts of western Africa. HEV is a recently identified hepatitis virus that is generally responsible for epidemics in underdeveloped areas such as Southeast Asia and Mexico. The major risk with this virus is the increased mortality (death rate) when it occurs in pregnant women. Hepatitis G virus is the most recently identified hepatitis virus. Currently, little is known about it.

   The clinical course, symptoms, and eventual outcome of hepatitis infection vary not only by etiologic agent but also by patient. There are three clinical courses:

Table 9–1 ■ Characteristics of Hepatitis Viruses*

	HAV	HBV	HCV	HDV	HEV
Source	F/O	Blood/body fluids	Blood/body fluids	Blood/body fluids	F/O
Chronic	No	Yes	Yes	Yes	No
Symptoms	Mild; >50% no jaundice	Mild–severe	Mild–severe	Often fulminant	Mild except in pregnancy
Vaccine	Yes; limited usage	Yes; recommended for all health care personnel	No	No	No
Markers	anti-HAV	HBsAg anti-HBc anti-HBe HBeAg anti-HBs	anti-HCV	anti-HDV	anti-HEV

* Abbreviations: F/O, fecal-oral; HBsAg, hepatitis B surface antigen; HbcAb, hepatitis B core antibody; HBsAb, hepatitis B surface antibody; HbeAg, hepatitis B early antigen.

- ■ Acute hepatitis that resolves without major damage to the liver
- ■ Acute hepatitis that progresses to fulminant hepatitis and death
- ■ Acute hepatitis that becomes chronic

Some patients with acute hepatitis may be asymptomatic, and the only means of detection will be an elevation in specific enzymes, bilirubin, or both. Others will present with generalized symptoms such as fever, sore throat, nausea, malaise, upper right quadrant pain, loss of desire to smoke, or anorexia. Still other patients may exhibit the classic sign of hepatitis—jaundice, a characteristic yellowing of the whites of the eyes and the skin. This icteric (yellow) condition is due to excess bilirubin in the blood. In general, most patients with hepatitis will resolve the infection and develop immunity without complications.

Patients with HAV infection, for example, are usually asymptomatic, and the infection rarely results in chronic or fulminant hepatitis. A few patients may develop *fulminant hepatitis*, in which there is massive and rapid destruction of hepatocytes, but this is a rare occurrence. HBV, HCV, and HDV are viruses associated with fulminant hepatitis. Infections with HCV and HDV are more likely to result in fulminant disease than HBV. Patients present with malaise, nausea, edema, and itching due to bile salts in the skin. There is bruising because of decreased levels of coagulation factors produced by the damaged liver. Eventually there is an increase in blood ammonia levels, leading to stupor, coma, and death.

Other patients will develop chronic hepatitis, in which there is a low rate of constant destruction of hepatocytes. This condition may eventually result in cirrhosis or hepatocellular carcinoma. HBV or HCV may cause chronic hepatitis. HCV, the more common cause of chronic hepatitis, often leads to cirrhosis and carcinoma of the liver.

In hepatitis, bilirubin and liver enzyme levels such as alanine transaminase (ALT) and aspartate transaminase (AST) are monitored in order to assess the patient's clinical status and the amount of damage to the liver. Testing for the presence of hepatitis or immunity to hepatitis also involves detection of specific serologic markers (see Table 9–1). These tests are most frequently performed in the serology or immunology section of the clinical laboratory. Depending on the viral agent suspected, tests are designed to detect either antibodies against the virus or specific viral antigens. The groups of tests used to determine the status of the patient are discussed in the Laboratory Tests section of this chapter.

Prophylaxis

Hepatitis B was the first virus for which a vaccine was developed. The vaccine uses an antigen from the virus to stimulate production of antibodies that protect the person from infection. This vaccine is now routinely given to health care workers to prevent HBV infection. A second type of prophylaxis for HBV infection, hepatitis B immune globulin (HBIG), is a product composed of antibodies to HBV. It is given to nonvaccinated persons who are exposed to the virus to help prevent infection.

Hepatitis A vaccine has recently become available for persons traveling to countries in which HAV is endemic and in which there is a significant risk of exposure to the virus. There is currently no vaccine for HCV. Hepatitis D can be prevented by preventing HBV. A vaccine for HEV is currently under development specifically for populations in endemic areas.

CIRRHOSIS

Cirrhosis *of the liver is a chronic condition in which there is repeated cell death and regeneration*. The liver loses its smooth surface, and develops macroscopic nodes and an abnormal structure at the cellular level. Cirrhosis is characterized by irreversible, progressive destruction of hepatocytes. This is followed by abnormal regeneration of the cells, increase in connective tissue, and subsequent loss of function. The entire underlying organization of blood vessels and ducts is destroyed. The liver cells become enlarged and retain secretory proteins. Impaired triglyceride metabolism also leads to fatty deposits within the liver (fatty metamorphosis). There are two major causes of cirrhosis: alcoholism and chronic hepatitis infection.

Cirrhosis is most commonly associated with chronic alcoholism because the liver is the principal organ for the metabolism of alcohol. Factors such as sex, body size, amount of ingested alcohol, the frequency of consumption, and relative nutritional status influence whether a person develops alcoholic liver disease. The severity and rapidity of development is complicated by the dietary deficiencies (decreased fat, protein, and carbohydrate consumption and decrease in intake of vitamin B_{12}) seen in this population. Anemia is often seen in patients with liver disease. Over 50% of patients with chronic liver disease or alcoholic cirrhosis have anemia—often due to underlying nutritional conditions. One reason is that these patients have abnormal intake of lipids, which alters the erythrocyte membrane.

There are several complications of liver cirrhosis. Patients with cirrhosis often have gastric and esophageal hemorrhages because the liver no longer manufactures the proteins needed for blood coagulation. Decreased levels of albumin lead to an imbalance in osmotic pressure, which in turn allows fluids to leak out of blood vessels into the abdominal cavity. Distention of the abdomen due to accumulation of fluid in the abdomen (*ascites*) results. The patient retains sodium, and has hypoalbuminemia and portal hypertension.

One type of cirrhosis, primary *biliary cirrhosis*, is due to an underlying autoimmune condition. This relatively rare condition appears in middle-aged women and is characterized by an inflammatory process affecting the bile ducts. This inflammation eventually leads to hepatic failure. Over 90% of the patients with this disease show the presence of antimitochondrial antibodies in the serum. Patients with this disease show jaundice, increased cholesterol, and malabsorption as part of the disease process.

METABOLIC DAMAGE

Most drugs and chemical toxins are metabolized by the liver and may be directly toxic to its cells. They may also indirectly interfere with the metabolic processes in the liver and cause a secondary injury. Often the damage is dose dependent. The variety of hepatotoxic drugs is wide; it includes antibiotics such as sulfonamides, anticonvulsants, antineoplastics, and acetaminophen.

CANCER

Hepatocarcinoma may be due to a primary tumor that originates in the liver, often caused by cirrhosis. Secondary tumors, in contrast, are the result of metastases from cancer in another organ. Breast, colon, and lung cancer are three of the common cancers that often spread to the liver. Patients with liver cancer show generalized symptoms such as weight loss, loss of appetite, hepatomegaly, and pain. Diagnosis is usually made by radiographic imaging. There is no effective treatment, and the prognosis for patients with liver cancer is poor.

DISEASES/CONDITIONS OF THE GALLBLADDER

Probably the most common disease of the gallbladder is **cholecystitis**, *or inflammation of the gallbladder*. Often, when a gallstone is present, the bile does not drain properly. As it remains in the gallbladder, bile becomes more concentrated and irritates the walls of the gallbladder. The patient experiences severe pain, usually under the right rib cage, after a meal that contains a high level of fats. Other patients have nausea and vomiting due to intolerance to fats in the diet. **Cholestasis** *commonly seen in parallel with cholecystitis, results from obstruction of the ducts with no bile draining into the intestinal tract.* The most common cause is gallstones in the bile duct or gallbladder (**cholelithiasis**). These gallstones are composed of precipitated cholesterol, calcium, bilirubin, and bile salts. While small stones may cause no problem for the patient, larger stones block the ducts. Characteristics of this condition may include jaundice, pale stools, and presence of bilirubin in the urine. The classic test for diagnosing gallbladder disease involves radiologic imaging wherein the patient ingests a radiopaque contrast dye. The gallbladder and location of any stones present will be seen.

LABORATORY TESTS

Diseases of the liver are most often diagnosed based on results of tests done in the chemistry section of the clinical laboratory. These tests are designed to detect elevations in enzymes or other constituents that reflect abnormal liver function. In addition, tests done in immunology, immunohematology (blood bank), or hematology may also be used to confirm the diagnosis of an underlying hepatic disease. The tests may provide a primary diagnosis and establish a baseline against which future results may be compared or used to monitor therapy and progress of the disease, and to provide a prognosis. The laboratory tests in this section are discussed in groups. One group deals with general liver function, another with adjunct or special tests for specific conditions, and the last with tests for agents of hepatitis.

LIVER FUNCTION TESTS

The primary tests that reflect liver function include enzyme assays (e.g., AST, ALT, and alkaline phosphatase), total protein and albumin, and bilirubin. Because the liver has a reserve ability to break down hemoglobin, bilirubin is not as sensitive a test for function as the other tests. Tests such as urine bilirubin, urine urobilinogen, and prothrombin time may be used as adjunct tests for integrity of liver function. It should be kept in mind that some of these enzymes and substances are found in tissues other than the liver and may be present in abnormal amounts due to a number of diseases. Therefore, the results of the laboratory tests are used in combination with the patient's clinical symptoms and history. In addition, results of the tests are often correlated with each other to identify significant liver problems.

Bilirubin

Bilirubin is a by-product of hemoglobin breakdown. Tests to determine bilirubin levels are often requested for the initial assessment of liver damage. As mentioned previously, bilirubin exists in two forms—conjugated and unconjugated. The **unconjugated** form represents the bilirubin prior to its entry into the liver. This form is not water soluble and cannot be excreted from the body. The **conjugated** form represents bilirubin after it has been acted upon by a liver enzyme (glucuronyltransferase). It is water soluble and can be excreted from the body by the kidney via the urine. The test for total bilirubin measures both types of bilirubin. A comparison of the values of total and unconjugated bilirubin helps determine where liver damage is occurring. For example, if the total bilirubin level is high but that of unconjugated bilirubin is less than normal, this indicates that the damage is occurring in the hepatocytes; the liver is unable to link bilirubin to the enzyme. If both values are increased above normal, there may be obstruction.

Enzyme Assays

There are many enzymes associated with the liver. Some are increased only in cases of obstruction, while others are markers of direct damage to the hepatocytes.

Aminotransferases *are responsible for moving amino acids from one compound to another.* A wide variety of transaminases exist in the body. There are two significant ones found in the serum as indicators of damage to hepatocytes—AST and ALT. *AST* is found in cardiac, hepatic, and skeletal muscle and brain and renal tissue. Significant elevations in plasma levels are found in cases of hepatic or myocardial damage or muscle necrosis. *ALT* is found in very high levels in liver tissue and very low levels in other tissues. Therefore, elevations in this enzyme generally reflect damage specific to the liver.

Gamma-glutamyl transpeptidase *(GGT) is a microsomal enzyme that is found throughout the body but has its highest concentration in the liver.* The enzyme is a good marker for liver damage. Elevated values are found in alcoholics with liver disease and there is slight elevation in biliary obstruction. Values are consistently higher in alcoholics with liver disease, while elevations are seen in only one fourth of those alcoholics with no underlying liver disease.

Aminoaciduria may be seen in some patients with liver disease. In acute hepatic necrosis, the liver cells undergo autolysis and release specific amino acids. Crystals of leucine and tyrosine are characteristically seen in the urine of patients with this condition. Occasionally these crystals are found in children with specific inborn errors of metabolism.

Tests for *total protein/protein electrophoresis/albumin* are used to measure the liver's ability to synthesize these proteins. Albumin is the most important because it is synthesized only in the liver. A decreased concentration most often reflects liver damage but may also be seen in patients with inadequate protein intake (malnutrition with or without alcoholic liver disease) or in patients who have renal damage that allows increased amounts of proteins to leak into the urine. **Protein electrophoresis** *is a method of quantitating the different proteins present in the serum.* The serum is placed on a special medium and exposed to an electric current, which causes the proteins to migrate in different patterns. Deficiencies or excesses of specific proteins can be visualized as well as measured.

Alkaline phosphatase *(ALP) is an enzyme found in many tissues, including the liver, so that elevated levels are not specific for liver disease.* Its primary use is to differentiate bone and liver disease from disease processes in other tissues. In liver diseases, ALP is characteristically elevated when the damage is due to obstruction, and is not in hepatocytes themselves.

Alpha-fetoprotein *(AFP) is a substance that reflects regenerative activity of the hepatocytes.* It is normally present in the fetus, infant, and pregnant women. Low levels can be found in most adults. It is increased in adults who have hepatocellular carcinoma. The level can be used as an indicator to monitor effectiveness of treatment. As the level goes down, the treatment is considered to be effective. AFP will also appear in increased amounts in non-neoplastic hepatic disease, such as chronic hepatitis.

Ceruloplasmin *is the protein responsible for transporting copper.* Decreased levels are a marker for Wilson's disease, an autosomal recessive condition that results in abnormal metabolism of copper and increased urine excretion of copper.

Alpha$_1$-antitrypsin *deficiency is an inborn error of protein metabolism that results in emphysema and cirrhosis.* The lack of alpha$_1$-antitrypsin allows other enzymes to damage structural proteins, resulting in lung and liver damage.

Ammonia

Bacteria in the intestine release ammonia from nitrogen-containing food. This ammonia is absorbed into the blood in the portal vein and transported to the liver. A healthy liver will convert the ammonia to urea for excretion through the kidneys into the urine. Elevated levels of ammonia are found in the blood either when the liver cells are damaged and cannot convert ammonia or when the blood in the portal vein is "shunted," or bypassed, around the liver so that cells do not have the opportunity to convert ammonia. Elevation of the blood ammonia level is seen in diseases such as cirrhosis, severe hepatitis, and hepatic coma.

ADJUNCT TESTS
Urine Bilirubin and Urobilinogen

Urine bilirubin and urobilinogen are adjunct tests that can help further determine where the damage is within the hepatic system. Bilirubin is not normally present in the urine but urobilinogen is. Therefore, changes in the values give valuable data. For example, the presence of bilirubin in urine and a decrease in urine urobilinogen indicates obstruction to the bile duct—no bilirubin is getting to the intestinal tract to be converted to urobilinogen. Conjugated bilirubin is backing up into the circulation and being excreted by the kidneys.

Prothrombin Time

The time it takes for plasma to clot reflects the level of specific coagulation factors present— the longer it takes to clot, the less the amount of one or more of the coagulation factors. In chronic liver disease, the level of vitamin K, which is needed for production of prothrombin and several other coagulation factors, is decreased. Therefore, the amount of these factors is also decreased. The prothrombin time (PT) is used as a screen to measure overall clotting ability. The longer the PT, the more advanced the liver disease and the poorer the prognosis for the patient. Increased PT time (time longer than reference value to clot) indicates decreased production of one or more of these factors.

Autoantibodies

Autoantibodies are antibodies directed against a person's own tissue. Primary biliary cirrhosis is a liver disease characterized by presence of an autoantibody directed against the mitochondria of the liver cell. About 90% of all patients with primary biliary cirrhosis have these antibodies. Patient serum is used in a test for confirming the presence of these antibodies.

TESTS FOR HEPATITIS

There are several different groups of tests that may be run when patients present with suspected or confirmed hepatitis. These panels of tests, which usually detect either viral antigens in the patient's blood or antibodies in the patient's serum against the viral agent, can be grouped as follows:

Table 9–2 ■ Expected Results for Acute Panel and Immune Status Panel Tests

Acute Panel

	Anti-HAV/IgM	Anti-HCV	Anti-HBc/IgM	HBsAg
HAV	+	−	−	−
HBV	−	−	+	+
HCV	−	+	−	−

Immune Panel

	Anti-HAV total	HBsAg	Anti-HBc total	Anti-HBs
Previous HAV	+	−	−	−
Previous HBV	−	−	+	+

* Abbreviations: HAV/IgM, hepatitis A virus, immunoglobulin M specific; HBc/IgM, hepatitis B core, immunoglobulin M specific; HBsAg, hepatitis B surface antigen; +, positive result; −, negative result.

- *Acute panel*—tests run when the patient presents with clinical symptoms suggesting hepatitis. These tests, designed to give clinical information as to the etiologic agent responsible, routinely detect exposure to HAV, HBV, or HCV. The panel usually consists of anti-HCV, HBsAg, anti-HBc/IgM, and anti-HAV/IgM (see Table 9–2).

- *Monitoring panel*—follows the course of the disease and recovery of the patient. It is commonly used in patients with chronic hepatitis B. HBsAg and anti-HBe markers help determine infectivity level of the patient.

- *Immunity panel*—used when a person has been exposed to blood or blood products (HBV) or to a fecally contaminated water or food source (HAV). The clinician wants to know if the patient has antibodies present that will protect him or her from developing the disease. The tests used for Hepatitis B are anti-HBc total, anti-HBs, and HBsAg (Table 9–2). Anti-HAV total may be tested for in suspected exposure to HAV.

Prior to receiving HBV vaccine, the patient may be tested for pre-existing antibodies to HBV. If these antibodies are present, there is no need to receive the vaccine. The test used is the one for anti-HBs, the marker of immunity to HBV.

PARASITES THAT INFECT THE LIVER

Of all the infectious agents to cause liver disease, parasites are probably one of the least common. There are, however, several different organisms that can be found in the liver and can cause damage to it. *The first such organism,* **Entamoeba histolytica**, *is a pathogenic parasite of the intestinal tract.* This ameba causes a secondary infection in the liver when it erodes the intestinal wall and travels through the portal vein to the liver. The patient experiences fever, weight loss, hepatomegaly, and pain. Production of proteolytic enzymes causes necrosis of the liver tissue, leading to amebic ulcers filled with pus and organisms. This condition is confirmed through use of liver scans or other diagnostic imaging techniques.

The adults of the sheep liver fluke *Fasciola hepatica* and the Chinese liver fluke *Opisthorchis sinensis* live in the bile ducts of the liver and cause damage through mechanical irritation, toxic metabolites, and occasionally obstruction. Neither organism is routinely seen in the United States. Diagnosis is made by finding the eggs of the adult in a patient's stool specimen.

Echinococcus granulosus *is a tapeworm whose natural life cycle involves sheep and dogs or other wild carnivores.* It is found in major sheep-raising areas of the world. In the United States, it is found primarily in states such as Arizona and New Mexico, where sheepherding is common. Humans can become accidentally infected and harbor the larval stage of the tapeworm, called the *hydatid cyst.* This fluid-filled structure often forms in the liver and may cause obstruction or pressure necrosis to bile ducts or blood vessels. Routine radiographs may show evidence of the cyst. Tests for antibodies may confirm the diagnosis. Adults of organisms such as the blood fluke live in veins of abdominal structures, but the liver serves as the site in which the larvae mature into adults.

CHAPTER SUMMARY

The liver is an organ that regulates many body processes and produces many vital proteins. It is involved in protein production, glucose metabolism and regulation, digestion of fats, and detoxiification of poisons or chemicals. It is susceptible to a variety of diseases that may cause transient or permanent damage. Hepatitis is a condition commonly caused by a number of different viral agents. Cirrhosis may result from chronic alcohol abuse or hepatitis. Disease of the gallbladder may affect digestion. Laboratory testing for diagnosis of liver disease includes immunogic tests for antigens and antibodies found in hepatitis. Chemistry tests for bilirubin, protein, and liver enzymes measure the amount of damage present in liver disease.

Review Questions

1. The conversion of glucose to glycogen is called
    a. gluconeogenesis
    b. glycogenolysis
    c. glyconeogenesis
    d. neoplasmagenesis

2. Bilirubin is a breakdown product of which substance?
    a. cholesterol
    b. alcohol
    c. hemoglobin
    d. bile salts

3. The following results were seen on a patient with upper right quadrant pain and loss of appetite.

    anti-HAV   =   anti-HBc IgM   +
    HBsAg   +   anti-HCV   =

    The most likely diagnosis is:
    a. previous HCV exposure
    b. chronic HBV
    c. acute HBV
    d. no evidence of current exposure

4. In a case of bile duct obstruction which set of urine results might be seen?

	urine bilirubin	urine urobilinogen
a.	↑	↑
b.	↓	↑
c.	↓	↓
d.	↑	↓

BIBLIOGRAPHY

Arias, I.M.: The Liver: Biology and Pathobiology, 23rd ed. New York, Raven Press, 1994.

Peters, R.L.: Liver Pathology. New York, Churchill Livingstone, 1986.

Targan, S.R. and Shanahan, F.: Immunology and Immunopathology of the Liver and Gastrointestinal Tract. New York, Igaku-Shoin, 1990.

Tavoloni, N. and Beck, P.D.: Hepatic Transport and Bile Secretion: Physiology and Pathophysiology. New York, Raven Press, 1993.

Vander, A.J., Sherman, J.H., and Luciano, D.S.: Human Physiology: The Mechanisms of Body Function. New York, McGraw-Hill, 1994.

Williams, J.W.: Hepatic Transplantation. Philadelphia, W.B. Saunders, 1990.

CHAPTER 10

The Central Nervous System

INTRODUCTION

ANATOMY OF THE CENTRAL NERVOUS SYSTEM

THE BRAIN
Brain Stem
Diencephalon
Cerebellum
Cerebrum

THE VENTRICLES

THE SPINAL CORD

THE MENINGES

CEREBROSPINAL FLUID
Formation and Flow
Regulation of Composition

DISEASES OF THE CENTRAL NERVOUS SYSTEM
Infectious Diseases
Noninfectious Diseases
Trends in Diagnosis

LABORATORY EVALUATION OF THE CEREBROSPINAL FLUID
Sample Collection
Analysis
　　Color and appearance
　　Cell count
　　Leukocyte differential
　　Gram stain and culture
　　Chemical analyses
　　Serologic examination
　　Other techniques

CHAPTER SUMMARY

REVIEW QUESTIONS

Objectives

1. Describe the major components of the central nervous system (CNS).
2. Identify the basic structural and functional units of the CNS.
3. Identify the major divisions of the brain and associate each with a basic function.
4. Describe the location of the brain, and the position of the major parts in relation to each other.
5. Describe the structure and function of the spinal cord and its position in relation to the brain.
6. Discuss the formation of cerebrospinal fluid (CSF), including its site of formation, its flow within the CNS, and its function.
7. Describe the basic biochemical and cellular composition of normal CSF.
8. Compare and contrast the function of the blood-brain barrier and the CSF-blood barrier.
9. List the common pathologic processes associated with the CNS.
10. Describe laboratory tests commonly performed on CSF and their diagnostic significance.

KEY TERMS

central nervous system	astrocytes	cerebral cortex	CSF-brain barrier
peripheral nervous system	ependymal cells	spinal cord	meningitis
neuron	choroid plexus	meninges	neurosyphilis
synapse	oligodendrocytes	dura mater	encephalitis
neurotransmitter	microglia	arachnoid mater	myelitis
cholinesterase	reticular formation	pia mater	encephalomyelitis
neuroglial cells	pineal body	subarachnoid space	multiple sclerosis
	cerebrum	blood-brain barrier	traumatic tap

Introduction

The central nervous system (CNS) can be compared to the CPU (central processing unit) of a computer. This is the organ system where information is received, processed, and acted upon. The CNS is composed of two major components, the brain and the spinal cord. The brain is the primary site of information processing, while the spinal cord serves in the role of a major communication trunk line.

The primary function of the **CNS** *is to coordinate and control various activities of the body.* This is known as the *integrative function* of the nervous system. Although the endocrine system assists in this task, the nervous system provides a much more rapid and precise response to the needs of normal body function. *This integrative function involves the receiving and processing of sensory input from various parts of the body through the* **peripheral nervous system** *and the processing of the information to produce a sensation or impression.* The short-term result is the addition of that sensation or impression to a memory bank. The ultimate result is the creation of either a conscious or a subconscious decision for an appropriate action or reaction.

When functioning properly, the CNS commands numerous bodily functions that are carried out without conscious effort—memories are stored, and motor control of the limbs and sensory organs allows us to perform everyday tasks. The number and variety of tasks and reactions that are simultaneously handled by the CNS would put the most sophisticated computer to shame. However, when the CNS is invaded by an infectious agent, traumatized, or rendered dysfunctional by organic disease or an inherited disorder, the ability of the body to function and react appropriately is significantly altered. Relatively minor damage to certain areas of the CNS may lead to coma and death.

ANATOMY OF THE CENTRAL NERVOUS SYSTEM

The **neuron,** *or nerve cell, is the basic functional and structural unit of the brain and the other components of the nervous system* (Fig. 10–1). The neuron is composed of a cell body with a nucleus, ribosomes, and the genetic information required for the synthesis of proteins. The neuron also possesses branching cytoplasmic extensions called *dendrites,* and a single long extension from the cell body called an *axon.* The axon branches at the end to form the structure referred to as the *axon terminal* or *terminus,* which culminates in rounded synaptic knobs. Axon terminals, or synaptic knobs, are the sites of release of the biochemicals that transfer messages along the neural pathways from neuron to neuron. Axons may vary in length and may also have branches referred to as *collateral axons.* While axons transfer information or stimuli from the neuron, the dendrites and cell body of the neurons provide receptor sites for the biochemicals released by the axons.

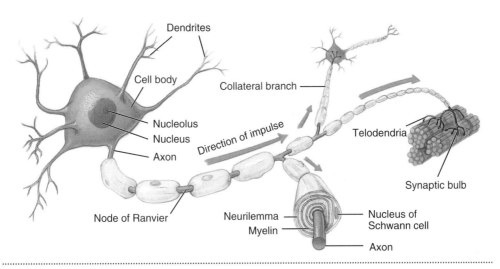

FIGURE 10-1

Schematic diagram of a neuron.
(From Applegate, E.J.: The Anatomy and Physiology Learning System. Philadelphia, W.B. Saunders, 1995, with permission.)

The space between the neurons that forms the juncture point for communication is called the **synapse**. Impulses can travel in both directions along the neuron (i.e., from the dendrite to the cell body to the axon terminal or in the opposite direction). In order for neurons to communicate with each other, biochemicals called *neurotransmitters* are required. **Neurotransmitters** *carry the impulse to the dendrite of the next neuron.* One of the best examples of a neurotransmitter is *acetylcholine*. In order to inhibit continuous stimulation of the neurons, most neurotransmitters are broken down by specific enzymes or inhibitors present in the synapse. *Cholinesterase, for example, is the enzyme that breaks down acetylcholine.*

Other types of cells are also found in the CNS and provide a number of important functions, such as metabolic support for the neurons, protection of the CNS from infection, production of myelin, and provision of structural support to the nervous tissue. *Collectively, these different types of cells are referred to as* **neuroglial cells**. There are four types of neuroglial cells:

- **Astrocytes**, *star-shaped cells commonly found between neurons and blood vessels, make up the major supporting tissue of the CNS and play a major role in the maintenance of the blood-brain barrier.*

- **Ependymal cells** *are epithelial cells that provide a membrane that covers some portions of the brain, such as the* **choroid plexus**, *and line the ventricles and spinal cord.* These cells play a role in the production of the cerebrospinal fluid (CSF) and in moving the CSF through the CNS.

- **Oligodendrocytes** *are cells that produce myelin sheaths, a lipid- and protein-containing protective wrapping, around the axons.*

■ **Microglia** *are specialized cells capable of phagocytizing bacteria and cellular debris.* These cells are scattered throughout the CNS and protect the CNS from infection.

THE BRAIN

The brain is located within the cranial vault (skull). It is one of the larger organs of the body and weighs approximately 1,400 g. The brain is composed of approximately 100 billion neurons and innumerable nerve fibers. The brain is divided into four major regions: (1) the brain stem, (2) the diencephalon, (3) the cerebrum, and (4) the cerebellum (Fig. 10–2).

BRAIN STEM

The brain stem is situated below the cerebrum (i.e., the uppermost and largest part of the brain) and diencephalon and in front of the cerebellum. It connects the cerebrum to the spinal cord. Damage to even a small area of the brain stem may lead to coma or death.

The brain stem is composed of the medulla oblongata, pons, midbrain, and reticular formation. Each of the areas of the brain stem, with the exception of the reticular formation, possesses ascending and descending neural pathways. These pathways are the neural fibers that carry impulses to and from the brain, via the spinal cord. Each of the areas also possesses unique structures that help to regulate or control various functions or bodily processes.

In addition to maintaining communication between the various parts of the body and the brain, the *medulla oblongata* is responsible for breathing, regulation of heart rate, vasoconstriction and vasodilation of blood vessels, coughing, sneezing, and swallowing. The *pons* possesses special *nuclei*, groups of neuronal cell bodies, that allow communication between the cerebrum and the cerebellum. The *midbrain* possesses *gray matter* (unmyelinated neurons), which is involved in visual and auditory functions and reflexes.

The **reticular formation,** *the most important area of the brain stem, is composed of a network of scattered neuronal cell bodies intermingled with bundles of gray matter.* This neuronal network interconnects various portions of the brain with the ascending and descending neural pathways. The reticular formation stimulates brain activity as sensory input is received. This is the portion of the brain upon which general anesthetics act to induce sleep. If the reticular formation is damaged, coma will usually result.

DIENCEPHALON

Located between the cerebral hemispheres and above the midbrain, the diencephalon is composed of the thalamus, hypothalamus, and pineal gland.

The *thalamus* consists of a cluster of nuclei and is the juncture point for the relay of sensory impulses to the cerebral cortex. The thalamus can register and produce a general awareness of pain or discomfort, although it cannot pinpoint the source.

The *hypothalamus* is connected via nerve fibers to the brain stem, thalamus, cerebral

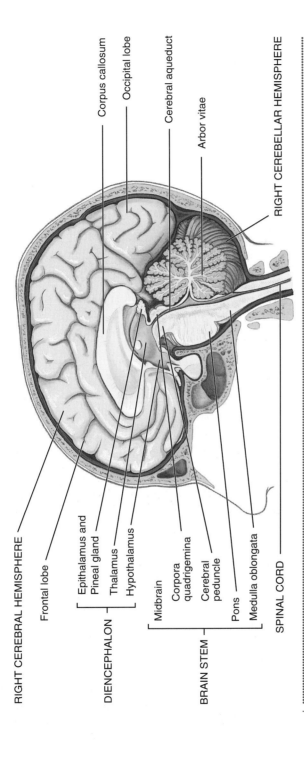

Corpus callosum

Occipital lobe

Cerebral aqueduct

Arbor vitae

RIGHT CEREBELLAR HEMISPHERE

RIGHT CEREBRAL HEMISPHERE

Frontal lobe

DIENCEPHALON — Epithalamus and Pineal gland

Thalamus

Hypothalamus

Midbrain

Corpora quadrigemina

Cerebral peduncle

BRAIN STEM — Pons

Medulla oblongata

SPINAL CORD

FIGURE 10-2

Major regions of the brain.
(From Applegate, E.J.: The Anatomy and Physiology Learning System. Philadelphia, W.B. Saunders, 1995, with permission.)

cortex, and pituitary gland. The hypothalamus is involved in a number of essential functions:

- Control of body temperature
- Regulation of water and electrolyte balance
- Control of hunger and thirst
- Regulation of heart rate and arterial blood pressure
- Generation of emotional responses, such as fear and anger
- Regulation of the pituitary gland

The **pineal body** is an endocrine gland that regulates melatonin and serotonin production. Its function is described more fully in Chapter 12.

CEREBELLUM

"Cerebellum" literally means "little brain." The cerebellum is located in the lower back portion of the cranial cavity beneath the occipital lobe of the cerebrum and posterior to the brain stem. It is composed of a thin layer of gray matter surrounding a larger area of *white matter*, or myelinated neurons. The primary function of the cerebellum is to compare incoming impulses with the impulse sent out from the brain and to make necessary corrections if a discrepancy is recognized. This part of the brain also plays a major role in the learning of motor skills, such as playing a musical instrument. The loss of balance or equilibrium and inaccurate movements observed in individuals consuming alcoholic beverages are prime examples of cerebelluar dysfunction, since the cerebellum is the portion of the brain that is most affected by alcohol.

CEREBRUM

The **cerebrum** *is the largest and uppermost portion of the brain.* It is divided into right and left hemispheres that are connected by a bridge of nerve fibers and separated by a membrane, the *dura mater. The cerebral hemispheres are composed of an outer layer of gray matter, the* **cerebral cortex,** *and the nerve fibers (white matter) that carry information to and from the cerebrum and interconnecting neurons.* One of the conspicuous features of the cerebrum is its numerous convolutions or folds, which increase the surface area of the cerebral cortex.

Each hemisphere is divided into lobes (Fig. 10–3), which are named for the bones of the skull under which they lie. The lobes include the following:

- The *frontal lobe*, which serves the primary motor area.
- The *parietal lobe*, located posterior to the frontal lobe, which functions as the primary area for receiving and interpreting sensory information such as touch. It is also a vital area for using and interpreting language.

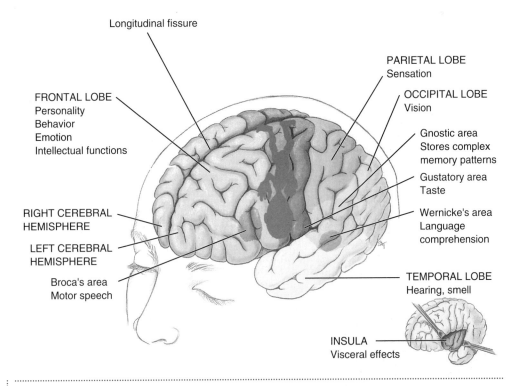

FIGURE 10-3

Lobes of a brain hemisphere.
(From Applegate, E.J.: The Anatomy and Physiology Learning System. Philadelphia, W.B. Saunders, 1995, with permission.)

■ The *temporal lobe*, which lies below the frontal lobe and is involved in interpretation of auditory (hearing) and olfactory (smell) input and in the storage of information (memory).

■ The *occipital lobe*, which is posterior to the parietal and temporal lobes and superior to the cerebellum. This area of the brain is involved in recognition and interpretation of visual images or stimuli.

THE VENTRICLES

Although not necessarily considered a part of the brain itself, the ventricles are located within the brain. These four interconnected cavities are the main sites of production of CSF. The lateral (first and second) ventricles extend into the cerebral hemispheres. The third ventricle is located in the center of the diencephalon, and the fourth ventricle is located in the brain stem at the base of the cerebellum. The fourth ventricle provides the opening to the central canal of the spinal cord and the subarachnoid space surrounding the brain, for distribution of CSF around the brain and spinal cord.

THE SPINAL CORD

The **spinal cord** *is a slender column of nerve tissue that extends from the base of the brain downward to approximately the second lumbar vertebra.* This places the end of the spinal cord approximately midway in what is commonly referred to as the "small of the back." The spinal cord is surrounded and protected by the vertebral column and is the junction for all nerves within the body.

The spinal cord is composed of 31 segments, each of which gives rise to a pair of spinal nerves. These nerves branch out to connect various parts and organs of the body to the CNS. The spinal cord might be compared to a major telephone trunk line, carrying signals from major stations out to individual telephones and similarly transmitting signals from the various parts of the body back to the brain for processing.

The spinal cord itself comprises a central area of gray matter (unmyelinated neurons) that resembles a butterfly with extended wings. This portion of the spinal cord is divided into three functional areas: the posterior horn, which contains sensory neurons; the anterior horn, which contains motor neurons; and the lateral horn (found in the thoracic and upper lumbar region), which contains the sympathetic autonomic neurons. The sympathetic autonomic neurons are those that are involved in preparing the body for some type of action or energy expansion.

The gray matter of the spinal cord is surrounded by white matter (myelinated nerve tissue). The white matter is divided into the ascending and descending nerve tracts. The ascending nerve tracts are composed of bundles of axons that carry impulses and sensory information from the parts of the body to the brain, while the descending tract transmits motor impulses from the brain to the muscles and glands.

THE MENINGES

The CNS is protected not only by the bones of the skull and vertebrae but also by a tough outer covering, the **meninges**. The meninges lies between the bones and the soft neural tissues.

The meninges consists of three layers of connective tissue—the dura mater, the arachnoid mater, and the pia mater (Fig. 10–4). *The* **dura mater** *is the outermost layer of the meninges and is attached to the inside of the skull.* It is very thick and fibrous and contains numerous blood vessels and nerves. The folds of the dura mater also extend down between the cerebral hemispheres and between the cerebrum and the cerebellum to help support and protect the special areas of the brain.

Although the dura mater extends down into the vertebral canal, it is not attached to the vertebrae. Instead, it is separated by the *epidural space.* This space is composed of loose connective and fat tissue that forms padding for the spinal cord.

The middle layer of the meninges is the **arachnoid mater,** *so named because it is a thin, spider-like covering.* It covers both the brain and spinal cord. *The innermost layer is the* **pia mater**, *which is actually attached to the surface of the brain and spinal cord.* It is a very thin layer and consists of nerves and blood vessels that help supply nutrients to the underlying nervous tissue.

Between the arachnoid and pia mater is a space called the **subarachnoid space**. This is a very vascular area that contains the *CSF.*

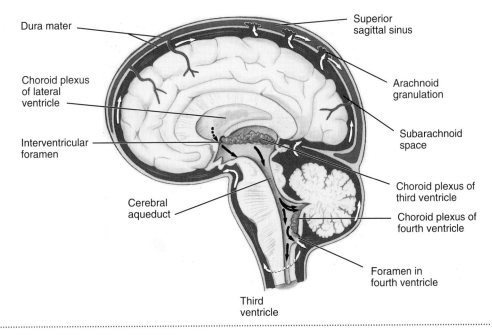

Dura mater

Superior sagittal sinus

Choroid plexus of lateral ventricle

Arachnoid granulation

Interventricular foramen

Subarachnoid space

Cerebral aqueduct

Choroid plexus of third ventricle

Choroid plexus of fourth ventricle

Foramen in fourth ventricle

Third ventricle

FIGURE 10-4

The meninges.
(From Applegate, E.J.: The Anatomy and Physiology Learning System. Philadelphia, W.B. Saunders, 1995, with permission.)

CEREBROSPINAL FLUID

FORMATION AND FLOW

The choroid plexuses, which are specialized capillary structures in the pia mater and in all the ventricles, produce CSF. Normal CSF is clear and colorless. Approximately 20 ml are produced each hour. Most adults have a total volume of 90 to 150 ml, while neonates have approximately 10 to 60 ml. The CSF represents a specialized filtrate of the plasma. It is formed through a combination of filtration of plasma and active secretion or transport of molecules across the blood-brain barrier. Although some constituents of normal CSF reflect their plasma concentrations, many are regulated by a selective process. Under normal conditions, when the CSF is formed it will contain less glucose, urea, and bicarbonate than plasma but have higher concentrations of sodium, magnesium, and chloride. Very little protein is found in normal CSF.

The CSF flows through the ventricles, into the subarachnoid space covering the brain and spinal cord, and through the central canal of the spinal cord. Most of the CSF ultimately flows to the uppermost part of the brain, where it is reabsorbed into the bloodstream through one-way valves in the larger veins in this area.

REGULATION OF COMPOSITION

Two major components of the CNS—the blood-brain barrier and the CSF-brain barrier—regulate the composition of the CSF. *The **blood-brain barrier** is composed of blood capillaries, whose endothelial cells are joined by tight junctions, and astrocytes, which almost completely surround the blood capillaries.* As a result, certain substances in the blood, such as lipid-soluble substances (i.e., heroin and alcohol) are able to move into the CSF rather easily by crossing the phospholipid membranes of the blood-brain barrier. Conversely, larger molecules, such as proteins, certain drugs, and most highly water-soluble substances, are restricted.

The **CSF-brain barrier** *is a manifestation of the special ependymal cells that line the choroid plexus.* These cells are also linked together by tight junctions, providing a barrier to many substances found in the capillaries. Water moves through this barrier by osmosis. Oxygen and carbon dioxide move across by diffusion. The movement of sodium and potassium, however, is actively regulated. Most large molecules, such as proteins and many antibiotics, are restricted from the brain by this barrier. Certain substances are actively (i.e., requiring ATP) secreted. The pH of the CSF is regulated by the generation of bicarbonate from carbon dioxide in the blood of the choroid plexus.

Several areas of the brain lack the CSF-brain barrier. An area in the fourth ventricle contains special receptors for carbon dioxide (influences respiration). In the third ventricle, neurons of the hypothalamus monitor CSF glucose levels (influences hunger and eating).

DISEASES OF THE CENTRAL NERVOUS SYSTEM

Various diseases may affect the CNS. Although some of these are not inherent to the CNS, they produce noticeable changes or alterations in the CSF, and all may produce neurologic signs and symptoms. Analysis of the CSF may be diagnostically significant in many of these disorders. It is of interest that the most common disease process associated with both alterations in the CSF and associated symptomatology are infections of the CNS. Examination of the CSF is requested by the physician for the primary purpose of detecting an infectious disease process.

INFECTIOUS DISEASES

Infectious diseases in the CNS usually occur as a result of invasion by a microorganism that crosses the blood-brain barrier, or as a direct insult to the CNS via skull fracture or trauma. Organisms found to invade the CNS are shown in Table 10–1.

Although symptoms of an infection may be quite profound, it is sometimes difficult to detect the organism present in the CSF by routine methods such as Gram stain and culture. Factors that contribute to the failure to detect the organisms include the small numbers of organisms necessary to cause pronounced symptoms, the small amount of fluid often submitted for analysis, and the inherent lack of sensitivity of the procedures mentioned. However, invasion of the CNS by microorganisms often produces chemical and hematologic changes in the CSF that are helpful in diagnosing the infection. Table 10–2 lists some of the chemical and hematologic changes associated with various infectious agents. In ad-

Table 10–1 ■ Organisms Associated with CNS Infection

Type of Organism	Name(s) of Organisms
Bacteria	*Haemophilus influenzae*
	Neisseria meningitidis
	Streptococcus pneumoniae
Fungi	*Cryptococcus neoformans*
	Candida albicans
Mycobacteria	*Mycobacterium tuberculosis*
Amebae	*Naegleria* species
	Acanthamoeba species
Viruses	Herpes simplex
	Epstein-Barr
Spirochetes	*Treponema pallidum*

dition, new methodologies for diagnosis of certain types of microorganisms are proving useful. One of the best examples of this is *polymerase chain reaction (PCR)* testing. Research using this technique has shown promise in identification of some organisms that have been particularly difficult to elucidate by more routine methods, such as mycobacteria and herpes simplex.

Infections are typically classified by the portion of the CNS affected by the organism. **Meningitis,** *or inflammation of the meninges, is usually caused by infection with bacteria or viruses.* Typical symptoms include headache (*cephalgia*), fever, and stiff neck (*nuchal rigidity*). The patient may also display *photophobia* (sensitivity to light), delirium, and contracted pupils. If the infection is severe, coma and death may result.

The CSF from *pyogenic* (pus-producing) bacterial meningitis will typically be cloudy and have increased numbers of neutrophils (Color Figure 24), markedly increased protein, and a decreased glucose level. Viral meningitis may present in much the same manner as bacterial meningitis, but the progression of the disease is less severe, and the CSF will contain increased numbers of lymphocytes and have a moderately elevated protein and usually a normal glucose level.

Neurosyphilis *is a progressive disorder resulting from infection of the CNS by Treponema pallidum.* The result of the infection is sometimes referred to as *tabes dorsalis.* The word "tabes" refers to a progressive wasting and, when combined with "dorsalis," indicates the sclerosis of the end of the spinal cord often associated with neurosyphilis. Symptoms of this disorder include loss of ability to coordinate muscle activities such as those involved in walking, some loss of sensation, and paralysis.

Encephalitis *is the result of infection of the nerve tissue of the brain.* It is usually caused by a viral infection, but may also result from infection with another type of infectious agent, as well as toxic substances. Patients display a variety of symptoms, including vomiting,

Table 10—2 ■ Chemical and Hematologic Findings Associated with Specific CNS Disorders

Disorder	*Chemical Findings**	*Hematologic Findings*
Bacterial meningitis	Glucose: ↓ Protein: ↑↑ Lactate: ↑	Increased neutrophils Increased cell count
Amebic meningoencephalitis	Glucose: ↓ or nor. Protein: ↑	Increased neutrophils Increased cell count
Viral meningitis or encephalitis	Glucose: nor. Protein: ↑ or nor. Lactate: nor.	Begins with increased neutrophils and converts to increased lymphocytes Increased cell count
Mycobacterial meningitis	Glucose: ↓ Protein: ↑ Lactate: ↑	May see increased lymphocytes and neutrophils Increased cell count
Neurosyphilis	Glucose: nor. Protein: var.; VDRL needed for confirmation	Usually increased lymphocytes with normal cell count
Fungal meningitis	Glucose: ↓ or nor. Protein: ↑ Lactate: ↑	Increased lymphocytes Increased cell count
Brain tumor	Glucose: nor. Protein: ↑	Normal cell count Typically increased lymphocytes May find tumor cells

* Key: ↓, decreased; ↑, increased; ↑↑, greatly increased; nor., normal range; var., variable

changes in levels of consciousness, increased blood pressure, seizures, nuchal rigidity, and decreased pulse. As with meningitis, encephalitis may culminate in coma or death.

Myelitis *is infection of the spinal cord, and* **encephalomyelitis** *is infection of both the brain and the spinal cord.* The organisms described previously may be implicated, and the symptoms are very similar.

Multiple sclerosis *(MS) is classified as a demyelinating disorder. The cause of MS is unknown, but it is believed to be of viral origin.* There is inflammation and an apparent immune response involved in the demyelination. Lesions that result in the area of demyelination contain myelin basic protein (MBP), proteolytic enzymes, macrophages, lymphocytes, and plasma cells. Manifestations of MS depend on the location of the lesions and the duration of the process. Typically, at some point in the progression of the disease, the patient will experience muscle weakness (*myasthenia*), poor muscle coordination (*ataxia*), speech impairment, and difficulties with vision.

The CSF may not reveal any particular diagnostic information in cases of MS. The findings are often similar to those seen with aseptic meningitis. However, CSF electrophoresis often reveals increased G class immunoglobulins (IgG). In addition, myelin basic protein (MBP) is elevated in most cases of MS; however, elevated MBP levels have also been found in other disorders.

NONINFECTIOUS DISEASES

Although often diagnosed by radiographic methods, *brain tumors* also often present diagnostic signs within the CSF. Although the spinal fluid is usually clear and colorless, xanthochromia (i.e., yellow or orange color) may occur with some types of tumors. In addition, protein levels and cell counts are often increased. CSF pressure is often elevated, and in some cases malignant cells will be found in the spinal fluid.

Hemorrhage within the CNS may show varying results on CSF analysis, depending on the size and location of the hemorrhage and how long it has been since the hemorrhage has occurred. Subarachnoid hemorrhage, when it occurs, must be distinguished from a *traumatic tap*. A **traumatic tap** *is a lumbar puncture in which capillaries or other vessels are punctured as the collecting needle is inserted into the subarachnoid space*. As a result of a traumatic tap, blood may be seen in the spinal fluid and confused with a hemorrhage within the CNS. There are two ways in which to differentiate a traumatic tap from subarachnoid hemorrhage. First, in a traumatic tap there is a decreasing amount of blood in subsequently collected tubes. Tube 1 will have more blood than tube 2, which will have more blood than tube 3. Conversely, in subarachnoid hemorrhage, the amount of blood in all tubes would be the same. Second, when the tubes are centrifuged, the supernatant will be generally clear in a traumatic tap, while it will appear *xanthochromic* (yellow or orange) in the case of subarachnoid hemorrhage. It is also not unusual to find *erythrophagia* (i.e., phagocytosis of erythrocytes by macrophages) upon microscopic examination of the spinal fluid from a patient with subarachnoid hemorrhage.

TRENDS IN DIAGNOSIS

Although many other disorders affect the CNS, those mentioned previously are examples of disorders or diseases in which the laboratory may play a major role in diagnosis. Newer radiologic methods, such as computed tomography (CT) and magnetic resonance imaging (MRI) have made it possible to diagnose many CNS disorders without performing such an invasive and potentially dangerous procedure as the lumbar puncture. It must be pointed out, however, that these new procedures are primarily utilized to identify lesions or abnormalities within the nerve tissues, such as tumors and hemorrhages.

New methodologies are continuously being developed to make laboratory diagnosis of infectious agents more specific, sensitive, and time efficient. For examples, latex agglutination tests for specific bacterial antigens are used as adjuncts for the Gram stain and culture of infectious agents.

LABORATORY EVALUATION OF THE CEREBROSPINAL FLUID

Examination of the CSF can provide important diagnostic information when there is reason to suspect there has been trauma or a nontraumatic insult to the CNS. Examples of disease processes or disorders that can be evaluated by examination of the spinal fluid include intracranial hemorrhage, infections, certain types of malignancies, demyelinating disorders such as multiple sclerosis, Guillain-Barré syndrome, and neurosyphilis. Many physicians rely on the laboratory evaluation of spinal fluid to diagnose the more commonly occurring disorders involving the CNS.

SAMPLE COLLECTION

Cerebrospinal fluid is collected by the physician using a procedure called the *lumbar puncture* (*spinal tap*). Depending on the age of the patient, the puncture is made between the third and fourth, or fourth and fifth, lumbar vertebrae. These vertebrae, located in the lower back, are just below the end or terminus of the spinal cord. This permits withdrawal of the fluid from the subarachnoid space while minimizing potential damage to the spinal cord.

There are a number of indications and contraindications for performing the spinal tap. The physician carefully evaluates the patient's history and condition and weighs the potential benefit against the potential damage that may result from collection of the spinal fluid. One of the primary contraindications for lumbar puncture is infection at the site of the puncture. Potential complications of lumbar puncture include headache, bleeding, and herniation that may result in paralysis or death of the patient.

Specimens are collected using sterile technique. After the needle is inserted into the subarachnoid space and before collection of the sample, the intracranial pressure is measured by connecting a sterile graduated manometer tube to the needle. Opening pressure should be between 90 and 180 mm of CSF. If the pressure is normal, up to 20 ml of fluid can be collected. If the opening pressure is greater than 200 mm of CSF, it is recommended that no more than 1 to 2 ml of fluid be removed. The normal closing pressure, after removal of 10 to 20 ml of CSF, should be approximately 45 to 90 mm. After the fluid has been collected and before the needle is removed, the closing pressure and amount of fluid withdrawn should be recorded.

The spinal fluid is collected into three or four successively numbered, sterile, screw-capped tubes. The first portion of the sample withdrawn is place in the tube labeled 1, the next portion of the sample in tube 2, and the last portion of the sample in tube 3. Each tube must be properly labeled and transported to the laboratory immediately.

Because the cellular components of spinal fluid break down rather quickly, and because of the circumstances that generally lead to the performance of a lumbar puncture, the cerebrospinal fluid examination is performed immediately. Each tube is sent to the appropriate area of the laboratory for testing. Tube 1 is most likely to be contaminated with bacteria from the surface of the skin and cells from the puncture; therefore, it is sent to chemistry for biochemical analysis, such as determination of glucose and protein levels. Tube 2 is least likely to be contaminated by bacteria and is sent to the microbiology area for culture and Gram stain. Tube 3 is sent to the hematology area for the cell count and differential because it is least likely to contain cells from trauma of puncture.

ANALYSIS

Like other body fluids, the CSF provides a sample for analysis that often reveals biochemical and cellular changes reflective of disease processes. Although obtaining the sample is considered to be a traumatic and invasive procedure, analysis of the cerebrospinal fluid often provides the clues or evidence needed by the physician to initiate appropriate treatment.

Although many tests can be performed on spinal fluid, there are several that are considered to be routine and are almost always requested (Table 10–3). Other test procedures are available and may be requested as needed for verification of diagnosis.

Color and Appearance

Normal CSF should be clear and colorless. Any coloration or cloudiness of the CSF is considered abnormal. Colors observed include white or pearlescent, red, pink, orange, and yellow. Red or pink indicates the presence of blood, while yellow or orange (xanthochromia) indicates the breakdown products of hemoglobin. CSF that appears white or pearlescent generally has increased numbers of leukocytes, lipids, or proteins. Hazy, cloudy, or turbid CSF may be due to increased numbers of blood cells, proteins, lipids, or bacteria.

Cell Count

Both leukocyte and erythrocyte counts are performed on the cerebrospinal fluid. Normal spinal fluid will usually contain fewer than five to eight leukocytes per cubic millimeter and fewer than one erythrocyte per cubic millimeter (these ranges vary from lab to lab). Increased numbers of leukocytes typically indicate an infectious process, while increased numbers of erythrocytes may indicate a hemorrhage or a traumatic lumbar puncture (see previous discussion on hemorrhage for differentiation).

Table 10–3 ■ **Commonly Requested Tests on CSF**

Color

Appearance

Cell count

Differential cell count

Gram's stain

Culture

Glucose determination

Protein level

Leukocyte Differential

When the leukocyte count is elevated, the leukocyte types are identified and counted by type. This procedure is referred to as the leukocyte or white cell differential. Most labs perform the differential while performing the cell count on the hemacytometer, differentiating only the polynuclear and mononuclear cells. A cytocentrifuged Wright-stained smear, however, provides more accurate results, especially when the cell count is increased. Under normal conditions, most of the leukocytes observed will be mononuclear. Most patients with bacterial infections will demonstrate increased numbers of neutrophils, while those with fungal, tubercular, and viral infections will have increased numbers of lymphocytes.

The differential may also reveal other cell types that may be of interest in diagnosing certain conditions. For example, the appearance of malignant cells in the cerebrospinal fluid may indicate the presence of a tumor within in the CNS or metastatic carcinoma. Plasma cells may be observed in several different disorders, including multiple sclerosis and tuberculous meningitis. The presence of macrophages often indicates hemorrhage, but may also be associated with certain types of infection. Cells associated with the CNS itself, such as ependymal cells, may also be found and associated with specific disorders or diagnostic procedures. Of course, it must also be remembered that any of the cells found in the peripheral blood may be found in the cerebrospinal fluid, and, because their presence is not considered normal, certain conclusions can be drawn about the type of disorder present.

Gram Stain and Culture

A Gram's stain is performed on almost all cerebrospinal fluid samples (Color Figure 24). The presence of even one organism is considered significant since the CSF is normally sterile. The physician will often act on the basis of Gram's stain results when an organism is observed using this procedure.

Cultures are also set up in order to retrieve and identify organisms present in the CSF. Obviously, standard culture procedures will isolate only bacterial pathogens and perhaps some of the fungal organisms that may be present in the cerebrospinal fluid. If the physician suspects a viral, mycobacterial, or rickettsial organism, it is important that special culture techniques be followed for isolation of these organisms.

Chemical Analyses

Chemical analyses are important in helping to establish a diagnosis. Through the years, a number of chemical tests have been proposed and used for analysis of spinal fluid. The two most reliable and useful tests are the protein and glucose determinations.

The spinal fluid *protein* is typically about 1/100th the concentration of protein in the blood; therefore, methods used for analysis of protein in the blood cannot be used accurately with CSF. Special techniques must be employed for determining protein concentrations in cerebrospinal fluid. Elevated protein levels are considered to be an important finding. Increased CSF protein may be due to damage to the CSF-brain barrier resulting in an increased permeability, decreased removal of protein from the cerebrospinal fluid, obstruction to the circulation of the cerebrospinal fluid, increased synthesis of immunoglobulins by the lymphocytes and plasma cells in the CNS, or increase in numbers of leukocytes and erythrocytes. Decreased protein levels are less commonly encountered. Examples of situations in which one might encounter decreased protein levels are removal of large amounts of CSF and leakage of CSF caused by trauma (e.g., rhinorrhea or otorrhea).

Glucose concentrations can be determined using the same methodologies as used for blood. The glucose concentration of the spinal fluid is typically about 65 to 70% of the blood glucose concentration (70 to 110 mg/dl). Typically, the most common finding is a low glucose concentration associated with most types of CNS infections. In order to properly evaluate the CSF glucose concentration, however, a blood glucose level should also be performed. If a patient is hyperglycemic (high blood glucose level), then the CSF glucose concentrations will likewise be elevated and an infection may be masked. Conversely, if the patient is hypoglycemic (low blood glucose), the physician may be misled by a low CSF glucose.

Lactate determination is considered to be of some use by physicians in differentiating bacterial, tuberculous, and fungal meningitis from viral meningitis. The lactate concentration in viral meningitis is generally normal or low in comparison to that in bacterial, tuberculous, or fungal meningitis. Unfortunately, the results of the test must be carefully weighed since a number of other CNS disorders and imbalances can affect the lactate test.

Other chemical analyses include glutamine (an indicator of excess ammonia in the CNS), lactate dehydrogenase, chloride, and bilirubin. Each of these tests provides information of limited use to the physician, and it is questionable whether or not the results are reliable indicators of specific disease processes associated with the CNS.

Serologic Examination

Serologic examination of the cerebrospinal fluid is typically involved with diagnosis of neurosyphilis. The Venereal Disease Research Laboratory (VDRL) test is most often utilized for this purpose, although a fluorescent treponemal antibody absorption (FTA-ABS) test for CSF has also been developed.

Other Techniques

Before leaving this discussion of laboratory tests, it is important to recognize other techniques that have been used and may still be used for cerebrospinal fluid analysis. These include counterimmunoelectrophoresis (CIE), latex agglutination tests for bacterial antigens (e.g., *Streptococcus pneumoniae*), enzyme-linked immunosorbent assay (ELISA), and limulus amebocyte lysate (used for detection of gram-negative bacteria). The nucleic acid probes using PCR are the newest of the techniques being investigated for identification of specific infectious agents.

CHAPTER SUMMARY

The central nervous system is a complex and extremely important organ system within the human body. The brain, through its ancillary parts, including the sections of the brain, the spinal cord, and the nervous tissue that spreads throughout the body, regulates and promotes homeostasis. The CNS is the conduit of information and the processing system of that information using electrical and chemical pathways.

When the CNS becomes injured or diseased, body function is affected. Depending upon the degree of injury or disease, an individual may be rendered unconscious, lose motor or sensory skills, or in extreme situations die.

The role of the clinical laboratory is to help physicians assess and diagnose dysfunction of the CNS so that appropriate treatment can be initiated as quickly as possible. It is often the responsibility of the laboratory to find the diagnostic clues by performing hematologic, chemical, microbiologic, and serologic procedures.

Review Questions

1. Which of the types of cells in the CNS play a major role in protecting the CNS from infection?
   a. neurons
   b. ependymal cells
   c. microglia
   d. astrocytes

2. Gray matter is composed of
   a. myelinated neurons
   b. nuclei
   c. descending neural pathways
   d. unmyelinated neurons

3. Which of the following is *not* a part of the diencephalon?
   a. thalamus
   b. reticular formation
   c. hypothalamus
   d. pineal gland

4. Cerebrospinal fluid is formed primarily in the
   a. cerebellum
   b. pineal gland
   c. ventricles
   d. brain stem

5. The portion of the CNS that is responsible for transmitting messages back and forth between various parts of the body and the brain is the
   a. brain stem
   b. cerebellum
   c. meninges
   d. spinal cord

6. The correct order of the layers of the meninges from outside in toward the brain is
   a. arachnoid mater, dura mater, pia mater
   b. dura mater, pia mater, arachnoid mater
   c. arachnoid mater, pia mater, dura mater
   d. dura mater, arachnoid mater, pia mater

7. A cerebrospinal fluid sample is accepted in the laboratory. The patient is a 4-year-old female with fever and a stiff neck. The cerebrospinal fluid is cloudy. The leukocyte count is 338 μl/mm, with large numbers of neutrophils. Rare erythrocytes are noted. The protein is elevated and the glucose concentration is decreased. This laboratory picture is *most consistent* with
   a. viral infection
   b. bacterial infection
   c. normal results for this age group
   d. subarachnoid hemorrhage

8. A patient is brought to the emergency room after having fallen about 30 ft from a ladder. The patient is unconscious and having some difficulty breathing. A spinal tap is performed and the samples of cerebrospinal fluid sent to the lab. Blood is observed in all tubes and the erythrocyte counts are increasingly lower in each successive tube counted. When the tubes are centrifuged, the supernatant is essentially clear and colorless. The leukocyte count is slightly elevated, but all other parameters are normal. This is *most likely* due to
   a. traumatic tap
   b. subarachnoid hemorrhage
   c. erythrophagia
   d. tumor within the CSF

9. Xanthochromia in a centrifuged sample of CSF is a good indication of
   a. traumatic tap
   b. subarachnoid hemorrhage
   c. erythrophagia
   d. tumor within the CSF

10. Usually three tubes of CSF are collected for testing in the laboratory. The tubes, if collected in the proper order, should be distributed as follows
   a. tube 1—microbiology; tube 2—chemistry; tube 3—hematology
   b. tube 1—chemistry; tube 2—hematology; tube 3—microbiology
   c. tube 1—chemistry; tube 2—microbiology; tube 3—hematology
   d. tube 1—hematology; tube 2—chemistry; tube 3—microbiology

BIBLIOGRAPHY

Aslandzadeh, J., Osmon, D.R., Wilhelm, M.P., Espy, M.J., and Smith, T.F.: A prospective study of the polymerase chain reaction for detection of herpes simplex virus in cerebrospinal fluid submitted to the clinical virology laboratory. Mol. Cell. Probes 6:367, 1992.

Baron, E.J., Peterson, L.R., and Finegold, S.M.: Bailey & Scott's Diagnostic Microbiology, 9th ed. St. Louis, Mosby–Year Book, 1994.

Gray, L.D., and Fedorko, D.P.: Laboratory diagnosis of bacterial meningitis. Clin. Microbiol. Rev. *5*:130, 1992.

Henry, J.B.: Clinical Diagnosis and Management By Laboratory Methods, 18th ed. Philadelphia, W.B. Saunders, 1991.

Hole, J.W., Jr.: Essentials of Human Anatomy and Physiology, 4th ed. Dubuque, IA, Wm. C. Brown Publishers, 1992.

Lin, J.J., Harn, H.J., Hsu, Y.D., Tsau, W.L., Lee, H.S., and Lee, W.H.: Rapid diagnosis of tuberculous meningitis by polymerase chain reaction assay of cerebrospinal fluid. J. Neurol. *242*:147, 1995.

Linné, J.J., and Ringsrud, K.M.: Basic Techniques in Clinical Laboratory Science, 3rd ed. St. Louis, C.V. Mosby, 1992.

Porth, C.M.: Pathophysiology: Concepts of Altered Health States, 4th ed. Philadelphia, J.B. Lippincott, 1994.

Ravel, R.: Clinical Laboratory Medicine: Clinical Application of Laboratory Data, 6th ed. St. Louis, C.V. Mosby, 1995.

Ringsrud, K.M., and Linné, J.J.: Urinalysis and Body Fluids: A Color Text and Atlas. St. Louis, Mosby–Year Book, 1991.

Seely, R.R., Stephens, T.D., and Tate, P.: Essentials of Anatomy and Physiology. St. Louis, Mosby–Year Book, 1991.

Strasinger, S.K.: Urinalysis and Body Fluids, 3rd ed. Philadelphia, F.A. Davis, 1994.

Vander, A.J., Sherman, J.H., and Luciano, D.S.: Human Physiology: The Mechanisms of Body Function. New York, McGraw-Hill, 1994.

Watson, M.A., and Scott, M.G.: Clinical utility of biochemical analysis of cerebrospinal fluid. Clin. Chem. *41*:343, 1995.

CHAPTER 11

The Hematopoietic and Lymphatic Systems

INTRODUCTION

HEMATOPOIETIC SYSTEM
Blood
    Composition
    Function
Bone Marrow
Blood Cells
    Erythrocytes
    Leukocytes
    Platelets

LYMPHATIC SYSTEM
Lymph
Lymph Nodes
Thymus
Spleen

PATHOLOGIC CONDITIONS
Anemia
    Iron-deficiency anemia
    Sickle cell anemia
Leukocytosis
    Neutrophilia
    Lymphocytosis

Leukemia
    Acute leukemia
    Chronic leukemia
Hemophilia

LABORATORY EVALUATION
Hematology Procedures
    Hemoglobin
    Hematocrit
    Erythrocyte count
    Leukocyte count
    Platelet count
    Peripheral blood smear
        examination
    Bone marrow examination
Coagulation Procedures
    Bleeding time
    Prothrombin time
    Activated partial
        thromboplastin time
    Factor assays

CHAPTER SUMMARY

REVIEW QUESTIONS

Objectives

1. Identify the primary components of blood.
2. Discuss the principal functions of blood and lymph.
3. Explain hematopoiesis.
4. Identify the cellular components of blood.
5. Describe the function of each blood cell.
6. Discuss the function of the lymph nodes, spleen, and thymus.
7. Identify the principal abnormality associated with anemia, leukemia, and hemophilia.
8. Identify the laboratory tests used in the evaluation of the hematopoietic and lymphatic systems.
9. Given clinical symptoms, laboratory data, or both, state the most likely hematopoietic abnormality.

KEY TERMS

blood	lymphocyte	sickle cell anemia	chronic leukemia
bone marrow	platelets	leukocytosis	hemophilia
erythrocyte	lymph	neutrophilia	hematocrit
neutrophil	lymph nodes	lymphocytosis	hemostasis
eosinophil	thymus	leukemia	hemoglobin
basophil	iron-deficiency	acute leukemia	prothrombin
monocyte	anemia		

Introduction

The hematopoietic and lymphatic systems are responsible for production of the blood cells of the body (e.g., erythrocytes, leukocytes, and platelets). The tissues of these systems provide the necessary environment for the differentiation of a common stem cell into specialized blood cells. In turn, the specialized blood cells are responsible for carrying out a variety of important functions, including the transport of oxygen and the defense from foreign substances (e.g., bacteria and viruses).

209

HEMATOPOIETIC SYSTEM

The primary purpose of the hematopoietic system is the production of the blood cells. Additionally, the hematopoietic system is composed of tissues and organs that are responsible for removing damaged or dying blood cells from the body. The following tissues and organs are included in the hematopoietic system: bone marrow, liver, spleen, thymus, lymph nodes, and the mononuclear phagocyte system.

BLOOD

Composition

Blood *is the fluid suspension that serves as the transport medium for the blood cells and a variety of chemical substances.* Blood circulates throughout the body via the circulatory system. Blood that circulates to the peripheral tissues and organs of the body provides nutrients to those tissues and helps maintain electrolyte balance throughout the body. Blood that circulates from the peripheral tissues to the excretory organs (e.g., kidney and lungs) provides a mechanism for the removal of harmful waste products that are formed by metabolic processes occurring at the peripheral tissues.

Blood is one of the largest tissues of the body. It makes up 8% of the body's weight. In the body of a normal adult man, there is approximately 6 liters of blood. Blood is composed of blood cells, chemical substances, and water. The amount of blood cells in whole blood is defined as the *packed cell volume* (PCV), or the percentage of blood cells in whole blood (Fig. 11–1). In normal individuals, the PCV is 45% and represents erythrocytes, leukocytes, and platelets. The remainder of the blood is composed primarily of water (90%). The chemical substances, which make up a relatively small portion of whole blood, include proteins (i.e., albumin, transferrin, and fibrinogen); glucose; lipids (i.e., cholesterol and triglycerides); hormones (i.e., cortisol, insulin, triiodothyronine, and thyroxine); and electrolytes (i.e., Na^+, K^+, Cl^- and HCO_3^-).

Function

The function of blood is related to its composition. The erythrocytes are responsible for the *transport of oxygen* to the tissues. Oxygen transport is accomplished by hemoglobin, the major erythrocyte protein. Each hemoglobin molecule is composed of four heme groups and four polypeptide chains (Fig. 11–2). The oxygen molecule is bound to an iron atom within a heme group. Within the alveoli of the lungs, oxygen is bound reversibly to the iron atoms. The alveoli represent areas of high oxygen concentration. Oxygen is released from the hemoglobin molecule at the peripheral tissues, which represent areas of low oxygen concentration. In this way, oxygen is transported to the metabolically active areas of the body.

Hemostasis is another function of the blood. Platelets and coagulation proteins within the blood are responsible for hemostasis. Platelets conduct a constant surveillance of the circulatory system, identifying small leaks or injury to the vessels. When platelets encounter injury, they adhere to the injured surface and activate other platelets in the area to form an initial platelet plug. The coagulation proteins circulate in an inert form, but become activated by substances released by the injured vessel. The activation of the coagulation proteins oc-

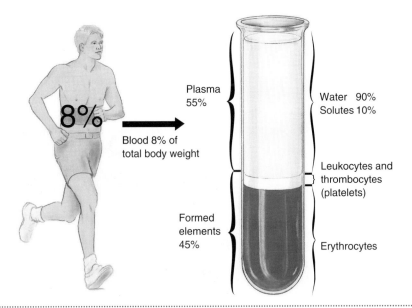

Plasma
55%

Blood 8% of
total body weight

Formed
elements
45%

Water 90%
Solutes 10%

Leukocytes and
thrombocytes
(platelets)

Erythrocytes

FIGURE 11-1

Composition of the blood.
(From Applegate, E.J.: The Anatomy and Physiology Learning System. Philadelphia, W.B. Saunders, 1995, with permission.)

curs in a cascade or waterfall manner (Fig. 11–3). The end result is the formation of fibrin. Fibrin creates a stable fibrin-platelet clot that prevents loss of excess amounts of blood and facilitates the repair of the injured vessel. This process is limited to the site of injury by regulatory proteins.

Leukocytes are responsible for the body's *defense against foreign substances* (i.e., bacteria, viruses, parasites, fungi, nonself tissue, or nonself blood cells). The defense process may be limited to the *phagocytosis* (killing and degradation) of the foreign substance by neutrophils, or it may involve the more complex interaction of monocytes and lymphocytes in the immune response. In either situation, the leukocytes use the blood and circulatory system as a rapid transport system.

Most leukocytes spend very little time in the circulatory system, leaving the system to enter the peripheral tissues and lymphoid organs in response to infections or inflammation within those tissues. Leukocytes leave the blood vessels and enter the tissues in response to chemical stimuli (e.g., complement and interleukin). The chemical stimuli, or *chemotaxins*, are substances that are released by other leukocytes already in the tissues, the invading organism, or the affected tissues. Monocytes and lymphocytes participate in the immune response. Monocytes are responsible for phagocytizing, processing, and presenting the foreign substance to the lymphocytes. In the humoral immune response, lymphocytes respond to the processed foreign substance and produce antibodies directed against it. The released antibodies will coat the substance and facilitate its removal from the body, thereby resolving the infection.

The transport function of the blood is vital to the body's well-being. As stated earlier, blood allows for the *transport of a variety of substances* throughout the body. Let's review a

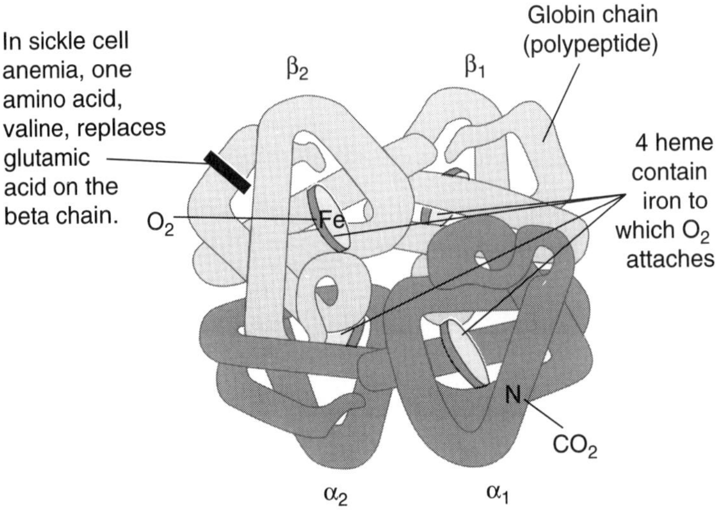

In sickle cell anemia, one amino acid, valine, replaces glutamic acid on the beta chain.

β_2 β_1

Globin chain (polypeptide)

4 heme contain iron to which O_2 attaches

O_2 Fe

N

CO_2

α_2 α_1

FIGURE 11-2

Structure of hemoglobin. Hemoglobin A, normal adult hemoglobin, is composed of two alpha (α) polypeptide chains, two beta (β) polypeptide chains, and four heme groups. Each heme group contains an iron atom.

(Modified from Gould, B.E.: Pathophysiology for the Health-Related Professions. Philadelphia, W.B. Saunders, 1997, with permission.)

few examples. Hormones (see Chapter 12) are transported from their site of synthesis to their target tissue via the blood. Nutrients from foodstuff are absorbed by the intestine into the blood and transported to their storage sites or utilization sites by the blood. For example, iron and vitamin B_{12} are absorbed by the intestine and are transported via the blood to their storage site (the liver) or to their utilization site (the bone marrow) for the production of blood cells. Glucose is transported via the blood to virtually all tissues of the body to provide an energy source for cellular functions. Lipids are absorbed from the intestine into the lymphatic vessels for transport to the venous circulation. Lipids that have entered the venous circulation are transported to their storage sites: the liver, adipose tissue, and other organs. In addition, metabolic waste products (e.g., carbon dioxide, sulfuric acid, and lactic acid) are transported from their source to the body's excretory organs for removal. For example, carbon dioxide is transported to the lungs for removal by exhalation.

Blood also helps *maintain the body's electrolyte balance* (pH 7.35 to 7.45). Overall, blood has a large buffering capacity due to the presence of hemoglobin, bicarbonate, phosphate, and plasma proteins. The erythrocyte plays an important role in removing acids from the peripheral tissues. The erythrocyte's hemoglobin serves as a carrier protein for hydrogen ions (H^+) or carbon dioxide and will transport them to the lungs for removal.

BONE MARROW

The bone marrow is located in the central "spongy" area of the trabecular bone. There are two types of marrow, red marrow and yellow marrow (Fig. 11-4). The red marrow represents hematopoietically active tissue and is composed of stem cells, committed progenitor cells, and developing hematopoietic cells (i.e., erythroblasts, myeloblasts, and megakaryoblasts). The yellow marrow is no longer capable of hematopoiesis and is composed primarily of adipocytes. The red marrow is infiltrated by an extensive capillary system and marrow sinuses. The marrow sinuses provide the means for mature hematopoietic cells to enter

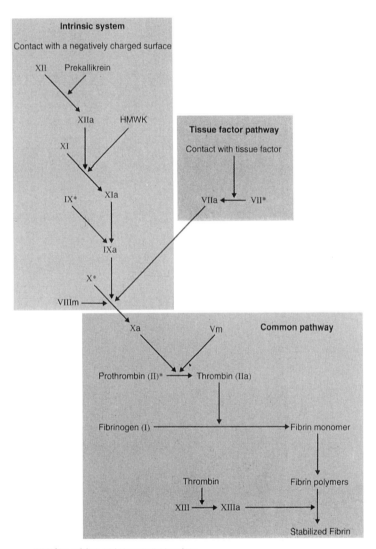

*requires calcium and phospholipid surface

FIGURE 11-3

The basic coagulation cascade. The coagulation cascade has three interacting pathways: intrinsic, extrinsic and common. The common pathway may be activated by either the intrinsic or extrinsic pathway.

(From Rodak, B.F.: Diagnostic Hematology. Philadelphia, W.B. Saunders, 1995, with permission.)

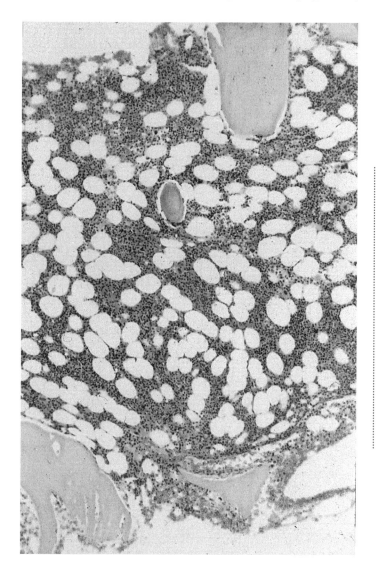

FIGURE 11-4
Fixed and stained bone
marrow tissue (hema-
toxylin and eosin, × 100).
The hematopoietic tissue
represents the red marrow,
while the adipose tissue
represents the yellow marrow. In the adult, the normal bone marrow displays
50% red marrow and 50%
yellow marrow.
(From Rodak, B.F.:
Diagnostic Hematology.
Philadelphia, W.B.
Saunders, 1995, with
permission).

the peripheral blood. In addition, the vascular system provides nutrients necessary for sustaining hematopoiesis.

The amount of red marrow varies during the course of one's life. In early childhood, red marrow comprises approximately 100% of the bone marrow tissue and is found in virtually every bone. By adulthood, the amount of red marrow has decreased and represents approximately 50% of the bone marrow tissue. The red marrow is confined to the flat bones of the skeleton (i.e., sternum, ribs, pelvis, and skull). At age 70, red marrow has decreased to approximately 30% of the bone marrow tissue.

Hematopoiesis requires a stem cell, a viable microenvironment, and hematopoietic growth factors. The *stem cell* is a self-perpetuating cell that is capable of differentiating along any of the hematopoietic cell lines (e.g., erythroid cell line, neutrophilic cell line). Reticular cells and macrophages help create and maintain the microenvironment. *Reticular cells* are responsible for creating the scaffolding or supporting network necessary for cell development. *Macrophages* play several roles in hematopoiesis. They provide the iron required for hemoglobin synthesis and they remove through phagocytosis the discarded erythrocyte nuclei and other debris, such as damaged or dying cells. Hematopoietic *growth factors* are responsible for triggering the stem cell to commit to one cell line or another (Table 11–1).

Hematopoiesis is divided into three compartments: the stem cell compartment, the progenitor cell compartment, and the morphologically identifiable cell compartment (Fig. 11–5). The *stem cell compartment* is composed of pluripotential stem cells, myeloid stem cells, and lymphoid stem cells. These cells are capable of self-renewal and may differentiate along several hematopoietic cell lines depending on the influence of hematopoietic growth factors and the microenvironment. The *progenitor cell compartment* is composed of cells that are committed to a hematopoietic cell line. Progenitor cells are named according to the hematopoietic cell line they are committed to (e.g., colony-forming unit–erythroid, or CFU-E, for the erythroid cell line). Progenitor cells will continue to differentiate into the morphologically identifiable hematopoietic cells. The *morphologically identifiable cell compartment* is composed of precursor cells developing along one specific cell line. These cells

Table 11–1 ■ Hematopoietic Growth Factors

Hematopoietic Cell Line	Hematopoietic Growth Factor	Growth Factor Class
Erythroid	Interleukin-3	Multilineage
	Granulocyte-monocyte colony-stimulating factor	Multilineage
	Erythropoietin	Lineage specific
Neutrophil	Interleukin-3	Multilineage
	Granulocyte-monocyte colony-stimulting factor	Multilineage
	Granulocyte colony-stimulating factor	Lineage specific
Monocyte	Interleukin-3	Multilineage
	Granulocyte-monocyte colony-stimulating factor	Multilineage
	Monocyte colony-stimulating factor	Lineage specific
Eosinophil	Interleukin-3	Multilineage
	Granulocyte-monocyte colony-stimulating factor	Multilineage
	Interleukin-5	Lineage specific
Basophil	Interleukin-3	Multilineage
	Granulocyte-monocyte colony-stimulating factor	Multilineage
Megakaryocyte	Interleukin-3	Multilineage
	Granulocyte-monocyte colony-stimulating factor	Multilineage
	Thrombopoietin	Lineage specific
Lymphoid	Interleukin-3	Multilineage

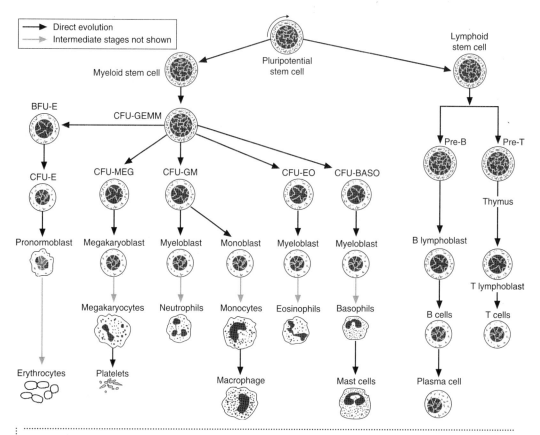

FIGURE 11-5

Hematopoiesis demonstrating the derivation of cells from the pluripotential stem cell. Note the three hematopoietic compartments: stem cell, progenitor cell, and morphologically identifiable cell. (Modified from Rodak, B.F.: Diagnostic Hematology. Philadelphia, W.B. Saunders, 1995, with permission.)

are readily identified on a Wright-stained bone marrow aspirate smear based on their morphologic features. These cells develop into the mature blood cells observed in the peripheral blood.

BLOOD CELLS

Erythrocytes

The mature erythrocyte is the most numerous peripheral blood cell. *The* **erythrocyte** *is an anuclear, biconcave-shaped cell that is approximately 7 microns (μ) in diameter* (see Color Figure 25). Its principle protein component is hemoglobin. Hemoglobin's main function is the transport of oxygen to the peripheral tissues. The biconcave shape of the erythrocyte provides a high surface area–to-volume ratio, which maximizes the oxygen-carrying capacity of the cell.

Leukocytes

There are five types of leukocytes: neutrophils, lymphocytes, monocytes, eosinophils, and basophils. Each leukocyte has a specific function, but generally the leukocytes' major role is defense of the body against invading organisms or foreign tissues.

Neutrophils.   The segmented neutrophil is the most numerous leukocyte in the peripheral blood (2.0 to 7.0 $\times$ 10⁹/l). *The segmented* **neutrophil** *is characterized by its nuclear shape and granulated cytoplasm* (see Color Figure 26). There are two types of cytoplasmic granules: azurophilic and neutrophilic. It is the *neutrophilic granules* that are specific for the neutrophils. The abundant number of neutrophilic granules in the cytoplasm results in an overall pinkish tan color to the cytoplasm. The granules contain various substances that are necessary to carry out the function of the neutrophil: phagocytosis of microorganisms (e.g., bacteria). The granular contents facilitate the killing and digesting of those microorganisms.

Eosinophils.   Eosinophils are a lesser component of the leukocyte population (0.0 to 0.45 $\times$ 10⁹/l). *Like the segmented neutrophil, the mature* **eosinophil** *contains a segmented nucleus.* The eosinophil possesses one type of granule, the eosinophilic granule. The *eosinophilic granules* are large granules that impart a characteristic red-orange color to the cytoplasm (see Color Figure 27). Eosinophils have important roles in allergic reactions and defense against parasitic infections. Both of these roles are facilitated by their granular contents.

Basophils.   Basophils are the least common leukocyte (0.0 to 0.2 $\times$ 10⁹/l) in the peripheral blood. *The* **basophil's** *segmented nucleus is often obscured by the large basophilic granules* (see Color Figure 28). These granules stain deep purple with Wright-Giemsa stain. Basophils act as mediators of inflammatory responses. The release of their granular contents results in the classic signs of an immediate hypersensitivity immune reaction, including vasoconstriction and bronchoconstriction.

Monocytes.   Monocytes represent between 4 and 10% (0.2 to 0.8 $\times$ 10⁹/l) of the leukocyte population. *The mature* **monocyte** *is characterized by a horseshoe-shaped or folded nucleus with abundant fine azurophilic granules in the cytoplasm* (see Color Figure 29). These granules give the cytoplasm an opaque grayish appearance. Monocytes leave the peripheral blood and enter the tissues, where they differentiate into *macrophages.* Macrophages or monocytes play a role in the phagocytosis of microorganisms. However, their principle role is in the immune response: phagocytizing, processing and presenting the foreign antigens to the lymphocytes.

Lymphocytes.   The lymphocyte is the second most numerous leukocyte in the peripheral blood (1.5 to 4.0 $\times$ 10⁹/l). **Lymphocytes** *possess a round or oval nucleus and light blue agranular cytoplasm* (see Color Figure 30). The function of the lymphocyte is dictated by its immunologic classification: B lymphocyte or T lymphocyte. Within the primary lymphoid tissues, the bone marrow or thymus, lymphocytes become immunologically competent. Immunocompetent bone marrow (B) lymphocytes are responsible for the humoral immune response that results in the formation of specific antibodies directed against a foreign substance. The antibodies facilitate the removal of the foreign substance from the body. In contrast, immunocompetent thymus (T) lymphocytes are involved in the cellular immune response. The cellular immune response results in the production of sensitized T lympho-

Table 11–2 ▪ Lymphokines and Their Activity

Lymphokine	*Activity*
Interleukin-2	Stimulates proliferation and activation of T lymphocytes
Interleukin-6	Stimulates proliferation of B lymphocytes and production of antibodies
γ interferon	Inhibits intracellular viral replication
Macrophage activation factor	Activates macrophages
Macrophage inhibition factor	Inhibits macrophage migration
Leukocyte chemotaxis factor	Promotes chemotaxis to the site of injury
Lymphocytotoxin	Kills nonlymphocytic cells

cytes, including helper T lymphocytes, suppressor T lymphocytes, and cytotoxic T lymphocytes, which release *lymphokines* (Table 11–2) that either directly or indirectly kill the foreign cells or organisms.

Platelets

Platelets, *the smallest cells in the peripheral blood, are round or oval anuclear cells with azurophilic granules in their cytoplasm* (see Color Figure 31). Platelets have an important role in hemostasis (coagulation). Platelets become activated by substances released by the injured tissue and aggregate with other activated platelets to form an initial platelet plug at the site of injury. Platelets are also involved in the formation of the more stable fibrin clot by providing a surface for several of the coagulation protein reactions to occur.

LYMPHATIC SYSTEM

The lymphatic system is composed of lymphatic vessels and lymphatic organs (i.e., lymph node and spleen) (Fig. 11–6). In addition to its role in hematopoiesis and the immune response, the lymphatic system plays an important role in homeostasis. This system provides a mechanism for substances that accumulate in extracellular spaces to re-enter the circulatory system.

LYMPH

Lymph is formed as a result of the pressure created by the heart's contractions. This pressure results in the filtering of plasma out of the capillaries and into the extracellular space between tissue cells. The filtered plasma is referred to as *interstitial fluid*. The majority of

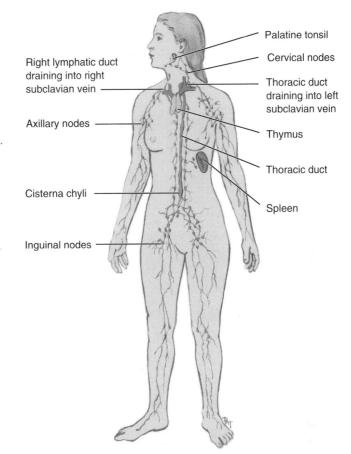

Palatine tonsil

Cervical nodes

Right lymphatic duct
draining into right
subclavian vein

Thoracic duct
draining into left
subclavian vein

Axillary nodes

Thymus

Thoracic duct

Cisterna chyli

Spleen

Inguinal nodes

FIGURE 11-6

The lymphatic system, depict-
ing its vessels and organs.
(From Applegate, E.J.: The
Anatomy and Physiology
Learning System. Philadelphia,
W.B. Saunders, 1995, with
permission.)

the interstitial fluid will re-enter the capillaries. However, some interstitial fluid cannot re-enter and becomes lymph. **Lymph** *is composed of excess interstitial fluid, large protein molecules, and other substances.*

Lymph enters the lymphatic system of capillaries, venules, veins, and ducts, which is similar to the circulatory system. Lymphatic capillaries are distributed throughout the tissue spaces. Because the endothelial cells of the lymphatic capillaries do not possess a tight "fit," excess fluid and large proteins easily enter these capillaries. Unlike the circulatory system, the flow of lymph is unidirectional. Lymph flows either to the right lymphatic duct or the thoracic duct depending on its site of origin (Fig. 11–7). Lymph from the right lymphatic duct enters the circulatory system at the right subclavian vein, while lymph from the thoracic duct enters at the left subclavian vein.

LYMPH NODES

Lymph nodes *are small, bean-shaped organs located throughout the body along the lymphatic vessels.* The lymph node consists of three components: the capsule, the cortex, and the medulla (Fig. 11–8). The *capsule* is an outer fibrous envelope that projects trabeculae of connective tissue into the node to form a fibrous supporting meshwork. The *cortex* is

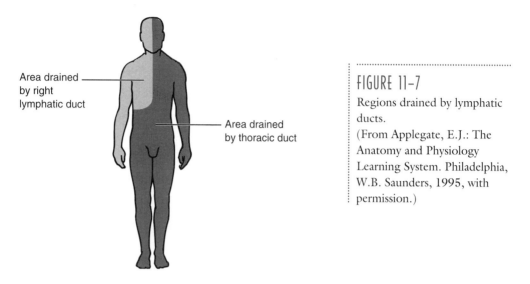

Area drained
by right
lymphatic duct

Area drained
by thoracic duct

FIGURE 11-7

Regions drained by lymphatic ducts.
(From Applegate, E.J.: The Anatomy and Physiology Learning System. Philadelphia, W.B. Saunders, 1995, with permission.)

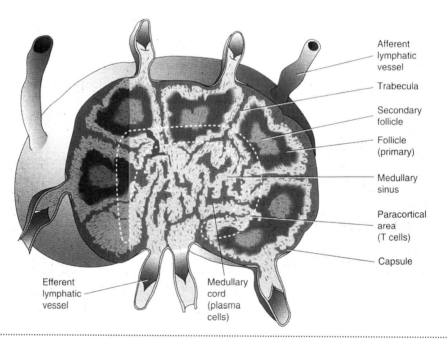

Afferent
lymphatic
vessel

Trabecula

Secondary
follicle

Follicle
(primary)

Medullary
sinus

Paracortical
area
(T cells)

Capsule

Efferent
lymphatic
vessel

Medullary
cord
(plasma
cells)

FIGURE 11-8

Histologic structure of a normal lymph node. The lymph node consists of the capsule, cortex, and medulla. The cortex is composed of primary and secondary follicles and the medulla consists of the medullary cords.
(From Rodak, B.F.: Diagnostic Hematology. Philadelphia, W.B. Saunders, 1995, with permission.)

located below the capsule and is subdivided into two parts: the superficial cortex, which is located just below the capsule, and the paracortex, which is located near the center of the node. Lymphoid follicles are located within the superficial cortex and are primarily composed of B lymphocytes. T lymphocytes are located in the paracortex. The *medulla* is the inner portion of the node that is created by smaller trabeculae that become flattened into medullary cords. Plasma cells, B lymphocytes, and macrophages are found in the medulla.

Lymph nodes act as filters. Afferent lymphatic vessels empty lymph into the node at various points on its periphery. Lymph is filtered as it passes through the node to the efferent lymphatic vessels located in the medulla. Macrophages within the node remove foreign substances from the lymph. A macrophage may phagocytose the foreign substance and present the processed substance on its surface for T-lymphocyte or B-lymphocyte recognition and the initiation of the immune response, either humoral or cell mediated. Thus, the lymph nodes play a major role in the immune response.

THYMUS

In addition to its role as an endocrine gland, the thymus is also a lymphoid organ. Like the lymph node, the thymus consists of a cortex and a medulla. The outer cortex is composed of small lymphocytes and a few macrophages. The inner medulla is composed of lymphocytes, medullary epithelial cells, and macrophages.

The **thymus** *is a primary lymphoid tissue.* Within the thymus, lymphocytes become immunocompetent T lymphocytes. The thymic hormone *thymosin* is critical to this differentiation process. The immunocompetent T lymphocytes leave the thymus and seed the T-lymphocyte compartments of the other lymphoid tissues (i.e., lymph node and spleen). Immunocompetent T lymphocytes are responsible for the cell-mediated immune response.

SPLEEN

The spleen is located in the upper left quadrant of the abdomen lateral to the stomach. Similar to the lymph node, the spleen is enclosed by a connective tissue capsule that extends trabeculae into the interior of the spleen, creating open spaces (Fig. 11–9). These spaces contain three types of splenic pulp: white pulp, red pulp, and the marginal zone. The white pulp consists of lymphoid follicles with germinal centers and the periarterial lymphatic sheaths. The periarterial lymphatic sheaths are composed of loose connective tissue that is packed with lymphocytes and macrophages. The sheaths surround arteries that enter the spleen. The white pulp is surrounded by the marginal zone. The marginal zone is a reticular meshwork of blood vessels, free cells, and narrow interstices. The red pulp consists of venous sinuses that are separated by cords. The cords are bands of reticular tissue and macrophages. The venous sinuses are thin-walled venous vessels that form an intricate network in the red pulp and begin the efferent circulation.

A rich supply of blood enters the spleen via the splenic artery. The blood flow through the spleen may take one of two pathways. The *rapid transit pathway* involves the direct transport of blood to the splenic sinuses or to that portion of the cords where there is free transfer to the sinuses. By this route, blood passes virtually unobstructed into the splenic collecting system and exits the spleen via the splenic veins. Only a small amount of blood

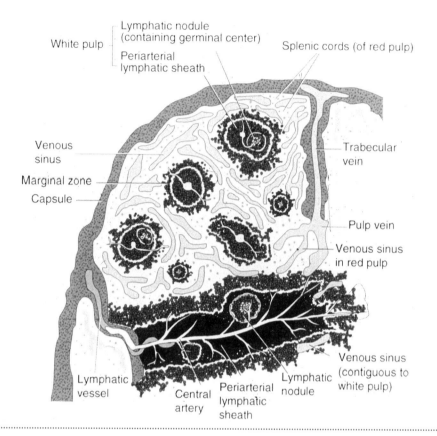

FIGURE 11–9

Schematic of the normal spleen.
(From Weiss, L., and Greep, R.O.: Histology. New York, McGraw-Hill, 1977, with permission.)

follows this pathway. The majority of blood entering the spleen follows the *slow transit pathway*. In this pathway, blood enters the cords (white, red, or marginal zone) and percolates through the macrophage-lined cords before penetrating the small pores through which it gains access to the splenic sinuses.

The splenic functions occur as a result of the flow of blood through the slow transit pathway. Splenic *"culling"* refers to the spleen's ability to remove senescent or imperfect erythrocytes by phagocytosis. The macrophages that line the cords provide this function. Splenic *"pitting"* refers to the spleen's ability to remove inclusions from intact erythrocytes and not destroy the cell. Again, it is the macrophages that line the cords that are responsible for this function. The third function performed during the slow transit pathway is the immunologic function. As blood flows through the cords, the macrophages will recognize and remove microorganisms. The immune response may be initiated as a result of the macrophage recognition.

PATHOLOGIC CONDITIONS

ANEMIA

Anemia *refers to a condition of diminished oxygen-carrying capacity of the blood and is characterized by a decreased erythrocyte count, decreased hemoglobin, or both.* This condition may result from decreased production of erythrocytes, decreased concentration of normal hemoglobin, or increased destruction of erythrocytes. Changes in erythrocyte morphology may provide clues as to the particular anemia the individual is expressing. For example, erythrocytes are hypochromic (decreased hemoglobin content) and microcytic (decreased size) in iron-deficiency anemia. In vitamin B_{12}–deficiency anemia, erythrocytes are macrocytic (increased in size) and oval or elliptical in shape.

Iron-Deficiency Anemia

Iron is an essential component of hemoglobin. If iron is deficient, the developing erythroblasts will be unable to synthesize adequate amounts of hemoglobin, resulting in the production of mature erythrocytes with decreased hemoglobin in their cytoplasm and an overall smaller size compared to normal erythrocytes. There are several possible causes for iron deficiency, including chronic blood loss (e.g., gastrointestinal bleeding), inadequate diet, increased requirements (e.g., pregnancy), and malabsorption from the intestinal tract. Typical clinical findings associated with iron-deficiency anemia are fatigue, weakness, and lethargy.

The diagnosis of iron-deficiency anemia is based on clinical and laboratory findings. The laboratory findings are decreased erythrocyte count, decreased hemoglobin, and decreased hematocrit. Examination of erythrocyte morphology reveals hypochromic and microcytic erythrocytes (see Color Figure 32). Iron-deficiency anemia is confirmed by decreased serum iron levels and decreased bone marrow iron stores. Treatment of iron-deficiency anemia must consist of two parts: (1) treating the cause of the anemia (e.g., gastrointestinal bleeding) and (2) replacing the iron. Iron supplements are given until iron stores have returned to normal, which takes typically 6 months.

Sickle Cell Anemia

Sickle cell anemia *is an inherited condition that leads to a decreased erythrocyte count.* In sickle cell anemia, hemoglobin S, an abnormal hemoglobin, is produced as the result of an amino acid substitution in the beta polypeptide chain. Unlike hemoglobin A (normal adult hemoglobin), hemoglobin S polymerizes and forms rods when deoxygenated. In the deoxygenated state, the erythrocyte's shape is distorted into a sickle (see Color Figure 33). The sickle cells become trapped in the small capillaries of the spleen and other organs and are removed from the circulation. Therefore, the observed anemia is the result of increased destruction of erythrocytes. Hypoxic conditions (i.e., acidosis, infection, dehydration, and strenuous exercise) typically promote sickle cell formation. During these instances, the individual will exhibit clinical findings that are common to all anemias, such as weakness and fatigue. There are also specific clinical findings associated with sickle cell anemia, such as painful infarctive crisis. The infarctive crisis represents the trapping of the sickle cells in the small capillaries of an organ and the subsequent blockage of normal blood flow to the area. If the blockage persists, the tissue will become necrotic.

A diagnosis of sickle cell anemia is based on clinical and laboratory findings. The laboratory findings are decreased erythrocyte count, decreased hemoglobin, and decreased hematocrit. Examination of erythrocyte morphology reveals the presence of sickle cells and target cells (see Color Figure 34). Hemoglobin electrophoresis is necessary to confirm the diagnosis. Hemoglobin electrophoresis is based on the separation of hemoglobins in an electric field on cellulose acetate at pH 8.6. Hemoglobins will migrate according to their electric charge at this pH. An individual with sickle cell anemia will exhibit hemoglobin S (70 to 95% of total hemoglobin) and hemoglobin F (5 to 30% of total hemoglobin). There is no cure for sickle cell anemia. Treatment is preventative to minimize the sickling episodes.

LEUKOCYTOSIS

Leukocytosis *is a leukocyte count greater than 11.0 × 10⁹/l.* Increased numbers of leukocytes are associated with a variety of conditions (Table 11–3). Depending on the cause of the infection, a specific leukocyte will be increased in numbers.

Table 11–3 ■ **Conditions Associated with Leukocytosis**

Leukocytosis with Neutrophilia

Bacterial infections

Inflammation

Hemolysis

Hemorrhage

Stress or anxiety

Vigorous exercise

Exposure to certain drugs or toxins

Chronic myelogenous leukemia

Leukocytosis with Lymphocytosis

Viral infections

Chronic inflammation

Autoimmune disorders

Cigarette smoking

Chronic lymphocytic leukemia

Neutrophilia

A neutrophil count greater than 7.0 × 10⁹/l represents a **neutrophilia**. Conditions associated with neutrophilia are given in Table 11–3. *Streptococcus pyogenes* pharyngitis is an example of a bacterial infection associated with neutrophilia. The bacteria invades the pharyngeal tissue. Chemotaxins released by the bacteria and the infected tissues stimulate the migration of neutrophils from the peripheral blood into the infected area. Peripheral blood neutrophils are increased in response to the released chemotaxins. The clinical findings include fever, chills, and sore throat (pharyngitis).

The diagnosis is based on clinical and laboratory findings. The typical laboratory finding is an increased leukocyte count with increased numbers of neutrophils. Peripheral blood smear examination reveals the presence of immature neutrophils (e.g., band neutrophils and metamyelocytes), as well as segmented neutrophils (see Color Figure 35A, 35B). The presence of immature neutrophils is referred to as a "shift to the left" and is indicative of the increased requirement for neutrophils. Confirmation of the diagnosis is based on positive identification of *Streptococcus pyogenes* through microbiologic techniques. Antibiotic therapy is used to treat *Streptococcus pyogenes*.

Lymphocytosis

Lymphocytosis *is characterized by a lymphocyte count greater than 4.0 × 10⁹/l.* Lymphocytes are typically increased in viral infections (Table 11–3). An example of a viral infection associated with lymphocytosis is infectious mononucleosis, which is caused by the Epstein-Barr virus. This virus invades the pharyngeal tissue and initiates the immune response involving B and T lymphocytes. The clinical findings of infectious mononucleosis are lethargy, fever, and sore throat. Physical examination reveals *lymphadenopathy* (enlarged lymph nodes).

The diagnosis of infectious mononucleosis is based on clinical and laboratory findings. The characteristic laboratory finding is an increased leukocyte count, usually 12.0 to 25.0 × 10⁹/l. The majority of these cells are lymphocytes. Peripheral blood smear examination reveals the presence of reactive lymphocytes. *Reactive lymphocytes* are lymphocytes that have been immune stimulated. They are larger than normal lymphocytes, with irregular-shaped nuclei and less condensed chromatin (see Color Figure 36). The reactive lymphocyte has abundant cytoplasm with a deep blue color (*basophilia*). To confirm the diagnosis, a monospot test is performed. The monospot test will detect the presence of heterophil antibodies formed in infectious mononucleosis. Treatment is not necessary since infectious mononucleosis is resolved by the body's immune response.

LEUKEMIA

Leukemia *describes a variety of neoplastic disorders associated with the malignant, uncontrolled growth of hematopoietic blood cells. The specific type of leukemia is defined by the predominant cell type involved.* For example, acute myeloblastic leukemia is identified by the uncontrolled proliferation of myeloblasts, while chronic lymphocytic leukemia is identified by the uncontrolled proliferation of mature lymphocytes. Leukemias are further classified as acute or chronic based on the invasiveness of the disease. Without treatment, acute leukemia is associated with a rapid disease course, and death occurs within several months of the diagnosis. Chronic leukemia is associated with a prolonged asymptomatic period. The disease course is usually defined in terms of years.

Acute Leukemia

Acute leukemia *is characterized by an increased leukocyte count with increased numbers of blast cells in the peripheral blood and bone marrow.* The blast cells infiltrate the bone marrow and replace the developing erythrocytes, leukocytes (primarily neutrophils), and megakaryocytes. As a result, the individual develops anemia (decreased erythrocyte count), neutropenia (decreased neutrophil count), and thrombocytopenia (decreased platelet count). The decreased peripheral blood cells account for the clinical findings observed in acute leukemia, such as weakness, fatigue, and pallor due to the anemia; recurrent infections due to the neutropenia; and easy bruising and frequent nosebleeds due to the thrombocytopenia. An individual may also experience bone pain due to increased bone marrow activity.

Acute leukemias are diagnosed based on clinical and laboratory findings. Typical laboratory findings include decreased erythrocyte count, decreased hemoglobin and hematocrit, and decreased platelet count. The leukocyte count is variable. Peripheral blood smear examination reveals the presence of blasts. The bone marrow examination reveals a hypercellular bone marrow with greater than 30% blasts (see Color Figure 37). The two basic forms of acute leukemia, acute myeloblastic leukemia and acute lymphoblastic leukemia, cannot be differentiated on the basis of their blast morphology alone. Special cytochemical stains are performed to differentiate the two leukemias. A myeloblast is differentiated from a lymphoblast based on its reaction pattern with special cytochemical stains. The myeloperoxidase and Sudan black B cytochemical stains will be positive if the cell is a myeloblast and negative if the cell is a lymphoblast. It is important to differentiate between the two leukemias in order to choose the most appropriate chemotherapeutic regimen.

Chronic Leukemia

Chronic leukemias *are identified by increased leukocyte counts and a prevalence of mature blood cells. Chronic leukemias are defined by the particular hematopoietic cell line that is most affected.* For example, chronic myelogenous leukemia is characterized by a proliferation of malignant neutrophils and neutrophil precursors in the peripheral blood and bone marrow (see Color Figure 38). Chronic lymphocytic leukemia is characterized by a proliferation of malignant mature lymphocytes (see Color Figures 39A, 39B, and 39C). Similar to the acute leukemias, clinical findings are associated with the malignant proliferation of hematopoietic cells in the bone marrow and a decrease in the production of normal hematopoietic blood cells. Therefore, clinical findings are related to anemia, neutropenia, and thrombocytopenia. In addition, chronic leukemias are associated with organomegaly, such as splenomegaly, hepatomegaly, or lymphadenopathy.

The diagnosis of a chronic leukemia is frequently made by accident during a routine physical examination. The diagnosis is based on clinical and laboratory findings. Laboratory findings associated with chronic myelogenous leukemia include increased leukocyte count (greater than $100 \times 10^9/l$), decreased erythrocyte count, decreased hemoglobin, decreased hematocrit, and decreased platelet count. Peripheral blood smear examination reveals the presence of an absolute neutrophilia with all stages of neutrophilic development present, increased basophils, and increased eosinophils. The bone marrow examination reveals a hypercellular marrow with all stages of neutrophilic development present, increased basophils, and eosinophils. There is decreased erythropoiesis and megakaryopoiesis. Laboratory findings associated with chronic lymphocytic leukemia include increased leukocyte count (10 to 150 × 10⁹/l), decreased erythrocyte count, decreased hemoglobin, decreased hematocrit, and decreased platelet count. Peripheral blood smear examination reveals the presence of an absolute lymphocytosis with mature lymphocytes. The bone marrow examination reveals a hypercellular marrow with an infiltration of malignant mature lymphocytes, resulting in decreased erythropoiesis, megakaryopoiesis, and myelopoiesis. The correct diagnosis of chronic leukemia is important to assure that the appropriate chemotherapeutic regimen is used.

HEMOPHILIA

Hemophilia *is an inherited (X-linked recessive) bleeding disorder associated with a deficiency in factor VIII.* Factor VIII plays an important role as a cofactor in factor IX's activation of factor X. A deficiency in factor VIII will result in decreased fibrin formation. Individuals with hemophilia have no problem forming an initial platelet plug; bleeding episodes are the result of a failure to form the subsequent stable fibrin clot. Therefore, an individual with factor VIII deficiency will experience bleeding episodes such as subcutaneous hematomas following minor trauma, hemarthrosis (bleeding into a joint), spontaneous intramuscular or intracranial hemorrhages, and delayed bleeding. These bleeding episodes may become life threatening.

A diagnosis of hemophilia is based on the clinical and laboratory findings. The typical screening tests for a bleeding disorder include a platelet count, bleeding time, prothrombin time, and activated partial thromboplastin time. All of the screening test results will be normal except the activated partial thromboplastin time, which is prolonged. To confirm the diagnosis, a factor VIII assay is performed to quantitate the activity of factor VIII. In a severe case of hemophilia, factor VIII activity will be less than 5%. Hemophilia is treated using cryoprecipitate that is rich in factor VIII activity or commercially prepared factor VIII concentrate. Treatment is generally limited to prevention when the individual may be undergoing a surgical procedure or therapy during a bleeding episode.

LABORATORY EVALUATION

The investigation of a disorder of the hematopoietic or lymphatic system begins with a series of screening tests designed to narrow the possibilities and focus the approach to further diagnostic testing. The *hematology screening tests* include hemoglobin determination, hematocrit determination, erythrocyte count, leukocyte count, platelet count, and peripheral blood smear examination. The bone marrow examination is an example of a follow-up diagnostic test. In addition, there are *coagulation screening tests* designed to identify possible bleeding disorders. This series includes a platelet count, peripheral blood smear examination, bleeding time, prothrombin time, and activated partial thromboplastin time. The factor assay is an example of a follow-up diagnostic test. The choice of screening tests is dependent on the patient's clinical presentation. For example, the physician would order the hematology screening tests on a patient who presents with weakness and fatigue, but the coagulation screening tests for a patient presenting with frequent bleeding episodes.

HEMATOLOGY PROCEDURES

Hemoglobin

The determination of an individual's hemoglobin concentration is an example of a screening test for anemia (decreased erythrocyte count) or polycythemia (increased erythrocyte count). The hemoglobin concentration in whole blood is determined using a spectrophotometric procedure. A known amount of the patient's whole blood is added to an optimal amount of cyanmethemoglobin reagent. The reagent releases hemoglobin from the erythrocytes and converts the released hemoglobin into cyanmethemoglobin. The absorbance of the cyanmethemoglobin is determined using a spectrophotometer. As defined by Lambert-Beer's Law, the absorbance of the cyanmethemoglobin is directly proportional to the hemoglobin concentration in whole blood. The reference ranges for hemoglobin are found in Table 11–4.

Hematocrit

The **hematocrit** *is a measure of the packed cell volume, reflecting the erythrocyte percentage in a known amount of whole blood*. It is a simple screening test for anemia and polycythemia. In this procedure, a capillary tube is filled with anticoagulated whole blood and centrifuged in a microhematocrit centrifuge for approximately 5 minutes at 10,000 to 15,000 *g*. The erythrocyte volume is expressed as a percentage of the total volume. The reference ranges are given in Table 11–4.

Erythrocyte Count

Together with the hemoglobin and hematocrit determinations, the erythrocyte count is used in the investigation of anemia and polycythemia. In the laboratory, the erythrocyte count is determined by automated cell counters. The majority of cell counters utilize the electrical impedance principle or Coulter principle for cell counting. Whole blood is diluted in an isotonic solution. Two electrodes that are separated by an aperture (opening) are suspended in the dilution (Fig. 11–10). The erythrocytes and other blood cells are drawn through the small aperture. As a blood cell passes through the aperture, it creates impedance, or increased electrical resistance. The amount of resistance encountered is proportional to the volume of the cell passing through the aperture. Using this characteristic, erythrocyte counts are determined by setting threshold limits based on the range in volumes for the erythrocyte population. For example, the lower threshold limit for erythrocytes is set at 36 fl on the Coulter S-Plus instrument, an automated cell counter. In normal conditions, the leukocyte count will not significantly affect the erythrocyte numbers. The reference ranges are found in Table 11–4.

Leukocyte Count

Like the erythrocyte count, the leukocyte count is determined by automated cell counters. Electrical impedance is a common method for counting leukocytes. Whole blood is diluted in isotonic diluent. A lysing agent is added to this dilution to hemolyze the erythrocytes and

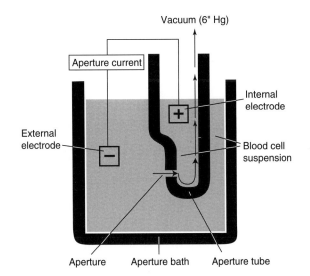

FIGURE 11-10

Coulter principle of cell counting.
(From Coulter Electronics: Coulter STKR Product Reference Manual (PN 4235547 E). Hialeah, FL, Coulter Electronics, 1988, with permission.)

Table 11-4 ■ **Hematology Reference Range***

Hematologic Parameter	*Reference Range*
Hemoglobin	
Adult man	13.3–17.7 g/dl
Adult woman	11.7–15.7 g/dl
Hematocrit	
Adult man	40–52%
Adult woman	35–47%
Erythrocyte count	
Adult man	$4.4–5.9 \times 10^{12}/l$
Adult woman	$3.8–5.2 \times 10^{12}/l$
Leukocyte count	
Adult man	$3.9–10.6 \times 10^{9}/l$
Adult woman	$3.5–11.0 \times 10^{9}/l$
Platelet count	$150–440 \times 10^{9}/l$

* Modified from McKenzie, S.B.: Textbook of Hematology, 2nd ed. Baltimore, Williams & Wilkins, 1996, with permission.)

eliminate their interference. To determine leukocyte numbers, the threshold limits are set at a lower limit of 35 fl and an upper limit of 450 fl on the Coulter S-Plus instrument. The total leukocyte count is the number of cells encountered between these two cell volumes. The reference ranges are found in Table 11–4.

Platelet Count

Changes in platelet numbers are observed in a number of different conditions (Table 11–5). Similar to the erythrocyte and leukocyte counts, a common method for the determination of platelet numbers is electrical impedance. Whole blood is diluted in isotonic diluent and the threshold limits are set at a lower limit of 2 fl and an upper limit of 20 fl on the Coulter S-Plus instrument. The platelet count is based on the number of cells encountered in this region. The reference range is found in Table 11–4.

Peripheral Blood Smear Examination

The examination of a Wright-stained peripheral blood smear is a valuable tool that is used to screen for illness, investigate hematologic and nonhematologic conditions, and monitor a patient's response to therapy. The peripheral blood smear examination includes an estimate of leukocyte numbers; observation for abnormal cells, abnormal erythrocyte distribution, and erythrocyte and platelet morphology; an estimate of platelet numbers; and a 100-cell leukocyte differential.

Evaluation of erythrocyte morphology includes observation of erythrocyte size, shape, and color and presence of inclusions. Normal erythrocyte morphology is described as normochromic (normal color/normal hemoglobin content) and normocytic (normal size and shape). Certain variations from normal are characteristic of specific anemias. For example, sickle cells are observed in sickle cell anemia and hypochromic, microcytic erythrocytes are observed in iron-deficiency anemia.

The 100-cell leukocyte differential determines the relative numbers of the different leukocytes. The observation of abnormal cells or cells not normally found in the peripheral blood is useful in the diagnosis of different disease states. In addition, certain morphologic changes are indicative of certain diseases (e.g., reactive lymphocytes in viral infections). The leukocyte differential reference ranges are shown in Table 11–6.

Table 11–5 ■ **Conditions Associated with Changes in Platelet Numbers**

Increased Concentration	*Decreased Concentration*
Following splenectomy	Immune thrombocytopenic purpura
Hemorrhage	Aplastic anemia
Iron-deficiency anemia	Acute leukemia
Chronic myelogenous leukemia	Vitamin B_{12}–deficiency anemia

Table 11—6 ■ Leukocyte Differential Reference Ranges*

Leukocyte	Reference Ranges	
	Relative (%)[†]	Absolute ($\times 10^9/l$)[‡]
Segmented neutrophil	54–62	2.0–7.0
Lymphocyte	20–40	1.5–4.0
Monocyte	4–10	0.2–0.8
Eosinophil	1–3	0–0.45
Basophil	0–1	0–0.2

* Modified from McKenzie, S.B.: Texbook of Hematology, 2nd ed. Baltimore, Williams & Wilkins, 1996, with permission.)

† Represents the relative number or percentage of a specific leukocyte in 100 leukocytes.

‡ Represents the actual number of a specific leukocyte in 1 liter of whole blood.

Bone Marrow Examination

Examination of the bone marrow provides additional information related to the bone marrow's hematopoietic activity and may identify the presence of benign or malignant changes (e.g., acute leukemia). The typical samples obtained for examination are a small portion of the liquid bone marrow (referred to as bone marrow aspirate) and a bone biopsy. Several bone marrow aspirate smears are prepared and stained with Wright-Giemsa stain. The bone biopsy is processed and thin sections of the bone are obtained. These sections are stained with a hematoxylin-and-eosin stain. The stained bone marrow aspirate smears and bone biopsy sections are examined to evaluate the cellularity of the marrow (e.g., normocellular, hypocellular, or hypercellular), determine a 500-cell differential, evaluate cellular morphology, observe for abnormal cells (e.g., malignant lymphocytes), and determine the myeloid:erythroid ratio.

Changes in the various cell populations within the bone marrow are identified by performing the 500-cell differential. These changes may be indicative of certain disease states. For example, the presence of 30% or more myeloblasts would indicate acute myeloblastic leukemia, while the presence of an increased number of segmented neutrophils and neutrophil precursors would be indicative of chronic myelogenous leukemia.

COAGULATION PROCEDURES

Bleeding Time

The bleeding time evaluates the components (the platelets and vascular system) involved in the formation of the initial platelet plug. The bleeding time is determined by placing a blood pressure cuff on the arm above the elbow and inflating it to 40 mm Hg to create venostasis. A small incision is made on the volar surface of the forearm. A stopwatch is started and blood is blotted away at 30-second intervals using filter paper. The bleeding time is the length of time required for bleeding to cease. The reference range is 1 to 9 minutes. A prolonged bleeding time is associated with thrombocytopenia (platelet count less than $100 \times 10^9/l$), platelet dysfunction (e.g., von Willebrand disease or Bernard-Soulier disease), or certain vascular bleeding disorders (e.g., Ehlers-Danlos syndrome).

Prothrombin Time

The prothrombin time evaluates the coagulation factors in the extrinsic and common pathways (factors VII, X, and V, prothrombin, and fibrinogen) (see Fig. 11–3). A deficiency in any of these factors will result in a prolonged prothrombin time. The prothrombin time is determined by adding an optimal concentration of thromboplastin-calcium reagent to a patient's platelet-poor plasma. The prothrombin time is the time required for a clot to form. The reference range is 11 to 15 seconds.

Activated Partial Thromboplastin Time

The activated partial thromboplastin time (APTT) evaluates the coagulation factors in the intrinsic and common pathways (factors XII, XI, IX, VIII, X, and V, prothrombin, and fibrinogen) (see Fig. 11–3). A deficiency in any of these factors will result in a prolonged APTT. The APTT is determined by adding an optimal concentration of activated partial thromboplastin reagent to a patient's platelet-poor plasma. Following a short incubation period, calcium is added to the mixture. The APTT is the time required for a clot to form. The reference range is 35 to 45 seconds.

Factor Assays

Factor assays are performed to confirm a specific factor deficiency and quantitate the activity level for the deficient factor. For example, a factor VIII assay is performed by first creating a factor VIII activity curve. This curve is plotted using the APTT clotting times obtained on several dilutions of normal reference plasma and factor VIII–deficient plasma. The clotting time will return to near normal as the concentration of normal reference plasma increases compared to the factor-deficient plasma in these dilutions. Next, the patient's plasma is mixed with factor VIII–deficient plasma and APTT clotting times are obtained for the dilutions. The patient's clotting times are compared to the factor VIII activity curve to determine the activity level of factor VIII in the patient's plasma. The activity level is expressed as a percentage of normal. Normal factor VIII activity is 50 to 150%.

CHAPTER SUMMARY

The hematopoietic and lymphatic systems are intricately involved in the body's homeostasis. Together, they are responsible for the production of blood cells. In turn, these blood cells perform a variety of functions necessary to maintain the body's homeostasis. The erythrocytes transport oxygen to and remove carbon dioxide from the tissues. The neutrophils provide a front-line defense mechanism against invading microorganisms. The lymphocytes within the lymphoid tissue respond to foreign substances through the immune response. The monocytes and macrophages that are found throughout the hematopoietic and lymphoid tissues serve many roles, but it is their ability to phagocytose a wide variety of substances, including cells, that is the key to their ability to serve in those roles. Finally, the platelets play a crucial role in maintaining vascular integrity through hemostasis. An abnormality in any blood cell, hematopoietic tissue, or lymphatic tissue will effect the body's homeostasis. Laboratory evaluation provides the necessary information to identify the blood cells, tissue, or both that are affected.

Review Questions

1. Which function is not performed by the blood?
    a. oxygen transport
    b. hemostasis
    c. glucose transport
    d. hematopoiesis

2. Which blood cell is responsible for the phagocytosis (killing and degradation) of bacteria?
    a. neutrophil
    b. platelet
    c. lymphocyte
    d. basophil

3. Which leukocyte is characterized by a segmented nucleus and the presence of large red-orange granules in the cytoplasm?
    a. monocyte
    b. basophil
    c. eosinophil
    d. neutrophil

4. Which lymphatic tissue/organ is responsible for the differentiation and maturation of pre-T lymphocytes into immunocompetent T lymphocytes?
    a. lymph node
    b. thymus
    c. spleen
    d. bone marrow

5. Splenic "culling" refers to the spleen's ability to
    a. remove senescent erythrocytes by phagocytosis
    b. inactivate viral particles through the immune response
    c. remove erythrocyte inclusions while maintaining the cell's integrity
    d. synthesize lymphokines

6. Which pathologic conditions is associated with an increased leukocyte count and the presence of 30% or more blasts in the bone marrow?

    a. infectious mononucleosis

    b. chronic leukemia

    c. acute leukemia

    d. bacterial infection

7. Which laboratory test is not considered a coagulation screening test?

    a. activated partial thromboplastin time

    b. bleeding time

    c. factor assay

    d. prothrombin time

BIBLIOGRAPHY

Butcher, E.C.: Leukocyte-endothelial cell recognition: Three (or more) steps to specificity and diversity. Cell *67*: 1033, 1991.

Cox, C.J., Habermann, T.M., and Payne, B.A.: Evaluation of the Coulter Counter Model S-Plus IV. Am. J. Clin. Pathol. *84*: 297, 1985.

Guyton, A.C.: Textbook of Medical Physiology, 9th ed. Philadelphia, W.B. Saunders, 1996.

Henderson, A.R., Tietz, N.W., and Rinker, A.D.: Gastric, pancreatic, and intestinal function. *In* Burtis, C.A., and Ashwood, E.R. (eds.): Tietz Fundamentals of Clinical Chemistry, 4th ed. Philadelphia, W.B. Saunders, 1996, p. 593.

Jagels, M.A., and Hugli, T.E.: Neutrophil chemotactic factors promote leukocytosis. J Immunol. *148*:1119, 1992.

McKenzie, S.B.: Textbook of Hematology, 2nd ed. Baltimore, Williams & Wilkins, 1996.

National Committee for Clinical Laboratory Standards: Activated Partial Thromboplastin Time Test (APTT), vol. 12, no. 23. Villanova, PA, 1992.

National Committee for Clinical Laboratory Standards: Determination of Factor VIII Coagulant Activity (VIII:C), vol. 6, no. 6. Villanova, PA, 1986.

National Committee for Clinical Laboratory Standards: One-Stage Prothrombin Time Test (PT), vol. 12, no. 22. Villanova, PA, 1992.

National Committee for Clinical Laboratory Standards: Procedure for Determining Packed Cell Volume by the Microhematocrit Method, vol. 5, no. 5. Villanova, PA, 1985.

National Committee for Clinical Laboratory Standards: Reference Procedure for the Quantitative Determination of Hemoglobin in Blood, vol. 4, no. 3. Villanova, PA, 1984.

Paraskevas, F., and Foerster, J.: The lymphatic system. *In* Lee, G.R., et al. (eds.): Wintrobe's Clinical Hematology, 9th ed. Philadelphia, Lea & Febiger, 1993.

Pruden, E.L., Siggaard-Andersen, O., and Tietz, N.W.: Blood gases and pH. *In* Burtis, C.A., and Ashwood, E.R. (eds.): Tietz Fundamentals of Clinical Chemistry, 4th ed. Philadelphia, W.B. Saunders, 1996, p. 506.

Rodak, B.F.: Diagnostic Hematology. Philadelphia, W.B. Saunders, 1995.

Rothstein, G.: Origin and development of the blood and blood-forming tissues. *In* Lee, G.R., et al. (eds.): Wintrobe's Clinical Hematology, 9th ed. Philadelphia, Lea & Febiger, 1993.

Williams, W.J., Beutler, E., Erslev, A.J., and Lechtman, M.A.: Hematology, 4th ed. New York, McGraw-Hill, 1990.

12 The Endocrine System

INTRODUCTION

HORMONES
Biosynthesis
Release and Transport
Degradation
Regulation of Secretion
Mode of Action of Hormones

ENDOCRINE GLANDS
Pineal Gland
Hypothalamus
  Hypothalamic hormones
Pituitary Gland
  Hormones produced by the
    anterior pituitary gland
  Hormones produced by the
    posterior pituitary gland
Thyroid Gland
  Thyroid hormones
Parathyroid Glands
Thymus
Pancreas
Adrenal Glands
  Hormones produced by the
    adrenal glands
Testes

Ovary
Other Endocrine Glands

PATHOLOGIC CONDITIONS
ASSOCIATED WITH THE
ENDOCRINE SYSTEM
Pituitary Gland Disorders
  Gigantism
  Acromegaly
  Dwarfism
Diabetes Insipidus
Thyroid Disorders
  Graves' disease
  Hashimoto's thyroiditis
  Cretinism
**Disorders of the Parathyroid
  Gland**
  Hypoparathyroidism
  Hyperparathyroidism
Adrenal Gland Disorders
  Addison's disease
  Cushing's syndrome
  Conn's syndrome
  Pheochromocytoma
Disorders of the Pancreas
  Diabetes mellitus
  Hyperinsulinemia

LABORATORY EVALUATION OF ENDOCRINE SYSTEM DISORDERS

Immunoassays
Stimulation Tests
Suppression Tests

CHAPTER SUMMARY

REVIEW QUESTIONS

Objectives

1. *Discuss the three classes of hormones.*

2. *Explain the feedback mechanism for regulation of hormone secretion.*

3. *Compare and contrast the mode of action of protein hormones and the mode of action of steroid hormones.*

4. *Identify the hormones released by the common endocrine glands.*

5. *Describe the physiologic effects of each hormone and the stimulus for its secretion.*

6. *Identify the laboratory tests used in the evaluation of endocrine abnormalities.*

7. *Given clinical symptoms, laboratory data, or both, state the most likely endocrine abnormality.*

KEY TERMS

hormones	prolactin	somatostatin	gigantism
specific effect	growth hormone	adrenal glands	acromegaly
global effect	vasopressin	aldosterone	Graves' disease
aromatic amine	oxytocin	cortisol	Hashimoto's thyroiditis
granule	thyroid gland	gonadal steroids	Conn's syndrome
feedback mechanism	parathyroid gland	testes	pheochromocytoma
pineal gland	parathyroid hormone	testosterone	insulin-dependent
hypothalamus	thymus	inhibin	diabetes mellitus
pituitary gland	thymosin	ovaries	non-insulin-dependent
thyroid-stimulating	thymostatin	estrogen	diabetes mellitus
hormone	pancreas	progesterone	radioimmunoassay
gonadotropin-releasing	insulin	renin	fluorescent immuno-
hormone	glucagon	erythropoietin	assay

Introduction

The endocrine system represents one of the body's communication systems. This system interacts with the other two communication systems, the nervous system and the immune system, to create homeostasis within the body (Fig. 12–1). Together, these systems influence physiologic responses and behavior through the effects of hormones released by the endocrine system, neurotransmitters released by the nervous system, and cytokines released by the immune system.

HORMONES

Hormones *are chemical substances that are synthesized by endocrine cells, but produce their effect on target cells located at a distance from the site of synthesis.* Only minute quantities of a hormone are needed to dramatically influence the physiologic functions of the body. Hormones may produce very specific or global effects. *Insulin is an example of a hormone that produces a* **specific effect**. It is responsible for decreasing blood glucose levels. *Growth hormone is an example of a hormone that produces a* **global effect**. Growth hormone promotes cell growth through its influence on the body's protein and carbohydrate metabolism and its stimulation of growth factors.

BIOSYNTHESIS

Based on their chemical structure, hormones are divided into three classes: aromatic amines, proteins, and steroids. The **aromatic amines,** *epinephrine* and *norepinephrine*, are synthesized from the precursor substance, tyrosine, in a series of enzymatic steps (Fig. 12–2). Depending on the enzymes present within the cell, either epinephrine or norepinephrine will be synthesized. *Thyroid hormones* have the same precursor substance as aromatic amines (tyrosine). Within the thyroid follicle, however, iodine is added to produce the thyroid hormones, triiodothyronine (T_3) and thyroxine (T_4) (Fig. 12–3).

The majority of hormones are proteins. The synthesis of *protein hormones* occurs within the membrane-bound ribosomes of an endocrine cell. The prehormone is the polypeptide chain that is initially produced by the membrane-bound ribosomes and processed within the endoplasmic reticulum (ER) to a prohormone. The prohormone is transported from the ER into the Golgi apparatus for the final processing steps. In the Golgi apparatus, the prohormone and the enzymes necessary for its conversion to mature hormone are packaged within secretory **granules** (Fig. 12–4).

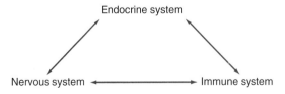

FIGURE 12-1

The three communication systems of the body are the endocrine system, nervous system, and immune system. These systems interact with one another to maintain the body's homeostasis.

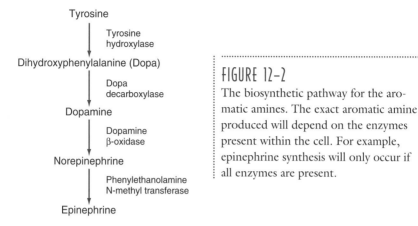

FIGURE 12-2

The biosynthetic pathway for the aromatic amines. The exact aromatic amine produced will depend on the enzymes present within the cell. For example, epinephrine synthesis will only occur if all enzymes are present.

All *steroid hormones* have the same precursor substance, cholesterol. Through a series of enzymatic steps, cholesterol is converted to a steroid hormone (Fig. 12–5). The specific steroid hormone synthesized is dependent on the enzymes present within the cell.

RELEASE AND TRANSPORT

The aromatic amines, epinephrine and norepinephrine, are stored within secretory granules until the cell is stimulated by a nervous impulse. Following stimulation, the contents of the secretory granules are released by *pinocytosis.* The secretory granule fuses with the cell membrane. The cell membrane is ruptured at this site and the contents are released into the surrounding area. The aromatic amines enter the bloodstream and are carried to their target cells. The aromatic amines are water soluble and are easily transported within the blood.

Protein hormones are stored in secretory granules within the cells where their synthesis occurred. These hormones are released from the cells following the appropriate stimulation. The secretory granules fuse with the cell membrane and, through the process of pinocytosis, release their contents into the bloodstream. Protein hormones are water soluble and are free to circulate within the blood to their target cells.

The steroid hormones are synthesized in response to stimulation. In other words, the rate of synthesis is equal to the rate of stimulation. Steroid hormones are not stored within the cells that synthesize them; rather, steroid hormones readily diffuse out of the cell. Steroid hormones are water insoluble and must be bound to a carrier protein for transport within the bloodstream.

The thyroid hormones are stored within the thyroid follicle. They are released in response to the appropriate stimulation. Thyroid hormones are water insoluble and must be transported within the blood bound to a carrier protein. The protein-bound thyroid hormones are readily transported via the bloodstream to their target cells.

DEGRADATION

The aromatic amines are converted to inactive hormones through oxidation or deiodination. These inactive hormones are either excreted in the urine by the kidneys or further degraded by the liver for excretion in the feces. The protein hormones are degraded by pro-

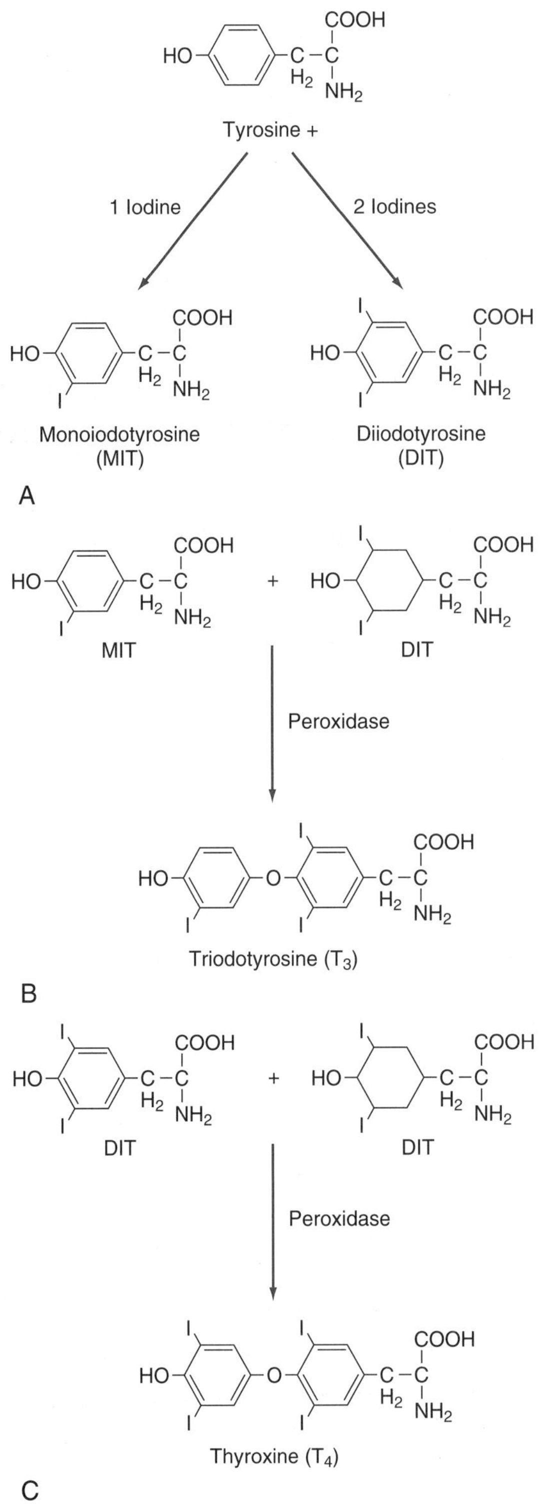

FIGURE 12-3

The biosynthetic pathway for the thyroid hormones. *A,* Within the thyroid follicle, the tyrosine molecules have been hydroxylated to the thyroglobulin. Iodine (I^0 or I^+) combines with the tyrosyl groups, forming monoiodotyrosine (MIT) if one iodine atom attaches or diiodotyrosine (DIT) if two iodine atoms attach. *B,* Triiodothyronine (T_3) is formed by the enzymatic coupling of MIT and DIT, catalyzed by the enzyme peroxidase. *C,* Thyroxine (T_4) is formed by the enzymatic coupling of two DIT molecules, catalyzed by peroxidase.

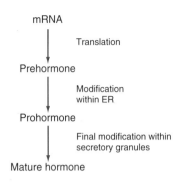

mRNA

   Translation

Prehormone

   Modification
   within ER

Prohormone

   Final modification within
   secretory granules

Mature hormone

FIGURE 12-4

The biosynthetic pathway of protein hormones. The biosynthesis of a protein hormone begins with the translation of the mRNA at membrane-bound ribosomes. The resulting prehormone enters the endoplasmic reticulum (ER) for initial processing to a prohormone. The prohormone leaves the ER and enters the Golgi apparatus. Within the Golgi apparatus, the prohormone and the enzymes necessary for its conversion to mature hormone are packaged into secretory granules. The prohormone is converted to mature hormone within the secretory granules.

teases within the blood or the tissues. These smaller polypeptides are filtered by the glomerulus and further degraded by the renal tubular cells. The degradation products are excreted in the urine.

    The steroid hormones, which are bound to carrier proteins, are converted to water-soluble inactive forms by hydroxylation, oxidation, or conjugation with glucuronic acid or sulfate. The inactive forms of the steroid hormones are excreted by the kidney. Within the peripheral tissue, active steroid hormones are converted to less active hormones by oxidation. The less active hormones are removed by the liver and converted to inactive forms.

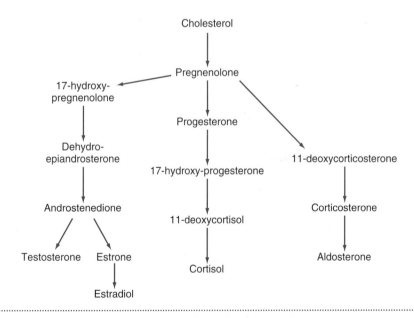

FIGURE 12-5

The biosynthetic pathway of steroid hormones. The exact steroid hormone produced depends on the enzymes present within the cell.

REGULATION OF SECRETION

The regulation of hormone secretion is critical to the maintenance of the body's physiologic equilibrium (homeostasis). The principal mechanism for regulating hormone secretion is the **feedback mechanism.** The feedback mechanism consists of two types: positive feedback and negative feedback. In the *positive* feedback mechanism, an increase in one hormone would result in the increase of a second hormone. For example, an increase in thyroid-stimulating hormone (TSH) results in an increase in the thyroid hormones (T_3 and T_4). In the *negative* feedback mechanism, an increase in one hormone causes a decrease in the second hormone. As an example, an increase in the thyroid hormone level causes a decrease in TSH. Frequently, the positive feedback mechanism and negative feedback mechanism pair to create a *feedback loop;* an increase in TSH results in an increase in thyroid hormone, which in turn causes a decrease in TSH (Fig. 12–6). Therefore, the feedback loop serves to regulate hormone concentrations within the body.

MODE OF ACTION OF HORMONES

Hormones act by binding to a specific receptor located on the cell membrane or within the cytoplasm of the target cell. Protein hormones recognize their target cells based on the presence of a specific membrane receptor. The protein hormone binds to its membrane receptor and, as a result, the enzyme adenylate cyclase is activated (Fig. 12–7). Adenylate cyclase is responsible for the formation of the second messenger, cyclic adenosine monophosphate (cAMP). cAMP, in turn, activates protein kinase, and protein kinase is responsible for the activation of the biochemical pathways within the cell that lead to the hormone's final effect.

Since steroid hormones and thyroid hormones are lipid soluble, they readily diffuse through the phospholipid membrane of the target cell. The steroid hormone binds to a specific receptor within the cytoplasm of the target cell (Fig. 12–8). The steroid hormone–receptor complex enters the nucleus and binds to the nonhistone protein of the chromatin. This binding results in the production of new messenger RNA (mRNA). The mRNA leaves the nucleus and enters the cytoplasm, where it attaches to ribosomes. The mRNA is translated into proteins that ultimately affect the final actions of the hormone.

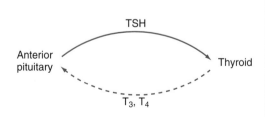

FIGURE 12-6

The feedback loop mechanism. In this example, TSH released from the anterior pituitary causes the release of increased amounts of thyroid hormones. The increased levels of thyroid hormones will feed back to the anterior pituitary and inhibit the release of TSH. The solid line depicts stimulation and the dotted line depicts inhibition.

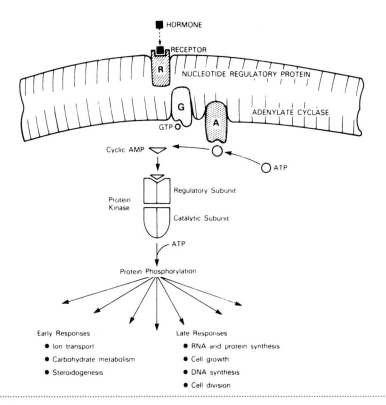

FIGURE 12-7

Protein hormone action through the second messenger cAMP. Hormone binds to its receptor on the cell's surface. This binding results in the activation of adenylate cyclase. Activated adenylate cyclase is responsible for the conversion of ATP to cAMP. cAMP activates protein kinase, which is responsible for the phosphorylation of a variety of enzymes that produce the effects of the hormone. (From Catt, K.J., Harwood, J.P., Clayton, R.N., et al.: Regulation of peptide hormone receptors and gonadal steroidogenesis. Recent Prog. Horm. Res. *36*:557, 1980, with permission of S. Karger AG, Basel, Switzerland.)

ENDOCRINE GLANDS

PINEAL GLAND

The **pineal gland** *(pineal body) is located in a pocket near the posterior end of the corpus callosum* (Fig. 12–9). The major hormone produced by the pineal gland is *melatonin* (Table 12–1). In humans, melatonin has a major role in the circadian timing system (i.e., sleep-wake rhythm and body temperature regulation). Melatonin induces sleep and lowers core body temperature. The secretion of melatonin is regulated by the hypothalamus through neuronal stimulation. The neuronal stimulation occurs in response to light (photosensitiv-

Molecular Pathway of Steroid Hormone Action

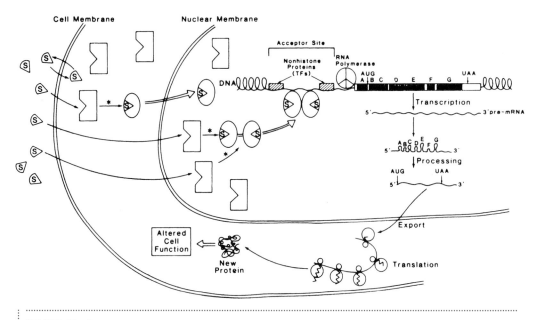

FIGURE 12-8

Steroid hormone action. Steroid hormone diffuses through the cell's membrane and binds to a specific intracellular receptor. The hormone-receptor complex enters the nucleus and binds to nonhistone protein. This binding results in the production of new messenger RNA. The messenger RNA enters the cytoplasm, attaches to ribosome, and is translated into a new protein. This protein affects the final actions of the hormone.

(From Clark, J., Schrader, W., and O'Malley, B.: Mechanisms of action of steroid hormones. *In* Wilson, J.D., and Foster, D.W. (eds.): Williams Textbook of Endocrinology, 8th ed. Philadelphia, W.B. Saunders, 1992, with permission.)

ity). Light suppresses melatonin synthesis and has a sustained effect on the timing of melatonin secretion. Therefore, the highest levels of melatonin are seen at night and only minimal levels are observed during the daylight hours. Secretion of melatonin is also affected by seasonal changes, primarily day length. During periods of short days and long nights, melatonin is secreted for long periods. Jet lag syndrome, delayed sleep phase syndrome, and seasonal affective disorders have been linked to disruptions in the circadian timing system involving melatonin.

HYPOTHALAMUS

The **hypothalamus** *is located behind the frontal lobe and below the thalamus.* It is divided into two parts by the third ventricle. Neuronal cell bodies, such as ventromedial nuclei and arcuate nuclei, that make up the hypothalamus are responsible for the synthesis of hypothalamic hormones. The secretion of these hormones is in response to stimulation by neuro-

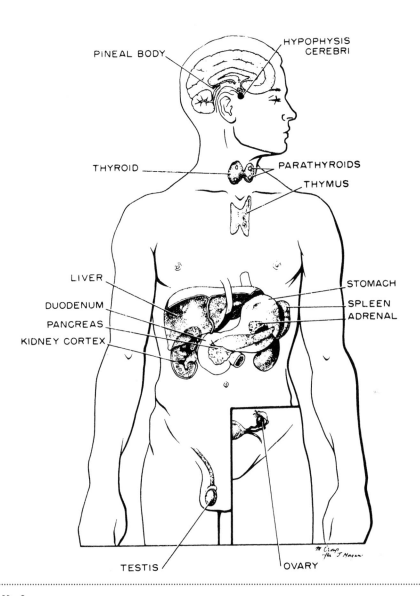

FIGURE 12-9

The major endocrine glands.
(From Turner, C.D.: General Endocrinology, 4th ed. Philadelphia, W.B. Saunders, 1966, with permission.)

Table 12-1 ■ Hormones, Their Sources, and Their Actions*

Endocrine Gland	Hormone	Nature of Hormone	Site of Action	Principal Actions†
Pineal gland	Melatonin	Indoleamine	Hypothalamus	Induction of sleep
Hypothalamus	Thyroid-releasing hormone	Protein	Anterior pituitary	Release of TSH
	Corticotropin-releasing hormone	Protein	Anterior pituitary	Release of ACTH
	Gonadotropin-releasing hormone	Protein	Anterior pituitary	Release of LH and FSH
	Growth hormone–releasing hormone	Protein	Anterior pituitary	Release of GH
	Somatostatin	Protein	Anterior pituitary	Suppression of GH
	MSH releasing hormone	Protein	Anterior pituitary	Release of MSH
	MSH release-inhibiting factor	Protein	Anterior pituitary	Suppression of MSH release
	Prolactin-releasing factor	Protein	Anterior pituitary	Release of PRL
	Prolactin release-inhibiting factor	Dopamine	Anterior pituitary	Suppression of PRL release
Anterior pituitary	TSH	Protein	Thyroid gland	Stimulates release of thyroid hormones
	ACTH	Protein	Adrenal cortex	Stimulates release of glucocorticoids
	FSH	Protein	Ovary and testis	Promotes development of gametes and secretion of gonadal hormones

Gland	Hormone	Chemical type	Target tissue	Function
	LH	Protein	Ovary and testis	Ovary—stimulates ovulation and formation of corpus luteum Testis—stimulates interstitial cells to secrete testosterone
	PRL	Protein	Mammary gland	Proliferation of mammary gland; initiation of milk secretion
	GH	Protein	Majority of body's cells	Growth of bone and muscle
	MSH	Protein	Skin	Dispersion of melanin, darkening of skin
Posterior pituitary	Vasopressin	Protein	Kidney	Promotes water reabsorption
	Oxytocin	Protein	Mammary gland, uterus	Stimulates lactation, stimulates contractions
Thyroid gland	T_3	Aromatic amine	General body tissue	Stimulates body's metabolic activity
	T_4	Aromatic amine	General body tissue	Same as T_3
	Calcitonin	Protein	Skeletal bone	Inhibits calcium reabsorption
Parathyroid gland	PTH	Protein	Skeletal bones, kidney, gastrointestinal tract	Promotes reabsorption of calcium, increases calcium uptake from GI tract
Thymus	Thymosin	Protein	T lymphocytes	Promotes differentiation of pre-T lymphocytes to mature T lymphocytes

(Table continues)

Table 12–1 ■ (Continued)

Endocrine Gland	Hormone†	Nature of Hormone	Site of Action	Principal Action†
	Thymostatin	Protein	Lymphocytes	Inhibits development and differentiation of lymphocytes
Pancreas	Insulin	Protein	Most cells	Promotes cellular uptake of glucose, regulates carbohydrate metabolism
	Glucagon	Protein	Liver	Glycogenolysis
Adrenal cortex	Aldosterone	Steroid	Kidney	Promotes sodium reabsorption by kidney
	Cortisol	Steroid	General body tissue	Regulates carbohydrate, fat, and protein metabolism
Adrenal medulla	Epinephrine	Aromatic amine	Sympathetic receptors, liver, muscle, adipose tissue	Increases heart rate and glucose levels
	Norepinephrine	Aromatic amine	Sympathetic receptors	Vasoconstriction, increases blood pressure
Testis	Testosterone	Steroid	Male accessory sex organs	Development of secondary sex characteristics
	Inhibin	Protein	Hypothalamus	Suppression of FSH release from anterior pituitary
Ovary	Estrogen	Steroid	Female accessory sex organs	Development of secondary sex characteristics
	Progesterone	Steroid	Female accessory reproductive structure	Prepares uterus for ovum implantation, maintenance of pregnancy

Kidney	Renin	Protein	Bloodstream	Maintains plasma sodium balance
	Erythropoietin	Protein	Bone marrow	Stimulates erythropoiesis
Heart	Atrial natriuretic factor	Protein	Vascular, renal, and adrenal tissue	Regulates blood pressure and blood volume
Gastrointestinal tract	Gastrin	Protein	Stomach	Stimulates secretion of HCl and increases intestinal motility
	Secretin	Protein	Pancreas	Stimulates secretion of pancreatic bicarbonate and digestive enzymes
	Cholecystokinin	Protein	Gallbladder, pancreas	Stimulates gallbladder contraction and secretion of pancreatic enzymes
Placenta	hCG	Protein	Ovary	Maintains the corpus luteum and progesterone production
	hPL	Protein	Mammary gland	Promotes growth and development of mammary glands

* From *In* Burtis, C.A., and Ashwood, E.R. (eds.): Tietz Fundamentals of Clinical Chemistry, 4th ed. Philadelphia, WB Saunders, 1996, with permission.)

† Abbreviations: ACTH, adrenocorticotropic hormone; FSH, follicle-stimulating hormone; GH, growth hormone; GI, gastrointestinal; hCG, human chorionic gonadotropin; hPL, human placental lactogen; LH, luteinizing hormone; MSH, melanocyte-stimulating hormone; PRL, prolactin; PTH, parathyroid hormones; T_3, triiodothyronine; T_4, thyroxine; TSH, thyroid-stimulating hormone.

transmitters from other neurons and chemical messengers (e.g., hormones) from the blood and cerebrospinal fluid.

Hypothalamic Hormones

There are nine hypothalamic hormones that are responsible for the regulation of anterior pituitary hormone secretion, as shown in Table 12–1. Three of the hypothalamic hormones, *thyroid-releasing hormone* (TRH), *corticotropin-releasing hormone* (CRH), and *gonadotropin-releasing hormone* (GnRH), are responsible for the release of specific anterior pituitary hormones. TRH stimulates the release of TSH, while CRH stimulates the release of adrenocorticotropic hormone (ACTH). GnRH stimulates the release of follicle-stimulating hormone (FSH) and luteinizing hormone (LH). The remaining six hormones are paired hormones, with one hypothalamic hormone promoting a hormone's release and a second hypothalamic hormone inhibiting the hormone's release. *Growth hormone–releasing hormone* (GH-RH) and *somatostatin* regulate the release of growth hormone (GH). GH-RH stimulates GH's release while somatostatin inhibits its release. *Melanocyte-stimulating hormone releasing factor* (MSH-RF) stimulates release of melanocyte-stimulating hormone (MSH), while *melanocyte-stimulating hormone release-inhibiting factor* (MSH-RIF) inhibits MSH release. Likewise, *prolactin-releasing factor* (PRF) stimulates the release of prolactin (PRL), while *prolactin-inhibiting factor* (PIF) inhibits its release.

PITUITARY GLAND

The **pituitary gland** *(hypophysis) hangs from the hypothalamus by the pituitary stalk (infundibulum)* (Fig. 12–9). The pituitary gland is composed of three parts: anterior lobe, intermediate lobe, and posterior lobe (Fig. 12–10). The anterior lobe and intermediate lobe

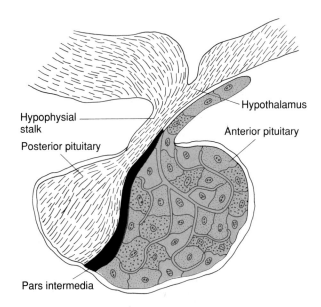

Hypophysial stalk
Posterior pituitary
Pars intermedia
Hypothalamus
Anterior pituitary

FIGURE 12–10

The pituitary gland. The pituitary gland is composed of the anterior lobe (anterior pituitary), intermediate lobe (pars intermedia), and posterior lobe. The anterior lobe and the intermediate lobe form the anterior pituitary. It hangs from the hypothalamus by the pituitary stalk (hypophysial stalk). (From Guyton, A.C.: Textbook of Medical Physiology, 9th ed. Philadelphia, W.B. Saunders, 1996, with permission.)

form the anterior pituitary gland (*adenohypophysis*). The posterior lobe represents the posterior pituitary gland (*neurohypophysis*).

Hormones Produced by the Anterior Pituitary Gland

The function of the anterior pituitary gland is regulated by hypothalamic hormones. The anterior pituitary gland produces and releases the following hormones, which are responsible for a number of the regulative processes of the body:

Anterior Lobe Hormones
- thyroid-stimulating hormone
- adrenocorticotropic hormone
- growth hormone
- follicle-stimulating hormone
- luteinizing hormone
- prolactin

Intermediate Lobe Hormone
- Melanocyte-stimulating hormone

Table 12–1 summarizes the functions of these hormones.

Thyroid-stimulating hormone is synthesized by the thyrotroph cells and released into the bloodstream following TRH stimulation. TSH's target organ is the thyroid gland. TSH stimulates the thyroid gland, resulting in the production and release of thyroid hormones (T_3 and T_4). Thyroid hormones are responsible for the regulation of the energy processes of the body.

The corticotroph cells synthesize and release *ACTH* into the bloodstream in response to CRH. The adrenal gland, specifically the adrenal cortex, is the target organ of ACTH. Following ACTH stimulation, the adrenal cortex produces and releases glucocorticoid hormones (e.g., cortisol). The glucocorticoids affect carbohydrate, fat, and protein metabolism.

Gonadotropin-releasing hormone is responsible for stimulating the gonadotroph cells to synthesize and release *FSH* and *LH*. The release of FSH from the anterior pituitary affects both sexes in a similar fashion. FSH promotes the development of the gametes and secretion of gonadal hormones from either the ovaries or the testes. The release of LH in women stimulates ovulation and the formation of progesterone-secreting luteal cells in the ovary. The release of LH in men stimulates the interstitial cells (Leydig cells) to secrete testosterone.

The synthesis of **prolactin** by the lactotroph cells is regulated by PRF and PIF. The release of PRL stimulates the production of milk within the mammary glands. In addition, PRL plays a role in growth, osmoregulation, fat and carbohydrate metabolism, reproduction, and parenting behavior.

The somatotroph cell's production and secretion of **growth hormone** is controlled by the regulatory hormones GH-RH and stomatostatin. GH does not have a specific target organ. It is responsible for stimulating growth in almost all cells of the body, including bone, muscle, brain, and heart. GH promotes cell growth through somatomedins or growth factors. It is the somatomedins that mediate the effects of GH on growth.

Within the intermediate lobe of the anterior pituitary, the melanotroph cells synthesize and release *MSH* under the influence of MSH-RF and MSH-RIF. MSH's role in humans is not well understood. It stimulates the melanocytes located between the dermis and the epidermis of the skin to produce melanin. In addition, alpha-MSH appears to influence learning and memory.

Hormones Produced by the Posterior Pituitary Gland

The posterior pituitary gland is composed of neural tissue and represents an extension of the brain. The pituitary stalk contains the axons of neuronal cell bodies within the hypothalamus. The terminals of these axons are located within the posterior pituitary. The cell bodies are responsible for the synthesis of the two hormones released by the posterior pituitary gland, vasopressin and oxytocin. Following their synthesis in the cell bodies, these hormones are transported down the axons and stored in the axonal terminals. When the cell bodies are stimulated by the appropriate neurotransmitter, the hormones are released from the terminals and enter the bloodstream.

Vasopressin (antidiuretic hormone) is responsible for the regulation of blood pressure and water balance. An increase in plasma osmolality results in the release of vasopressin. In response to vasopressin, the kidney reabsorbs water and blood pressure rises. This concept is discussed further in Chapter 7.

Oxytocin promotes uterine contractions during the birth process and stimulates milk ejection from mammary glands during lactation. The stimulus for oxytocin release during the birth process is unknown. However, the stimulus for oxytocin release that stimulates milk ejection is the suckling of the breast.

THYROID GLAND

The **thyroid gland** *consists of two lobes located on either side of the neck* (Fig. 12–9). The structural unit of the thyroid is the follicle. The follicle is composed of a single layer of follicular epithelial cells surrounding the colloid, a secretory substance whose major constituent is thyroglobulin (Fig. 12–11).

Thyroid Hormones

The follicular epithelial cells synthesize and release the two most important hormones, T_4 and T_3, in response to TSH. The precursor substance for these hormones is the amino acid tyrosine, which is part of the thyroglobulin. Iodine is necessary for the synthesis of these hormones; T_4 contains four iodine atoms and T_3 contains three iodine atoms (Fig. 12–3). T_4 and T_3 are responsible for the body's metabolic activity, including the increase of energy production and an increase in the rate of protein synthesis.

The parafollicular cells are located within the interstitium and are responsible for the synthesis of calcitonin. *Calcitonin* is responsible for decreasing the reabsorption of calcium and phosphate from the bones to the blood, and thereby lowering the blood levels of these minerals. Through this process, calcitonin helps maintain a stable, strong bone matrix and

FIGURE 12-11

Microscopic appearance of the thyroid gland. The follicle is composed of colloid surrounded by follicular epithelial cells.
(From Guyton, A.C.: Textbook of Medical Physiology, 9th ed. Philadelphia, W.B. Saunders, 1996, with permission.)

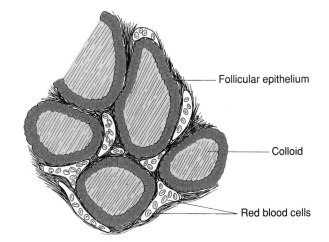

prevents the loss of these minerals from the bones until there is a real need. The presence of increased levels of calcium in the blood results in the secretion of calcitonin from the parafollicular cells.

PARATHYROID GLANDS

The **parathyroid glands** *are located on the posterior surface of the thyroid gland* (Fig. 12–9). Two parathyroid glands are present on each thyroid lobe. The hormone secreted by the parathyroid gland is **parathyroid hormone** (PTH). PTH has an antagonist role in the regulation of calcium in the blood. It serves to elevate blood calcium levels; therefore, it is secreted when blood calcium levels are low. PTH acts on the bones, small intestine, and kidneys. It promotes the reabsorption of calcium from the bone into the blood, increases the uptake of calcium from the small intestine, and increases the reabsorption of calcium from the kidney. Its overall effect is to raise blood calcium levels and lower blood phosphate levels. Calcitonin and PTH work together to maintain homeostasis of blood calcium and phosphate levels. Adequate blood calcium levels are essential for hemostasis and normal activity of neurons and muscle cells.

THYMUS

The **thymus** *gland is located in the upper chest cavity, below the thyroid gland* (Fig. 12–9). During fetal development and infancy, the thymus is large and active. In the adult, little thymic tissue is present since the thymus shrinks with increasing age. The principal thymic hormones are thymosin and thymostatin. **Thymosin** is responsible for the differentiation of pre-T lymphocytes into mature T lymphocytes, which are immunocompetent cells. Mature T lymphocytes are responsible for cell-mediated immunity. **Thymostatin** inhibits the development and differentiation of lymphocytes within the thymus.

PANCREAS

The **pancreas** *is located in the upper left quadrant of the abdominal cavity* (Fig. 12–9). The endocrine cells of the pancreas are the *islets of Langerhans*, which produce hormones that regulate blood glucose levels and maintain the blood glucose within normal range. There are three types of cells that make up the islets of Langerhans: alpha cells, beta cells, and delta cells. The *alpha cells* synthesize insulin, the *beta cells* synthesize glucagon, and the *delta cells* synthesize somatostatin.

Insulin *is a glycoprotein responsible for lowering the blood glucose level.* Insulin increases cellular uptake of glucose from the blood. A deficiency of insulin or lack of insulin receptors on cells leads to increased blood glucose levels (*hyperglycemia*).

Glucagon has the opposite effect on blood glucose levels. The secretion of glucagon causes the liver to convert glycogen to glucose (glycogenolysis), hence increasing blood glucose levels. Hypoglycemia stimulates the secretion of glucagon.

The release of **somatostatin** affects insulin levels by inhibiting insulin secretion. Therefore, elevated somatostatin levels will cause increased blood glucose levels (hyperglycemia). Somatostatin has other hormonal actions, including inhibition of gastrin, inhibition of the release of GH, and inhibition of the secretion of exocrine pancreatic enzymes.

ADRENAL GLANDS

The **adrenal glands** *are located on top of the kidneys* (Fig. 12–9). Each adrenal gland consists of two parts, the *adrenal medulla* and the *adrenal cortex*, which have well-defined functions.

Hormones Produced by the Adrenal Glands

The adrenal cortex is an *endocrine gland*. It is responsible for the production and secretion of adrenal steroid hormones. Steroid hormones fall into three categories: *glucocorticoids*, *mineralocorticoids*, and *sex steroids*. The adrenal cortex is composed of three distinct layers: zona glomerulosa, zona fasiculata, and zona reticularis (Fig. 12–12). The outer layer, or

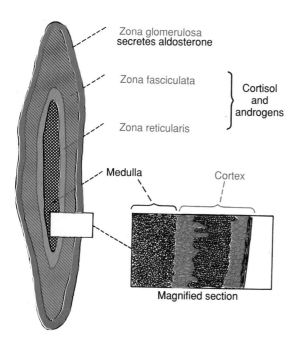

Zona glomerulosa secretes aldosterone

Zona fasciculata
Zona reticularis
} Cortisol and androgens

Medulla   Cortex

Magnified section

FIGURE 12-12

Adrenal gland. The adrenal cortex, which is composed of the zona glomerulosa, zona fasciculata, and zona reticularis, surrounds the adrenal medulla.
(From Guyton, A.C.: Textbook of Medical Physiology, 9th ed. Philadelphia, W.B. Saunders, 1996, with permission.)

zona glomerulosa, is the site of mineralocorticoid synthesis. The primary mineralocorticoid is **aldosterone**. The release of aldosterone is stimulated by decrease serum sodium levels. Aldosterone promotes the reabsorption of sodium in the kidneys. Aldosterone's action is discussed in detail in Chapter 7.

The middle layer of the adrenal cortex is the *zona fasiculata.* Within the zona fasiculata, glucocorticoid synthesis is stimulated by ACTH from the anterior pituitary gland. The principal glucocorticoid is **cortisol.** The glucocorticoids are responsible for regulating carbohydrate, fat, and protein metabolism. In addition, they have anti-inflammatory and immunosuppressive functions.

The *zona reticularis* represents the inner layer of the adrenal cortex. Glucocorticoids and minute amounts of **gonadal** (sex) **steroids** (androgen, estrogen, and progesterone) are synthesized in this layer. The adrenal sex hormones appear to influence sexual differentiation and bodily changes that occur at puberty.

The adrenal cortex surrounds the adrenal medulla. The chromaffin cells of the adrenal medulla more closely resemble nerve cells than endocrine cells. The adrenal medulla synthesizes *epinephrine* (adrenaline) and *norepinephrine* (noradrenaline), which are released in response to stimulation of the sympathetic nervous system and are not under hormonal influence. Epinephrine (EPI) is released following stress associated with environmental extremes, physical exertion, or fear. EPI acts to increase heart rate and blood glucose levels, thereby increasing the amount of work the muscles can do. Norepinephrine acts to increase blood pressure and constrict blood vessels.

TESTES

The **testes** *are located in the scrotum* (Fig. 12–9). *They secrete two hormones, testosterone and inhibin.* **Testosterone** is secreted by the interstitial cells (*Leydig cells*) when stimulated by LH from the anterior pituitary gland. Testosterone promotes the maturation of the sperm, a process that begins at puberty and continues throughout life. During puberty, testosterone stimulates the development of the male secondary sex characteristics, including growth of reproductive organs, growth of facial and body hair, growth of the larynx and deepening of the voice, and growth of skeletal muscles. Testosterone also stops growth of the long bones by promoting the closure of the epiphyseal discs of the long bones.

Inhibin is secreted by the sustentacular cells of the testes. Its release is stimulated by increased levels of testosterone. Inhibin decreases the secretion of FSH from the anterior pituitary gland. It is the interaction between the anterior pituitary hormones, testosterone, and inhibin that maintains spermatogenesis at a constant rate. The role of testosterone and inhibin in the reproductive system is discussed in detail in Chapter 13.

OVARY

The **ovaries** *are located in the pelvic cavity, one on either side of the uterus* (Fig. 12–9). *They produce the sex steroid hormones estrogen and progesterone.* **Estrogen** is produced by the follicle cells and released by the stimulation of FSH from the anterior pituitary gland. Estrogen promotes the maturation of the ovum within the ovarian follicle and stimulates growth of blood vessels in the endometrium in preparation for possible implantation of a fertilized egg. Estrogen also is responsible for the development of the female secondary sex characteristics, including development of the duct system within the mammary glands, uterine growth, and the deposition of fat subcutaneously in the hips and thighs. Growth is stopped by the action of estrogen on the epiphyseal discs of the long bones. Estrogen is also believed to have a beneficial effect by lowering serum levels of cholesterol and triglycerides, and thereby decreasing the risk of atherosclerosis and coronary heart disease.

Progesterone is secreted by the corpus luteum in response to stimulation by LH from the anterior pituitary gland. Progesterone promotes the storage of glycogen and continued growth of the blood vessels in the endometrium. The secretory cells of the mammary gland develop under the influence of progesterone. A detailed discussion of the roles of estrogen and progesterone in the reproductive system is found in Chapter 13.

OTHER ENDOCRINE GLANDS

There are a number of organs or body tissues that have an endocrine gland component. These include the kidneys, heart, stomach, duodenum, and placenta. The kidneys produce renin and erythropoietin. **Renin** acts as a catalyst in the conversion of angiotensinogen to angiotensin. The renin-angiotensin-aldosterone feedback system is responsible for maintaining plasma sodium balance. **Erythropoietin** *is a glycoprotein hormone that stimulates erythropoiesis (development of erythrocytes) in the bone marrow.*

Within the heart, the granular cells secrete *atrial natriuretic factor* (ANF). This hormone regulates blood pressure, blood volume, and the excretion of water, sodium, and potassium through its actions on the kidneys and adrenal glands. The role of ANF is discussed in more detail in Chapter 7.

Cells within the walls of the stomach produce and secrete gastrin in response to distention caused by the presence of food. **Gastrin** stimulates the release of hydrochloric acid from the parietal cells of the stomach, stimulates secretion of pancreatic enzymes, and increases intestinal motility. The duodenum secretes two hormones, secretin and cholecystokinin. Secretin release is stimulated by the movement of partially digested food into the duodenum. **Secretin** stimulates the secretion of pancreatic bicarbonate and plays a role in other functions involved in digestion, including stimulation of hepatic bile flow and the potentiation of cholecystokinin-stimulated pancreatic enzyme secretion. **Cholecystokinin** (CCK) is released by cells that line the duodenum in response to the presence of food, in particular fats and fatty acids. Like gastrin, CCK functions to stimulate gallbladder contraction, pancreatic enzyme secretion, and inhibition of gastric emptying. The role of these hormones is discussed in detail in Chapter 9.

The placenta produces several different hormones: *human chorionic gonadotropin* (hCG), *human placental lactogen* (hPL), *estrogens*, and *androgens*. hCG is released by the placenta to maintain the corpus luteum and progesterone production during early pregnancy. hPL is released by the placenta to promote growth and development of the mammary glands. The role of the placenta and its hormones is discussed in detail in Chapter 13.

PATHOLOGIC CONDITIONS ASSOCIATED WITH THE ENDOCRINE SYSTEM

PITUITARY GLAND DISORDERS

Gigantism

Gigantism *is a disorder seen in children that is caused by hypersecretion of GH.* In this condition, individuals experience excessive growth, and a height of greater than 8 feet may be observed. Typically, it is associated with an adenoma of the somatotroph cells of the anterior pituitary gland. In this disorder, although there is hypersecretion of GH, hyposecretion of other pituitary hormones also occurs. An increased level of GH is a common laboratory finding in gigantism. With early detection, the effects of GH can be minimized by surgical removal or irradiation of the tumor.

Acromegaly

Acromegaly *is the result of excessive GH production and release in the adult.* As in gigantism, the excess GH is the result of an adenoma of the somatotroph cells. Abnormal growth is associated with the hands, feet, and facial cartilage and soft tissue since the epiphyses of the long bones have been fused. The physical features are a prominent forehead, widened teeth, change in hat or glove size, and development of a husky voice. These features progress slowly and are frequently overlooked by the individual, the family, and the physician. Clinical features include headaches, sweating, weakness, lethargy, and disturbances in vision. Several complications have been observed in acromegaly, including atherosclerosis, hypertension, diabetes mellitus, and heart failure. Heart failure is a frequent cause of death.

Diagnosis of acromegaly is based on radiographic and laboratory studies. Radiographs or computed tomography scans reveal abnormalities in the sella turcica, the pocket where the pituitary sits, indicating the presence of an adenoma. Laboratory indicators of acromegaly include elevated levels of GH, insulin-like growth factor, or both. (*Insulin-like growth factor* is produced by the liver in response to GH stimulation.) As in the case of gigantism, treatment of acromegaly involves the elimination of the tissue producing the excess growth hormone through surgery or radiation therapy.

Dwarfism

Dwarfism is associated with decreased levels of GH. These decreased levels of GH may be the result of a deficiency in the release of GH-RH from the hypothalamus or a lack of synthesis or release of GH from the pituitary. In children, decreased levels of GH cause severe retardation of growth. Individuals are short but retain normal proportions. Dwarfism is not associated with abnormalities of intellectual development, unlike cretinism, a hypothyroidism that includes mental retardation. If hyposecretion of GH is associated with panhypopituitarism, other conditions will also be apparent, including lack of sexual development, hypothyroidism, and hypoadrenocorticism. As a result, hypoglycemia may be observed.

The diagnosis of dwarfism is based on clinical and laboratory findings. Laboratory testing includes the stimulation tests and insulin tolerance test, which are discussed later in this chapter. If isolated GH deficiency is diagnosed, it is treated with exogenous recombinant growth hormone. For panhypopituitarism, replacement therapy using those hormones stimulated by the missing pituitary hormones (i.e., thyroid hormones and adrenocortical hormones) is necessary.

DIABETES INSIPIDUS

Hyposecretion of antidiuretic hormone (ADH) results in *diabetes insipidus.* This condition is characterized by severe polyuria (10 to 12 L/day), excessive thirst, and polydypsia. Diabetes insipidus is a rare condition associated with the destruction of the posterior pituitary or hypothalamus secondary to neurosurgical procedures, tumors, trauma, a degenerative process, or an infiltrative process. The diagnosis of diabetes insipidus is based on clinical and laboratory findings. The laboratory test used in this diagnosis is the overnight water deprivation test, which assesses the patient's ability to concentrate urine. In a normal individual, the urine osmolality would be increased in excess of 800 mOsm/kg. An individual with hyposecretion of ADH would show failure to concentrate urine and the urine osmolality would be less than 800 mOsm/kg. Treatment of diabetes insipidus involves replacement therapy of ADH with arginine vasopressin or desmopressin (DDAVP).

THYROID DISORDERS

Graves' Disease

One of the most common forms of hyperthyroidism is Graves' disease. **Graves' disease** *is an immunologic disorder that affects thyroid hormone production.* Autoantibodies directed against the TSH receptors in the thyroid cells bind to those receptors and stimulate the synthesis and release of thyroid hormone. The incidence of Graves' disease in the United States is 0.4%, and it is six times more prevalent in women than in men. Clinical features are an enlarged thyroid gland (goiter), bulging eyes (exophthalamus), and pretibial edema. Symptoms associated with increased levels of thyroid hormones are nervousness, irritability, fatigue, heat intolerance, and weight loss.

Diagnosis of Graves' disease is based on clinical presentation and laboratory findings. Thyroid function is assessed by a panel of laboratory tests, including T_3, T_4, TSH, TRH stimulation, and thyroid-stimulating immunoglobulins. The results of the thyroid function tests in various thyroid diseases are found in Table 12–2.

Several modes of treatment exist: (1) eliminating excess thyroid tissue by surgery or radioiodine, (2) inhibiting thyroid hormone synthesis using thyroid-blocking drugs, (3) inhibiting thyroid hormone release, and (4) suppressing symptoms of hyperthyroidism.

Hashimoto's Thyroiditis

Hashimoto's thyroiditis *is the most common cause of hypothyroidism. This condition is associated with a massive diffuse infiltration of the thyroid by lymphocytes and the presence of autoantibodies directed against the thyroid tissue.* The net result is a destruction of the thyroid

Table 12–2 ■ Laboratory Results for Thyroid Function Tests in Selected Diseases of the Thyroid*

Disease State	Thyroid Function Tests				
	T_3	T_4	TSH	TRH	TSI
Graves' disease	Elevated	Elevated	Decreased	Blunted	Elevated
Hashimoto's thyroiditis	Decreased	Decreased	Elevated	Elevated	†
Cretinism	Decreased	Decreased	Elevated	Elevated	†

* Abbreviations: T_3, triiodothyronine; T_4, thyroxine; TSH, thyroid-stimulating hormone; TRH, thyroid-releasing hormone; TSI, thyroid-stimulating immunoglobulin
† not applicable.

gland. The incidence of Hashimoto's thyroiditis in the United States is 1 to 2%, with a high prevalence in women. The clinical findings are an enlarged thyroid gland (goiter), fatigue, slowing of mental and physical performance, change in personality, and cold intolerance. The clinical findings are the result of insufficient levels of thyroid hormones needed to maintain adequate metabolic activity at the cellular level. Severe hypothyroidism leads to myxedema, which is characterized by pallor, skin edema of the face and hands, and apathy.

The diagnosis of Hashimoto's disease is based on the clinical manifestations and laboratory findings. The results of the thyroid function tests are found in Table 12–2. Treatment of hypothyroidism is through thyroid hormone replacement, typically with L-thyroxine.

Cretinism

Cretinism is a result of thyroid hormone insufficiency in infancy. It may be acquired or congenital. Congenital hypothyroidism may be the result of (1) lack of a thyroid gland, (2) insensitivity of the thyroid gland to TSH, (3) rare enzymatic defects, or (4) thyroid dysfunction. Acquired cretinism is associated with lack of iodine in the diet. Lack of appropriate levels of thyroid hormones leads to mental retardation, dwarfism, and diminished sexual organ development. Clinical features include puffy face, open mouth with protruding tongue, hoarse cry, short thick neck, narrow forehead, and short legs. Early diagnosis of hypothyroidism in the newborn is imperative to prevent the physical and mental developmental problems associated with this condition.

All 50 states require screening of newborns for early diagnosis of hypothyroidism. The typical screening test is total T_4; TSH levels are used for confirmation. The entire thyroid function panel results are listed in Table 12–2. Treatment is accomplished by replacement therapy (e.g., thyroid hormone replacement).

DISORDERS OF THE PARATHYROID GLAND

Hypoparathyroidism

Hypoparathyroidism is usually detected in childhood, and is characterized by an inability to maintain serum calcium levels without calcium supplements. Decreased parathyroid function may be the result of accidental injury associated with thyroid or other neck surgery or idiopathic atrophy of the parathyroid. The clinical findings are manifestations of the hypocalcemia, including numbness and tingling of the extremities and around the mouth, muscle cramps, convulsions, irritability, emotional lability, and depression. If the calcium levels are less than 6 mg/dl, the patient will experience laryngeal stridor and grand mal seizures. The diagnosis is based on laboratory findings, including decreased calcium, increased phosphorus, and decreased PTH. Treatment is accomplished with calcium replacement.

Hyperparathyroidism

In hyperparathyroidism, there is excess production and release of PTH. The most common cause of primary hyperparathyroidism is a parathyroid tumor (e.g., parathyroid adenoma) or a response to decreased calcium levels observed in vitamin D deficiency and chronic renal disease. The excess blood calcium levels are the result of the demineralization of the bone by the lytic action of PTH. The clinical manifestations of hyperparathyroidism are the result of excessive blood calcium levels. The individual may present with weakness, fatigue, renal stones, other renal disease, peptic ulcers, pancreatitis, and bone pain. The central nervous system (CNS) may also be affected. The presence of mental status changes (e.g., easily confused, irritable) is indicative of CNS involvement. Hyperparathyroidism is typically found in adults.

The diagnosis of hyperparathyroidism is based on clinical and laboratory findings. Laboratory findings include an elevated serum calcium level, decreased serum phosphorus level, and elevated PTH level. Therapy for primary hyperparathyroidism is surgical removal of the parathyroid.

ADRENAL GLAND DISORDERS

Addison's Disease

Addison's disease represents a condition of primary adrenal insufficiency due to an autoimmune abnormality. The individual has circulating adrenal antibodies that destroy the adrenal cortex and lead to *hypocortisolism*. The majority of the adrenal cortex must be destroyed before symptoms will appear. The clinical features of hypocortisolism are weight loss, weakness, loss of appetite, nausea, irritability, and hypotension (low blood pressure). Acute adrenal insufficiency is a life-threatening condition that is precipitated by stress. Signs of acute adrenal insufficiency include hypotension, hypoglycemia, extreme weakness, epigastric pain, and coma. Without immediate therapeutic intervention, the individual may die.

Diagnosis of Addison's disease is based on clinical manifestations and laboratory studies. Changes associated with routine clinical chemistry tests are decreased serum sodium, decreased serum bicarbonate, decreased serum glucose, elevated potassium, and elevated blood urea nitrogen levels. Specific laboratory studies for Addison's disease would reveal decreased serum cortisol and elevated serum ACTH levels. The treatment protocol for Addison's disease is replacement therapy, including cortisol and fluids.

Cushing's Syndrome

Cushing's syndrome is the result of increased cortisol levels (*hypercortisolism*). There are four possible causes of hypercortisolism: (1) excessive production of cortisol by an adrenal adenoma or carcinoma, (2) excessive production of ACTH by a pituitary adenoma, (3) production of ectopic ACTH by a tumor of nonendocrine tissue, and (4) exogenous administration of cortisol. The classic features of Cushing's syndrome are a round, moon-shaped face with acne-like eruptions; weight gain in the face, neck, shoulders ("buffalo hump"), and abdomen; and purplish bruises. The individual may also complain of weakness, loss of strength, amenorrhea, impotence, and bone pain. As a result of Cushing's syndrome, the individual experiences a decreased ability to fight infections and poor wound healing.

Laboratory diagnosis of Cushing's syndrome includes measurement of serum cortisol levels, plasma ACTH levels, and 24-hour urinary free cortisol level. The dexamethasone suppression test is useful in differentiating pituitary adenoma from adrenal adenoma as the etiology. The typical results of these studies are found in Table 12–3.

Treatment of Cushing's syndrome involves elimination of the tissue causing the elevated cortisol level, such as surgical removal of the adrenal or pituitary tumor or radiation or chemotherapy to destroy the tissue.

Conn's Syndrome

Conn's syndrome *is a form of primary hyperaldosteronism.* The most common cause of Conn's syndrome is an aldosterone-secreting adrenal adenoma. The clinical findings are associated with the effects of the excess aldosterone. Hypertension is caused by sodium and water retention. Muscle weakness, electrocardiogram changes, glucose intolerance, polyuria, and polydypsia are the result of decreased serum potassium levels (hypokalemia).

Table 12–3 ■ **Laboratory Diagnosis of Cushing's Syndrome**

Laboratory Tests	Adrenal Adenoma	Pituitary Adenoma	Ectopic ACTH Production
Serum cortisol	Elevated	Elevated	Elevated
Plasma ACTH	Decreased	Normal to elevated	Normal to elevated
24-hr urinary free cortisol	Elevated	Elevated	Elevated
Dexamethasone suppression	No suppression	Suppression	No suppression

Laboratory diagnosis of Conn's syndrome includes decreased serum potassium, increased serum sodium, increased serum aldosterone, and increased urinary aldosterone levels. Conn's syndrome is treated by surgical removal of the tumor.

Pheochromocytoma

Pheochromocytoma *is a rare tumor of the adrenal medulla or sympathetic ganglia.* The tumor produces and releases large quantities of catecholamines (epinephrine and norepinephrine). The individual's clinical findings are hypertension, increased heart rate, tightness in the chest, headache, sweating, pallor, and nervousness. These findings correspond to the release of large quantities of catecholamines. Although pheochromocytoma may occur in any age group, it is more typical in the third to fifth decades of life.

Laboratory diagnosis involves identification of increased urinary excretion of catecholamines and catecholamine metabolites (metanephrine and vanillylmandelic acid). Pheochromocytoma is treated by surgical removal of the tumor.

DISORDERS OF THE PANCREAS

Diabetes Mellitus

The characteristic finding in diabetes mellitus is hyperglycemia. Hyperglycemia may result from a deficiency of insulin or an insulin insensitivity of the tissues. There are two major types of diabetes mellitus, type I and type II.

Type I diabetes mellitus, also referred to as **insulin-dependent diabetes mellitus (IDDM), is the result of an absolute deficiency of insulin.** IDDM represents approximately 10% of the diabetes mellitus cases and is usually diagnosed by age 20. The clinical features include weight loss, polyuria, polyphagia, hyperglycemia, glucosuria, ketonemia, and ketonuria. Individuals with uncontrolled type I diabetes mellitus may experience diabetic ketoacidosis, which may lead to coma and death. The complications of IDDM are cataracts, neuropathy, kidney disease, and atherosclerosis. Laboratory findings may include elevated blood glucose, presence of glucose in the urine (glucosuria), and presence of ketones in the blood, urine, or both (ketonemia and ketouria). Treatment is accomplished by administration of exogenous insulin.

Type II diabetes mellitus is also referred to as **non-insulin-dependent diabetes mellitus (NIDDM).** This is the most common form of diabetes mellitus, representing 90% of all cases, and is typically observed in individuals over the age of 40. NIDDM is the result of an underproduction of insulin or insulin insensitivity at the target tissues. The characteristic findings are hyperglycemia and glucosuria. Patients with NIDDM may develop some of the same complications associated with IDDM. However, NIDDM is not associated with ketonemia or ketouria. Treatment of NIDDM is restriction of caloric intake and weight loss. Some cases may require the use of hypoglycemic drugs to lower blood glucose levels.

Hyperinsulinemia

Hyperinsulinemia is the result of insulin-producing tumors of the pancreas (insulinomas). The insulinoma causes excessive or inappropriate release of insulin into the peripheral blood, resulting in decreased blood glucose levels. The symptoms are related to the low glucose levels in the brain. Individuals experience weakness, headache, blurred vision, fainting, convulsions, and coma. These episodes are precipitated by fasting. Laboratory diagnosis is based on the observation of low blood glucose levels and elevated plasma insulin levels following an overnight fast. The treatment of hyperinsulinemia is surgical removal of the insulinoma.

LABORATORY EVALUATION OF ENDOCRINE SYSTEM DISORDERS

Traditionally, laboratory investigation of endocrine abnormalities was performed by bioassays. Bioassays involved the exposure of a live animal or living tissue culture to the patient's serum or urine and the observation of a change that was characteristic of the hormone being assayed. An example of a classic bioassay was the hCG bioassay. In the hCG bioassay, a patient's urine was injected into a rabbit. After 48 hours, the rabbit's ovaries were observed for the formation of a corpus luteum, which is caused by an elevation of hCG. This was the basis of the early pregnancy test. Bioassays, however, are cumbersome and prone to many nonspecific interferences. They are not cost-effective for the clinical laboratory setting but are still useful in research investigations.

Today, immunoassays, stimulation tests, and suppression tests are used to evaluate the function of the endocrine system and its hormones. These procedures have fewer nonspecific interferences and are easily adapted to the clinical laboratory setting.

IMMUNOASSAYS

Immunoassays are based on the principle of antigen-antibody binding. In hormone testing, the hormone serves as the antigen and the antibody is a specific antibody directed against that hormone. In pregnancy testing, hCG produced by the patient serves as the antigen and anti-hCG in the assay kit serves as the antibody. Hormone levels are determined by identifying antigen-antibody binding and the amount of antigen-antibody complexes formed. Detection of antigen-antibody complexes is accomplished by several different techniques using a variety of labels or tags.

The first immunoassay technique, the radioimmunoassay (RIA), was developed in 1960 by Yalow and Berson. In the RIA, the specific antibody is tagged with a *radioactive isotope* (i.e., ^{125}I or ^{56}Co). In this test system, the patient's serum is incubated with the radiolabeled antibody. If the antigen is present, antigen-antibody binding will take place. The unbound radiolabeled antibody is removed and the quantitation of antigen-antibody complexes is determined by measuring the amount of radioactivity present using a *gamma counter*. Since the original RIA technique was introduced, other radiometric methods have been developed to improve sensitivity and specificity of the assay. These include the competitive protein-binding technique and immunoradiometric assay (IRMA).

Because of the restrictions on the use of radioactive substances, and other disadvantages associated with their use, radioimmunoassays have been replaced with other immunoassay methods. Instead of radioactive isotopes as labels, antigens and antibodies may be labeled with an enzyme. In *enzyme-labeled immunoassays*, the quantitation of antigen-antibody binding is based on the spectrophotometric determination of a color change. An example of an enzyme immunoassay is the enzyme-linked immunosorbent assay (ELISA). In the ELISA, the patient's hormone is bound to an enzyme-labeled antibody and the unbound enzyme-linked antibody is removed from the system. In order to detect antigen-antibody binding, a chemical substrate is added to the test system. The enzyme catalyzes a reaction involving the substrate from which a colored product is formed as a result of that reaction. The intensity of the color, measured by a spectrophotometer, is directly proportional to the amount of hormone present in the patient's serum.

Another label that has proven useful in hormone testing is the fluorescence label. Two popular fluorescent immunoassays are the substrate-labeled fluorescent immunoassay and the fluorescence polarization immunoassay. The common fluorescent label used in these immunoassays is fluorescein isothiocynate (FITC). Immunoassay methods are available for the determination of specific hormones of interest in the investigation of endocrine abnormalities. Most immunoassay methods have been adapted to automated instruments.

STIMULATION TESTS

In endocrine abnormalities, there are a number of potential reasons for a hormone's hyposecretion. The hormone's altered level may be the result of an abnormality at any point in its particular feedback loop. Stimulation tests are designed to help identify where in the feedback loop the problem lies.

The *ACTH stimulation test* is a good example. This stimulation test is useful in identifying the reason for a decreased serum cortisol level. In the ACTH stimulation test, the patient is given synthetic ACTH. In a normal individual, synthetic ACTH will stimulate the adrenal cortex to produce cortisol. Peak levels will be observed within 30 minutes. If the patient's decreased serum cortisol level is the result of adrenal insufficiency, synthetic ACTH stimulation will cause no significant increase in serum cortisol.

SUPPRESSION TESTS

Suppression tests assist in the identification of the cause of a hormone's hypersecretion. An example of a suppression test is the *dexamethasone suppression test*. This test is useful in identifying the cause of an elevated serum cortisol level. In the dexamethasone suppression test, the individual is given dexamethasone, a potent synthetic glucocorticoid. In a normal individual, dexamethasone will provide negative feedback to the anterior pituitary, resulting in decreased ACTH release. The decreased ACTH levels will feed back to the adrenal cortex and there will be decreased production of cortisol. Therefore, a normal individual will have decreased levels of serum cortisol following the dexamethasone suppression test. If the individual's elevated serum cortisol is the result of excess production by an adrenal tumor, the decreased ACTH levels will have no effect on the adrenal tumor and no suppression of serum cortisol will be observed. If the individual's elevated serum cortisol level is the result of excess production of ACTH by the anterior pituitary, dexamethasone will suppress serum cortisol levels. Therefore, the dexamethasone suppression test will allow differentiation of excess cortisol levels due to adrenal tumor, ectopic ACTH production, and pituitary production of excess ACTH.

CHAPTER SUMMARY

The endocrine system is one of the body's communication systems. From their synthesis within the various endocrine glands to their transport to target cells, hormones communicate the body's physiologic status and influence homeostasis. Endocrine abnormalities arise from excess production of a hormone (hypersecretion) or decreased production of a hormone (hyposecretion). An understanding of the feedback mechanism affecting the hormone's synthesis and release is necessary for the delineation of the cause of the abnormal hormone level. Laboratory evaluation provides critical data needed for this delineation. Immunoassays are used to determine hormone and hormone metabolite levels, while stimulation or suppression tests are used to identify the cause of the endocrine abnormality.

Review Questions

1. Cholesterol is the precursor substance for
   a. epinephrine
   b. thyroid-stimulating hormone
   c. testosterone
   d. insulin

2. Which hormones are released into the bloodstream by pinocytosis?
   a. norepinephrine and epinephrine
   b. thyroxine and triiodthyronine
   c. estrogen and progesterone
   d. oxytocin and cortisol

3. Which hormone's mode of action is through cAMP, a second messenger?
   a. aldosterone
   b. thyroxine
   c. cortisol
   d. prolactin

4. Growth hormone is synthesized and released by the
   a. hypothalamus
   b. pituitary
   c. adrenal cortex
   d. thyroid gland

5. Which abnormality is associated with excess production of thyroid hormones?
   a. Graves' disease
   b. Conn's syndrome
   c. cretinism
   d. acromegaly

6. The dexamethasone suppression test is useful in the diagnosis of
   a. Addison's disease
   b. pheochromocytoma
   c. Cushing's syndrome
   d. dwarfism

BIBLIOGRAPHY

Avery, D., and Dahl, K.: Bright light therapy and circadian neuroendocrine function in seasonal affective disorder. *In* Schulkin, J. (ed.): Hormonally Induced Changes in Mind and Brain. San Diego, Academic Press, 1993, p. 357.

Bennett, B.D., and Wells, D.J.: Endocrinology. *In* Bishop, M.L., Duben-Engelkirk, J.L., and Fody, E.P. (eds.): Clinical Chemistry: Principles, Procedures, Correlation, 3rd ed. Philadelphia, J.B. Lippincott, 1996, p. 399.

Blalock, J.E.: A molecular basis for bidirectional communication between the immune and neuroendocrine systems. Physiol. Rev. *69:*1, 1989.

Brown, G.M.: Day-night rhythm disturbance, pineal function and human disease. Horm. Res. *37:*105, 1992.

Brown, R.E.: An Introduction to Neuroendocrinology. Cambridge, England, Cambridge University Press, 1994.

Carson-Jurica, M., Schraeder, W.T., O'Malley, B.W., et al.: Steroid receptor family: Structure and function. Endocr. Rev. *11:*210, 1990.

Cavallo, A.: The pineal gland in human beings: Revelance to pediatrics. J. Pediatr. *123:* 843, 1993.

Donnelly, J.G.: Carbohydrates and alterations in glucose metabolism. *In* Bishop, M.L., Duben-Engelkirk, J.L., and Fody, E.P. (eds.): Clinical Chemistry: Principles, Procedures, Correlation, 3rd ed. Philadelphia, J.B. Lippincott, 1996, p. 293.

Dunn, A.J.: Psychoneuroimmunology for the psychoneuroendocrinologist: A review of animal studies of nervous system-immune system interactions. Psychoneuroendocrinology *14:*251, 1989.

Endres, D.B., and Rude, R.K.: Mineral and bone metabolism. *In* Burtis, C.A., and Ashwood, E.R. (eds.): Tietz Textbook of Clinical Chemistry, 2nd ed. Philadelphia, W.B. Saunders, 1994, p. 685.

Fajans, S.S., and Vinik, A.I.: Insulin-producing islet cell tumors. Endocrinol. Metab. Clin. North Am. *18:*45, 1989.

Friedman, M.H., and Lapham, M.E.: A simple rapid method for the laboratory diagnosis of early pregnancies. Am. J. Obstet. Gynecol. *21:*405, 1931.

Guyton, A.C.: Textbook of Medical Physiology, 9th ed. Philadelphia, W.B. Saunders, 1996.

Hall, N.R.S., and O'Grady, M.P.: Regulation of pituitary peptides by the immune system: Historical and current perspectives. Prog. Neuroendocrinimmunol. *2*:4, 1989.

Kaplan, L.A., and Pesce, A.J.: Clinical Chemistry: Theory, Analysis, and Correlation, 3rd ed. St. Louis, C.V. Mosby, 1996.

Karlsson, F.A., Kampe, O., Winquist, O., et al.: Automimmune endocrinopathies 5. Autoimmune disease of the adrenal cortex: Pituitary, parathyroid glands, and gastric mucosa. J. Intern. Med. *234*:379, 1993.

McDougall, R.: Graves' disease: Current concepts. Med. Clin. North Am. *75*:79, 1991.

Plata-Salaman, C.R.: Immunomodulators and feeding regulation: A humoral link between the immune and nervous systems. Brain Behav. Immun. *3*:193, 1989.

Sacks, D.B.: Carbohydrates. *In* Burtis, C.A., and Ashwood, E.R., (eds.): Tietz Fundamentals of Clinical Chemistry, 4th ed. Philadelphia, W.B. Saunders, 1996, p. 351.

Sakiyama, R.: Thyroiditis: A clinical review. Am. Fam. Physician *38*:227, 1993.

Whitley, R., Meikle, A.W., Watts, N.B., et al.: Endocrinology. *In* Burtis, C.A., and Ashwood, E.R. (eds.): Tietz Textbook of Clinical Chemistry, 2nd ed. Philadelphia, W.B. Saunders, 1994, p. 1645.

Whitley, R., Meikle, A.W., Watts, N.B., et al.: Endocrinology. *In* Burtis, C.A., and Ashwood, E.R. (eds.): Tietz Fundamentals of Clinical Chemistry, 4th ed. Philadelphia, W.B. Saunders, 1996, p. 617.

Wilson, J.D., and Foster, D.W. (eds.): Williams Textbook of Endocrinology, 8th ed. Philadelphia, W.B. Saunders, 1992.

Yalow, R.S., and Berson, S.A.: Immunoassay of endogenous plasma insulin in man. J. Clin. Invest. *39*:1157, 1960.

The Reproductive System

INTRODUCTION

EMBRYOLOGY OF THE GONADS

CENTRAL NERVOUS SYSTEM
CONTROL OF REPRODUCTION

THE MALE REPRODUCTIVE SYSTEM
Spermatogenesis
Hormonal Control of
  Spermatogenesis
Semen
Disorders of the Testes and
  Male Reproductive Tract

LABORATORY TESTING OF MALE
FERTILITY
Semen Testing
Other Male Fertility Tests

THE FEMALE REPRODUCTIVE
SYSTEM
The Oviduct
The Ovary
  Follicular development
  Abnormalities of ovarian
    function
The Uterus
Hormonal Control of the
  Menstrual Cycle

LABORATORY TESTS OF FEMALE
FERTILITY
Progesterone Withdrawal Test
Ovarian Function Tests

CHAPTER SUMMARY

REVIEW QUESTIONS

Objectives

1. Describe the embryology of the reproductive system for both men and women.

2. Explain the mechanism by which the central nervous system controls reproduction.

3. Describe the male reproductive tract.

4. Explain the phenomenon of spermatogenesis and its hormonal control.

5. Describe some common disorders of the male reproductive tract and causes of male infertility.

6. Describe the characteristics of a normal semen collection.

7. Describe laboratory diagnostic tests of male fertility.

8. Describe the female reproductive tract.

9. Describe ovarian follicular development, some common abnormalities of ovarian function, and tests of ovarian function.

10. Explain the hormonal control of the menstrual cycle.

11. Describe some common abnormalities of the menstrual cycle and laboratory tests of menstrual cycle disorders.

KEY TERMS

ova	seminiferous tubules	isthmus	menopause
spermatozoa	epididymus	fimbriae	corpus luteum
müllerian ducts	spermatocytes	infundibulopelvic ligaments	corpus albicans
wolffian ducts	spermatids	ovary	Turner's
Leydig cell	spermiogenesis	hilum	syndrome
müllerian inhibitory factor	androgens	stroma	amenorrhea
Sertoli cell	5'-dihydrotestosterone	primordial oocytes	nulliparous
labioscrotal folds	semen	primordial follicles	uterus
oocytes	azoospermic	granulosa cells	endometrium
pituitary-gonadal-	cryptorchidism	theca interna	follicular phase
hypothalamic axis	anorchia	theca externa	secretory phase
follicle-stimulating	Kallman's syndrome	menarche	zona pellucida
hormone	orchitis	follicular atresia	zygote
luteinizing hormone	varicocele	antrum	human chorionic
spermatogenesis	oviduct	stigma	gonadotropin

Introduction

Human reproduction is a highly synchronized phenomenon involving both the central nervous system and the endocrine glands. These two systems are intimately related and influence each other greatly. The hypothalamus is the major organ that coordinates and integrates patterns of emotional behavior and endocrine activity. Humans are able to reproduce all year long, and therefore the seasons have no effect on reproductive capacity. Men produce sperm throughout their reproductive lives, which begin at puberty, and the production of viable sperm is temperature sensitive. The testicles are therefore located outside the body, where they are maintained at 2° to 3° F below the body temperature. Each normal ejaculate contains over 100 million sperms, and even though only one sperm is required for fertilization, individuals with sperm counts less than 20 million/ml are known to be sterile. The production of sperm does not follow a cyclic pattern as we find in women. The reproductive life of a woman is restricted to the period between puberty and menopause. During each ovarian cycle, usually only one, and rarely more than one, egg is released. Additionally, hormones are released that prepare the uterine lining for pregnancy. There is a time-limited window within which implantation of a fertilized egg can occur.

Several defects of normal reproductive function can lead to infertility. In men, the defect may involve either the sperm count, the semen volume, the motility of the sperm, or the sperm's ability to penetrate an egg. In women, inability to ovulate or disorders of endometrial growth may lead to infertility. There are a number of laboratory tests that may be used to diagnose the cause of a couple's infertility.

EMBRYOLOGY OF THE GONADS

All female gametes, called **ova** *(singular: ovum) or eggs, contain identical sex chromosomes, termed the X chromosomes. The male gametes, however, are equally divided between the X chromosome– and Y chromosome–carrying* **spermatozoa** *(singular: spermatozoon), or sperms.* The sex of an individual is therefore determined at fertilization, by the genotype of the sperm. Although the genotype is set at this stage, sexual differentiation of the gonads and the internal and external genitals is an ongoing process until about the 12th week in the male and the 14th week in the female during the life of the embryo.

The most important period of human development is undoubtedly between weeks 4 and 8 of embryonic life, because it is at this time that the major internal and external organs start their development. This period, therefore, is a very critical time when exposure of the developing embryo to exogenous substances might lead to the development of congenital

270

malformations. Some of these substances include high doses of naturally occurring hormones or over-the-counter medicines. This is also the time when technically the developing individual could be referred to as an "embryo." After the eighth week, "fetus" is the preferred term.

During the fifth week of embryonic life, the sex organ becomes visible but is undifferentiated, and the embryo could potentially develop into either sex, depending on, and sometimes in spite of, its genotype. By the seventh week of intrauterine life, the embryo has two sets of reproductive tracts that extend from the gonads to the urinary tract. *One set, the* **müllerian ducts,** *can potentially develop into the female reproductive tract, consisting of the ovaries, the oviducts (fallopian tubes), and the uterus. The other set, the* **wolffian ducts,** *can potentially develop into the male reproductive system, consisting of the epididymus, the vas deferens, and the vesicles* (Figs. 13-1*A* and 13-1*B*). It is important to remember that at this point in the fetus's life it is capable of developing into either a male or a female.

The decision for the embryo to develop into a male, and therefore retain the testes, is first made by a specific gene (called *SRY*) found on the Y chromosome. In the presence of functional testes, two testicular secretions are produced: (1) testosterone, synthesized by the **Leydig cells;** and (2) the **müllerian inhibitory factor** (MIF), synthesized by the **Sertoli cells.** In response to the latter, the müllerian structures degenerate while the wolffian ducts complete their development. MIF acts alone to cause the regression of the female müllerian ducts but, together with testosterone, supports the development of the vas deferens and related internal structures of the male reproductive tract. Only testosterone is involved with the development of the external genitalia. It is a common occurrence for genetic females exposed to androgens during the fetal period to develop external male genitals. By the same token, genetic males who are deficient in testosterone production may have female external genitalia. After directing the completion of the internal and external male characteristics, testosterone production by the embryonic testis is switched off until shortly before the onset of puberty.

Unlike the male, female development is not contingent upon the presence of an ovary. The development of female characteristics, both internally and externally, begins once the *SRY* gene signal is not received (signifying the absence of the Y chromosome). Although the embryo may wait for an extra 2 weeks for the signal to arrive, the absence of the *SRY* signal causes the internal ducts always to develop along female lines whether or not the undifferentiated gonads have developed into ovaries. Externally, the development of the penis is repressed and the vestigial structure becomes the clitoris. The **labioscrotal folds** become organized as the minor and major labia in the female. The regression of the male wolffian ducts is completed by the end of the first trimester of pregnancy. The ovary begins its development right away so that, by the time a female baby is born, the ovary contains its full complement of **oocytes.** However, follicular maturation does not commence until the onset of puberty.

CENTRAL NERVOUS SYSTEM CONTROL OF REPRODUCTION

Every component of reproductive activity depends on an interplay of neural and endocrine events. The most obvious role of the brain or the central nervous system as it influences human sexuality is exemplified in courtship. However, the role of the central nervous system extends beyond that; it regulates the **pituitary-hypothalamic-gonadal axis** in such a way

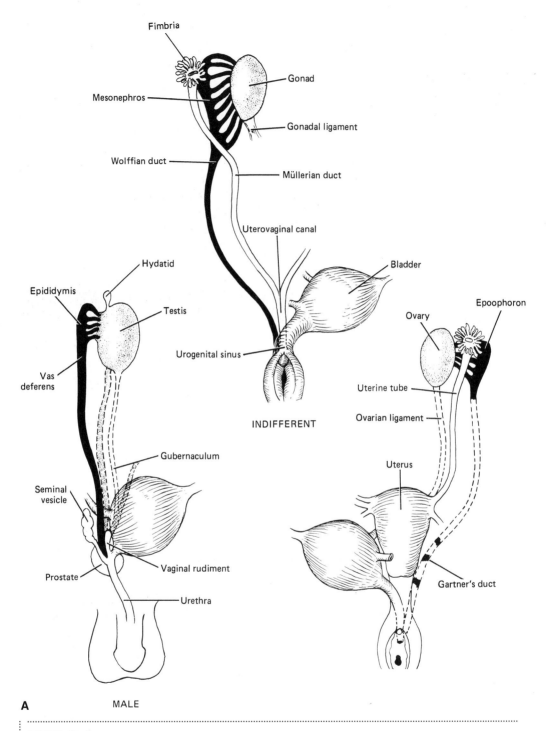

A   MALE

FIGURE 13-1

Embryonic differentiation of the male and female reproductive systems. *A*, Differentiation of the internal organs. *B*, Differentiation of the external genitalia. (From Ganong, W.F.: Review of Medical Physiology, 18th ed. Norwalk, CT, Appleton & Lange, 1997, with permission.) *Illustration continued on opposite page*

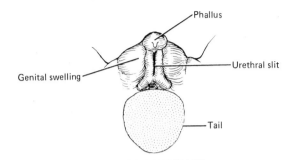

Phallus

Urethral slit

Genital swelling

Tail

INDIFFERENT STAGE

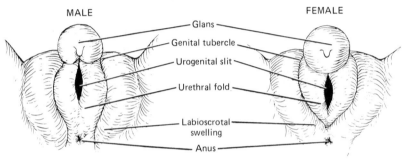

MALE   FEMALE

Glans

Genital tubercle

Urogenital slit

Urethral fold

Labioscrotal
swelling

Anus

SEVENTH TO EIGHTH WEEK

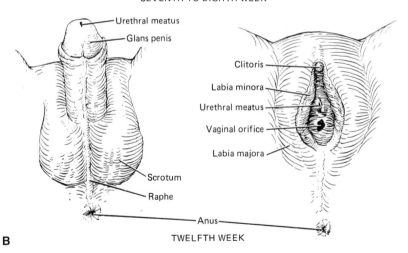

Urethral meatus

Glans penis

Clitoris

Labia minora

Urethral meatus

Vaginal orifice

Labia majora

Scrotum

Raphe

Anus

B   TWELFTH WEEK

FIGURE 13-1 *(Continued)*

as to integrate reproductive behavior with a viable reproductive cycle. It determines not only the onset of puberty, ovarian development, and the menstrual cycle but also the end of the reproductive life of a woman.

In response to neural signals, the hypothalamus produces a single releasing factor called gonadotropin-releasing hormone (GnRH), which controls the synthesis and release of the pituitary glycoprotein hormones **follicle-stimulating hormone** (FSH) and *luteinizing hormone* (LH). GnRH travels through the hypophyseal-portal venous system to the anterior pituitary, where it enhances the release of LH and FSH (Fig. 13–2). Although there may be overlap, it is now firmly established that each of these gonadotropins has specific roles and acts in distinct target cells in the reproductive system. FSH induces ovarian follicular maturation in women and catalyzes the conversion of testosterone to estradiol in both sexes. LH initiates **spermatogenesis** and stimulates the production of testosterone in men and induces ovulation and corpus luteum development in women. The sex steroids modulate the release of GnRH, and thereby LH and FSH, through a series of complex feedback mechanisms on the hypothalamus.

THE MALE REPRODUCTIVE SYSTEM

The testis lies in a thin membranous sac, the *tunica vaginalis*, formed by the perineum during descent from the abdominal cavity (Fig. 13–3*A*). The testis is encapsulated by a thick fibroelastic tissue that invades the testis, forming segments called septa and creating pyramidal lobules (Fig. 13–3*B*). Each lobule is made up of a series of convoluted **seminiferous tubules,** which are lined with primordial germ cells. Through the process of spermatogenesis, these germ cells are transformed into immotile sperm, which are carried in a fluid secreted by the Sertoli cells and drained into the *rete testis*. Near the top part of the testis, the sperm are carried by the efferent ducts to the caput (latin for "head") end of the **epididymis**. The sperm suspension undergoes concentration in the caudal (latin for "tail") end of the epididymis. Passage through the long epididymal tubes provides time for the sperm to mature and acquire the ability to fertilize an egg—a phenomenon called *capacitation*.

From the epididymides, the sperm pass into the vasa deferentia (singular: vas deferens) and, during ejaculation, peristaltic contractions propel the sperm along the tubes. Contractions of the prostate and Cowper's glands and the seminal vesicles provide the secretions that form the bulk of the ejaculate, which empties into the urethra, a single duct in the penis.

SPERMATOGENESIS

Although the fetal testes develop earlier than the fetal ovaries, no spermatogenesis takes place until shortly before adolescence. As puberty approaches, the germinal epithelium begins to respond to the pituitary hormones FSH and LH. The Sertoli cells in the testis nourish and support spermatogenesis and are under the control of FSH and testosterone. Scat-

FIGURE 13-2

Principal hormones that regulate the male and female reproductive systems.
(From Applegate, E.J.: The Anatomy and Physiology Learning System. Philadelphia, W.B. Saunders, 1995, with permission.)

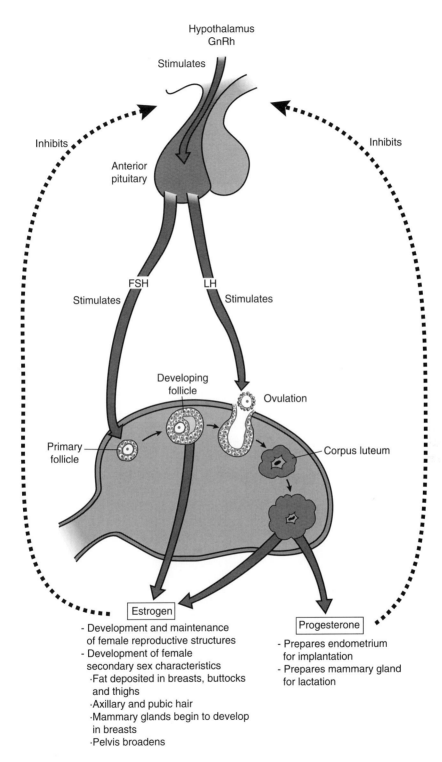

Hypothalamus
GnRh

Stimulates

Inhibits

Anterior
pituitary

Inhibits

FSH   LH

Stimulates   Stimulates

Developing
follicle

Ovulation

Primary
follicle

Corpus luteum

Estrogen

- Development and maintenance
  of female reproductive structures
- Development of female
  secondary sex characteristics
  ·Fat deposited in breasts, buttocks
   and thighs
  ·Axillary and pubic hair
  ·Mammary glands begin to develop
   in breasts
  ·Pelvis broadens

Progesterone

- Prepares endometrium
  for implantation
- Prepares mammary gland
  for lactation

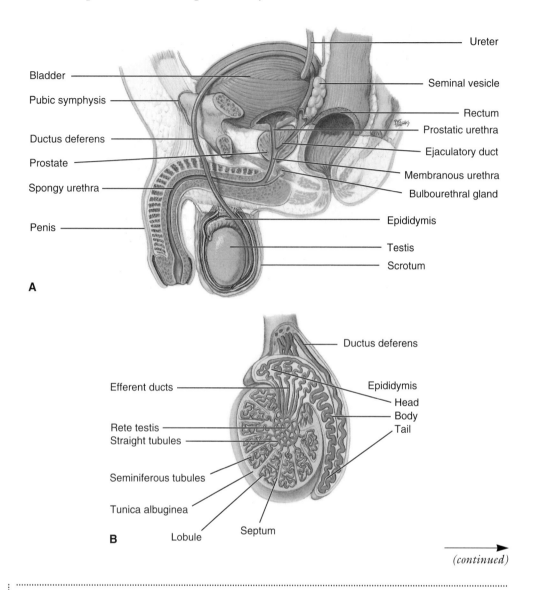

A, Structures that make up the male reproductive system. B, Sagittal section of a testis and epididymis. C, Schematic diagram of spermatogenesis.

(continued)

FIGURE 13-3

A, Structures that make up the male reproductive system. B, Sagittal section of a testis and epididymis. C, Schematic diagram of spermatogenesis.
(From Applegate, E.J.: The Anatomy and Physiology Learning System. Philadelphia, W.B. Saunders, 1995, with permission.) *Illustration continued on opposite page*

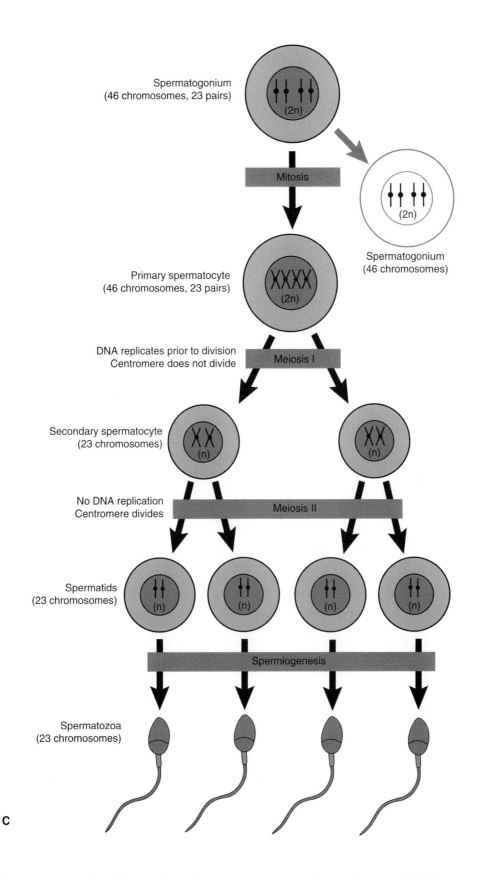

Spermatogonium
(46 chromosomes, 23 pairs)

(2n)

Mitosis

Spermatogonium
(46 chromosomes)

(2n)

Primary spermatocyte
(46 chromosomes, 23 pairs)

(2n)

DNA replicates prior to division
Centromere does not divide

Meiosis I

Secondary spermatocyte
(23 chromosomes)

(n)

(n)

No DNA replication
Centromere divides

Meiosis II

Spermatids
(23 chromosomes)

(n)

(n)

(n)

(n)

Spermiogenesis

Spermatozoa
(23 chromosomes)

C

tered in between the seminiferous tubules are the Leydig cells, which, in response to LH, synthesize and secrete testosterone. Under the control of these hormones, spermatogenesis commences after puberty with no sudden cessation of reproductive function, as is the case in women at menopause.

The whole process of spermatogenesis takes between 68 and 72 days. All stages of the phenomenon occur simultaneously in the seminiferous tubules; spermatogenesis does not follow a cyclic pattern. The process involves the maturation of a diploid (having a full set of chromosomes) spermatogonium through a series of mitotic divisions, giving rise to primary spermatocytes. These primary spermatocytes undergo the process of meiosis, giving rise first to secondary **spermatocytes** and then to **spermatids,** which now contain the haploid number of chromosomes (a half-set). *The morphologic and functional maturation of the spermatids into motile sperm is called* **spermiogenesis** (Fig. 13–3C).

HORMONAL CONTROL OF SPERMATOGENESIS

All steroid hormones are synthesized using cholesterol as precursor, and the biosynthetic pathway in all endocrine organs is essentially similar. The steroid hormones differ from one another only because of the different enzymes contained in the different cells in which they are produced. In addition to testosterone, the testis produces other **androgens** (e.g., androstenedione) and small amounts of estrogens. The spermatogenic function of the testis is under the control of FSH, which acts directly on the seminiferous tubules. Episodic LH production, in contrast, acts in the Leydig cells to stimulate testosterone production, which exerts a feedback on the hypothalamus to cause a reduction of pituitary LH, but not FSH. FSH is independently controlled by a substance called *inhibin*, secreted by the seminiferous tubules.

Testosterone has a *diurnal pattern*, with the peak level in the early morning and the trough level in the late afternoon or early evening. Testosterone, the daily output of which is about 4 to 9 mg in the normal adult man, may be metabolized by two different pathways. In the tissues that respond to testosterone (e.g., the prostate), the steroid is metabolized to a physiologically active metabolite called **5′-dihydrotestosterone** (DHT) as well as estradiol and androstanediol. Even though plasma DHT constitutes only about 10% of the plasma androgen levels, it is DHT, rather than testosterone, that is responsible for the development of the external genitalia and secondary sexual characteristics. Testosterone may also be metabolized in some tissues to produce a number of metabolites, such as androsterone, that are generally inactive or less active than testosterone itself. In the liver, the metabolites are converted into water-soluble compounds suitable for excretion by the kidney.

SEMEN

Semen *is a mixture of sperm and secretions from the Cowper's and prostate glands and the seminal vesicles.* An average ejaculate volume is 2 to 3 ml, containing approximately 100 millions sperm/ml and a variety of other components (Table 13–1). *Individuals with the complete absence of sperm in the semen are called* **azoospermics** *and are sterile.* It is still not fully understood why *oligospermics* (with sperm counts of less than 20 million/ml) and 40 to 50% of men with 20 to 40 million sperm/ml in their ejaculate are also relatively infertile, even though only one sperm is required to fertilize an egg.

Table 13–1 ■ Composition of Human Semen

General Characteristics

Color: White, opalescent

Specific gravity: 1.028

pH: 7.35–7.50

Sperm count: 100 million/ml (<20% abnormal forms)

Other Components

Seminal vesicles (60% of total volume)
Fructose (1.5–6.5 mg/ml)

Phosphocholine

Ascorbic acid

Prostaglandins

Prostate gland (20% of total volume)
Spermine

Citric acid

Phospholipids

Cholesterol

Acid phosphatase

Hyaluronidase

Buffers
Phosphate

Bicarbonate

DISORDERS OF THE TESTES AND MALE REPRODUCTIVE TRACT

During the normal fetal development of the male, the testes develop in the abdomen and spontaneously descend into the scrotum outside the body. *The failure of the testes to descend is referred to as* **cryptorchidism** *and is found in about 10% of newborn babies.* Because spermatogenesis is temperature sensitive, irreversible damage to the spermatogenic stem cells may take place, leading to sterility, if steps are not taken to correct the problem before puberty. Gonadotrophic treatment is effective in some cases, but the majority of the cases of cryptorchidism may require surgery. *Congenital* **anorchia** *is a rare disorder and a variant of* *cryptorchidism, in which both testes are missing in normal males with the 46,XY genotype.* As can be expected, congenital anorchism leads to a severe testosterone deficiency.

The cause of primary *testicular hypofunction* include abnormal testicular development as a result of chromosomal aberration or diseases of or injury to the testes, such as an infection, trauma, or a tumor. Testicular hypofunction may lead to failure of spermatogenesis and eventually sterility. The laboratory findings include increased serum gonadotropin (FSH, LH) levels. The substrates for androgen production may also be inadequate, or the testes may be unable to respond appropriately to the gonadotropins, and so decreased serum androgen levels are a common finding. Secondary testicular hypofunction may be caused by a disease of the pituitary gland (infection or tumor), leading to decreased levels of FSH and LH. In this case, although the testes are functionally normal, the low gonadotropin levels lead to decreased serum androgen levels. If testicular hypofunction begins prior to puberty, it prevents the development of secondary sexual characteristics. If the hypofunction occurs after puberty or in adulthood, then the secondary sexual characteristics may regress only slowly, and these changes may be less obvious: the deep voice may remain but there may be decreased beard and axillary hair growth.

The cause of a primary *testicular hyperfunction* may be a testicular tumor. An increase in the size of tissue that normally produces testosterone may result in increased androgen production and decreased serum pituitary gonadotropin levels. A secondary cause of testicular hyperfunction may be the inability of the hypothalamus to respond to circulating gonadotropins. In this case levels of serum androgens, as well as serum gonadotropins, may all be elevated. The increased production of androgens has little effect in adult men, but in prepubertal boys it may lead to sexual precocity (e.g., an enlarged penis) and early closure of the long bones, which invariably results in short stature.

LABORATORY TESTING OF MALE FERTILITY

The cause of infertility in about 25 to 40% of infertile men is *idiopathic* (no known identifiable cause). The causes that can be identified may be divided into pretesticular, testicular, and post-testicular factors. Pretesticular causes involve the hypothalamus, pituitary glands or both. For example **Kallman's syndrome** *is a hypothalamic disease that leads to an increased gonadotropin (FSH and LH) and a deficiency of GnRH.* Kallman's syndrome is second only to Klinefelter's syndrome as a cause of hypogonadism. The differential diagnosis includes delayed puberty. For cases involving the pituitary gland, the defect may involve production of LH, FSH, prolactin, or glucocorticoids. The incidence of primary endocrine defects in infetile men is less than 5%, and such defects are rare in men with a sperm concentration of greater than 5 million/ml.

Testicular causes of infertility include **orchitis** *and* **scrotal varicocele,** *which is the most common cause of infertility in men.* The post-testicular causes of infertility may involve disorders of (1) sperm production; (2) sperm transport; (3) sperm motility or function, such as capacitation; or (4) sexual dysfunction. In the latter, a decreased sex drive, erectile dysfunction, or failure of intromission may all play significant parts.

SEMEN TESTING

Technically, semen analysis is not a test of fertility, but when carefully performed it can provide some vital information on the functional status of androgen production, spermatogenesis, and the patency of the reproductive tract. The specimen must be assessed within 1 to 2 hours of collection. For the assessment of semen volume to be meaningful, it is important to remember that, with each day of abstinence (up to 1 week), semen volume increases by about 0.4 ml, sperm count by 10 to 15 million/ml, and the total sperm count by 50 to 90 million per ejaculate. Sperm motility and morphology appear to be unaffected by 5 to 7 days of abstinence, but longer periods lead to impaired motility. The minimum number of specimens to define good or poor quality of semen is three samples collected over a 6- to 8-week period with a consistent sexual abstinence of 2 to 3 days. Semen volume per se, however, affects fertility only when it falls below 2 ml (due to the inadequate buffering of vaginal acidity) or when the volume is greater than 5 ml.

By far, sperm motility is the single most important measure of semen quality and may be a compensatory factor in men with low sperm counts. Sperm motility is usually rated in two ways: the number of motile sperm as a percentage of the total, and the quality of forward progressive sperm movement (i.e., how fast and how straight the sperm swim). Ideally, at least 50% of the sperm should have good forward progression. The presence of leukocytes in semen should be noted because excessive leukocytes (> 1 million/ml) may indicate an infection that may contribute to reduced fertility.

If no sperm are observed in the semen, a qualitative test for fructose is performed. A low ejaculate volume and lack of fructose may suggest congenital absence of the vas deferens and seminal vesicles or obstruction of the ejaculatory ducts. Fructose is androgen dependent and is produced in the seminal vesicles.

OTHER MALE FERTILITY TESTS

Because of the episodic nature of LH secretion and its short half-life, a single LH determination is of very little use in testing for endocrine defects in infertile men. Testosterone is secreted episodically in response to LH pulses, and therefore has a diurnal pattern with an early morning peak. Serum FSH has a longer half-life; therefore, most clinicians request only FSH and testosterone levels, and the time of collection is important.

The *postcoital test* is used to assess the ability of sperm to penetrate and progress through cervical mucus. Cervical mucus is examined about 2 to 8 hours after intercourse at the time of expected ovulation. The presence of greater than 10 to 20 motile sperm per high-power field is generally accepted as a normal postcoital test, and the assumption is made that the semen and mucus are normal.

THE FEMALE REPRODUCTIVE SYSTEM

The female reproductive system is made up essentially of the ovaries, the oviduct (fallopian tubes), and the uterus (Fig. 13–4*A*).

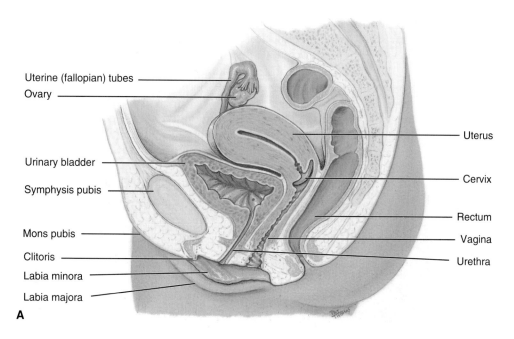

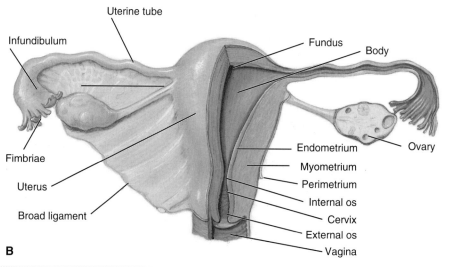

FIGURE 13-4

A, Structures that make up the female reproductive system. *B*, The oviduct or uterine tube. (From Applegate, E.J.: The Anatomy and Physiology Learning System. Philadelphia, W.B. Saunders, 1995, with permission.)

THE OVIDUCT

The **oviduct,** which is approximately 12 cm long, extends from the cavity of the uterus to the ovaries, where it opens up like a funnel (Fig. 13–4*B*). Structurally, the oviduct may be divided into four distinct segments:

- The intrauterine portion, referring to the portion embedded within the uterine wall.
- The **isthmus,** which is about 1 to 2 cm long, has the narrowest lumen, and is made up of a heavy muscular wall.
- The ampulla, which is 5 to 8 cm long.
- The infundibulum, which ends in tentacle-like structures called **fimbriae.**

The oviduct is lined by a mucous membrane of a single layer of columnar cells. The appearance of these cells changes with the menstrual cycle, indicating that they respond to hormones of the menstrual cycle. Some of the cells are secretory and others have cilia. The latter are believed to be used to sweep an egg or zygote down into the uterine cavity. The **infundibulopelvic ligaments** hold the fimbrae in place, close to the ovary.

THE OVARY

The **ovary** *is a complex, heterogeneous organ that, at the* **hilum,** *is penetrated by blood vessels, nerves, and the lymphatic vessels.* The ovary in the normal adult woman, which has a combined weight of about 14 g, contains several follicles in varying stages of maturation or degeneration. The ovary undergoes continuous differentiation, so that the morphology of the ovary changes considerably between birth and maturity of the individual. The ovary is a solid mass at birth and consists of basically two types of cells: (1) morphogenically undistinguished cells called **stroma** and (2) the more specialized **primordial oocytes,** in which development has been arrested at the prophase of the first meiotic cell division. The oocytes remain at this arrested stage until shortly before puberty, when a pulsatile release of GnRH from the hypothalamus causes the first ovulation. During this period when the oocytes are held in suspended animation, however, the ovary continues to grow in size, and the stroma becomes differentiated in association with the oocytes to form complex bodies called **primordial follicles,** which are embedded inside the ovary.

At birth, a primordial follicle is essentially "empty," being separated from the surrounding stroma by an inconspicuous but definite basal membrane (Fig. 13–5). It is the proliferation of the **granulosa cells** inside the primordial follicles that constitutes ovarian growth. The primary follicle, with only a single layer of granulosa cells, is about 40 μm in diameter. As it matures and acquires more layers of granulosa cells, it becomes a secondary follicle in which a distinct bilayer of cells organize themselves into the **theca interna** and **theca externa,** which surround the follicles. As follicular maturation proceeds, the follicles enlarge about 200- to 400-fold (from 40 μm to 10,000 to 20,000 μm) but the diameter of the oocytes increases only about 10-fold (from 15 to 20 μm to 150 μm).

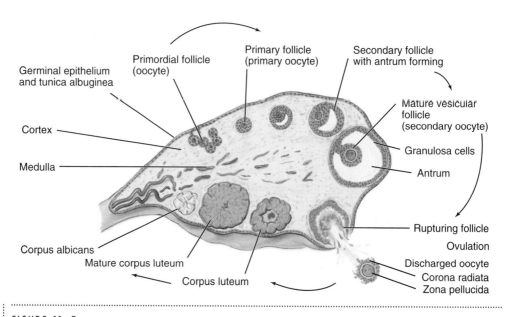

FIGURE 13-5

The ovary, showing the different stages in the development of the oocyte.
(From Applegate, E.J.: The Anatomy and Physiology Learning System. Philadelphia, W.B.
Saunders, 1995, with permission.)

Follicular Development

The time of the first menstruation (**menarche**) *is usually around 12 to 14 years of age, even though some girls may start menstruation as early as 9 or 10 years old.* At around this time, all maturing follicles undergo a degenerative process called **follicular atresia.** It has been estimated that 99.9% of all follicles present at birth are destined to degenerate. Fetal ovaries may contain over 800,000 potential eggs and, even though only about 400 of these may be released in a woman's reproductive lifetime, the ovaries may become depleted of eggs by the time she reaches menopause. One of the associated changes during the reproductive life of the female is the progressive decline in ovarian weight; at about the fourth decade of life the ovaries may weigh only about 5 g.

During the reproductive life, however, follicular maturation is the most conspicuous observation during the ovarian cycle. The primordial follicles increase in size and, as the granulosa cells increase, the innermost three or four layers become adherent to the ovum. As the follicle approaches maturity, a fluid-filled cavity called an **antrum** appears and the follicle forms a bulge from the surface of the ovary. It is at this point, called the **stigma,** that follicular rupture will occur and the egg will escape at ovulation. Follicular maturation is dependent on gonadotropic stimulation from the pituitary gland. That is why women whose follicular development is hampered can be made to ovulate with exogenous gonadotropic hormones (FSH and LH). The maturation events leading to ovulation may be completed in about 10 to 12 days.

Beginning with the menarche and continuing until **menopause,** one (rarely, more than one) out of a large number of maturing follicles may ovulate in a given cycle, with the remaining follicles undergoing follicular atresia. During the next 3 to 4 days after ovulation, capillaries invade the follicle and it becomes filled with a yellow carotenoid material and is referred to as a **corpus luteum.** The corpus luteum synthesizes the pregnancy-maintaining steroid called progesterone. If pregnancy does not take place, then the corpus luteum is transformed into a non-steroid-producing body composed of white scar tissue called the **corpus albicans,** and the cycle starts all over again.

Abnormalities of Ovarian Function

Normal ovarian function results in two major classes of products: steroid hormones and ova. The ovarian steroid hormones are estrogens (principally estradiol and estrone), progesterone, and androgens. The estrogens are produced largely during the follicular phase of the cycle, whereas progesterone is produced in large amounts during the luteal phase of the cycle. The androgens act principally as precursors for estrogen synthesis, when they stimulate the development of secondary sexual characteristics. During the reproductive life, they participate in gamete transport in the oviduct as well as preparing the endometrium for implantation of a fertilized zygote.

Defects in ovarian function may produce drastic effects in a woman. Ovarian estrogens not only affect the development of secondary sexual characteristics at puberty but, in combination with progesterone, may determine the woman's fertility. Laboratory tests of ovarian activity involve the measurement of estradiol and progesterone. Defects in ovarian function may be described as primary if the defect is at the level of the ovary itself. However, if the defect is primarily due to an aberration at a level other than the ovary, it is described as secondary. Primary *ovarian hypofunction* may be caused by abnormal ovarian development, as is seen in **Turner's syndrome** or during the normal process of menopause. Estradiol and progesterone levels are usually decreased, whereas FSH and LH levels are increased. Secondary ovarian hypofunction may be caused by a tumor or necrosis of the pituitary gland, in which case there may be decreased pituitary FSH and LH as well as ovarian estradiol and progesterone levels. If the reduced ovarian function begins prior to puberty, it may result in delayed or absent menarche. After puberty, it may result in secondary **amenorrhea.**

In the presence of an estrogen-producing tumor in the ovary, there is increased estradiol and decreased FSH and LH; this constitutes primary *ovarian hyperfunction.* Secondary ovarian hyperfunction may be idiopathic and results in sexual precocity in prepubertal girls. It is usual to find increased estradiol and elevated FSH and LH levels, revealing an inability of the pituitary gland to respond to the rising estradiol level. If ovarian hyperfunction occurs after puberty, it may cause irregular uterine or postmenopausal bleeding.

THE UTERUS

The uterus weighs 50 to 70 g in the female who has never borne a child (**nulliparous**), and weighs more than 80 g in the adult parous woman. It is supported in the abdominal cavity by a number of ligaments, some of which (e.g., broad ligaments) may in fact provide very little support but may enclose the vessels of the lymphatic and vascular system. *The* **uterus** *is a muscular organ located between the bladder and the rectum.* In pregnancy, the enlarging uterus squeezes on the bladder, explaining why pregnant women tend to urinate more frequently. The uterus is composed of three layers: (1) the peritoneum, the outer serosal layer; (2) a layer of smooth muscle; and (3) the endometrium. The **endometrium** responds to changes in ovarian steroids, which are carried to the uterus by two sets of minute arterial branches. Straight arterioles bring in nutrients to the basal layer of the endometrium, which is not shed during menstruation. It is from this layer that the endometrium regenerates itself after menstruation. The spiral or coiled arterioles supply the outer functional layer of the endometrium, respond to circulating ovarian hormones, and therefore participate in the mechanism of shedding off the functional endometrial layer during menstruation.

HORMONAL CONTROL OF THE MENSTRUAL CYCLE

Commencing at puberty and continuing until menopause, women undergo monthly reproductive cycles that prepare them for pregnancy. The rise of estrogen in the blood, produced predominantly by the developing follicles, exerts *positive feedback* on the amount of LH released by the pituitary gland. Unlike a negative feedback mechanism, the rising estrogen levels cause the LH levels to rise as well. In response to GnRH, both LH and FSH are released. These two gonadotropins produce cyclic changes in the ovaries, not only in terms of follicular maturation, but also on the steroid hormone synthetic capacity. It is now known that LH acts on the theca cells to produce androgens such as testosterone, which serve as substrates for granulosa cells to use for the production of estrogens under the stimulation of FSH. Therefore, the phenomenon of follicular maturation involves two cells, two gonadotropins, and two steroids.

The menstrual cycle may be divided into two distinct phases: the **follicular** *(proliferative) and* **secretory** *(luteal) phases* (Fig. 13–6). The follicular phase represents the first half of the menstrual cycle, which culminates with ovulation around day 14 or 15. Under the influence of FSH and LH, a number of follicles begin to mature, but only one follicle will be selected to suddenly undergo a growth spurt leading to follicular rupture at the stigma, expelling the ovum, which is surrounded by the **zona pellucida**. During the follicular phase, when the preceding month's corpus luteum ceases to function, estrogen and progesterone levels are relatively low and constant, and the LH level is low, but the FSH level is rising. This is responsible for stimulating the follicles to mature and synthesize estradiol. The increasing estradiol causes reduction in pituitary FSH release while it triggers a rise in LH through positive feedback. Estradiol reaches a maximum about a day before the LH peak, and it is now known that it is the fall in estradiol rather than the rise that triggers ovulation. That is why missing one day of the oral contraceptive pill will result in ovulation. After ovulation, the resulting corpus luteum produces progesterone, which is the predominant hormonal influence during the luteal phase of the cycle. Progesterone reaches a maximum about 8 to 9 days after the LH peak (days 23 to 25 of the cycle). As estradiol and progesterone levels increase, FSH and LH decline throughout the luteal phase.

The ovarian hormones estradiol and progesterone produce dramatic changes in the endometrium. The rising estradiol level during the follicular phase causes increased vascularity and starts the process of endometrial thickening. The continuity of the columnar cells of the epithelium is interrupted by crypts called *glands*, which are straight. During the first

FIGURE 13-6

The menstrual cycle.
(From Applegate, E.J.: The Anatomy and Physiology Learning System. Philadelphia, W.B. Saunders, 1995, with permission.)

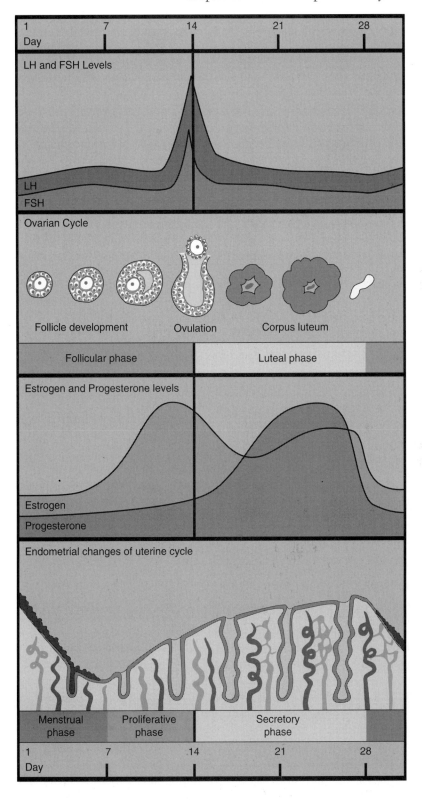

few days of the cycle, fertility is low because of the reduced and inadequate endometrial "ripening." During the luteal phase, progesterone stimulates further development of the glands, which now appear to be more tortuous and have increased secretory activity, hence the name secretory phase. To adequately prepare and enrich the endometrium, the secretory phase should be at least 10 to 14 days long. If a fertilized ovum (zygote) implants in the enriched luteal-phase endometrium, the resulting placental tissue synthesizes a new peptide hormone called **human chorionic gonadotropin** (hCG), which maintains the corpus luteum throughout pregnancy as a source of both estrogen and progesterone. If implantation does not occur, the progesterone-producing corpus luteum deteriorates toward the end of the cycle and is transformed into the corpus albicans, which does not produce hormones. The "progesterone withdrawal" leads to menstruation, which is provoked by vasoconstriction of the spiral blood vessels, restricting the blood supply to the endometrium. At the conclusion of menses, clotting factors seal off exposed bleeding sites, and the resumption of follicular development and estrogen production restores the endometrium. Menstruation, which takes 3 to 5 days, completes a menstrual cycle; during this period, only FSH levels may be elevated.

LABORATORY TESTS OF FEMALE FERTILITY

When it is determined that a couple's infertility is not due to the male partner, a series of tests may be conducted to ascertain what part of the female reproductive tract is defective. The tests are designed to determined if the woman can menstruate or ovulate. The failure of menstruation (amenorrhea) is a significant cause of infertility.

PROGESTERONE WITHDRAWAL TEST

The progesterone withdrawal test will confirm whether the uterus is capable of menstruating. Progesterone is administered over a 5- to 10-day period, and menstruation should take place in about 15 to 20 days, confirming that the ovaries are producing enough estrogen to build up the endometrial lining and that the uterus is capable of responding to estrogen and progesterone stimulation. In this case, the amenorrhea may be due to a failure of ovulation. However, ovarian function is modulated by hypothalamic-pituitary function. Two conditions must exist before the pituitary will release an LH surge: a responsive hypothalamus and the maturing ovarian follicles must release enough estradiol to induce the pituitary LH output.

If the progesterone withdrawal test is negative, the patient may be given a combined estrogen and progesterone test. If menstruation ensues, it proves that the uterus is capable of menstruating and the reason for the amenorrhea is that the ovaries may not be producing adequate amounts of estrogen. Serum estradiol may be measured to confirm this diagnosis.

Ovarian Function Tests

The failure to ovulate plays a significant role in infertility. The GnRH test is designed to assess the ability of the pituitary gland to respond to chemical signals coming from the hypothalamus. Administration of a synthetic GnRH should result in a rise in LH and FSH if the pituitary is responsive. The failure to observe an increase in FSH and LH elevation in response to GnRH is evidence of reduced pituitary function.

In some women, the failure to ovulate is due to weak signals between the hypothalamus and the ovary, principally the failure of the hypothalamus to produce a pulsating burst of GnRH. In the hypothalamic function test, an estrogen antagonist (clomiphene citrate) is administered; this blocks estrogen-induced negative feedback on GnRH release from the hypothalamus. The result is increased LH and FSH release. The inability to see a rise in these gonadotropins is indicative of a hypothalamic disease. Women with this kind of defect generally benefit from therapy with GnRH. GnRH is typically administered by intravenous or intramuscular injection.

Ovarian failure, resulting in the depletion of eggs, may be caused by a number of conditions, including infection, chemical toxins, medications, immunologic dysfunction, and genetic abnormalities. When this happens, the pituitary gland may produce increased FSH to force the ovary to manufacture estrogen and to ovulate. Although a few anovulatory women will have normal menstrual periods, most are amenorrhic. Women with anovulatory menstrual periods do not experience the typical menstrual discomforts often found in ovulatory women: breast soreness, mood swings, or cramping.

Elevated levels of various hormones can reveal the source of ovarian dysfunction. Excessive prolactin can suppress pituitary output (LH and FSH) and can act directly on the ovary to suppress follicular growth. Elevated FSH almost always indicates ovarian failure. In the presence of excessive hair (hirsutism) or male secondary sex characteristics (enlarged clitoris or ambiguous genitalia), elevated levels of testosterone, dehydroepiandrosterone sulfate (DHEAS), or adrenal androgens may indicate a congenital enzymatic defect, polycystic ovaries, or a tumor in the pituitary gland, adrenal gland, or ovary. Testosterone or adrenal androgens can suppress ovulation.

CHAPTER SUMMARY

Human reproduction is a highly synchronized phenomenon that requires every part of the system to work properly before a fertilized egg can implant in a well-nourished endometrium. The implantation event itself can occur only within a small window of opportunity during the menstrual cycle. An imbalance in the interplay of these events can lead to infertility, and there are many tests available to diagnose where the defect might be located, be it in the male or female reproductive system. The window of opportunity refers not only to the implantation event but also to female reproductive function as a whole. Female fertility is restricted to only the period between puberty and menopause, whereas male reproductive function is not limited after puberty. Synchronization of the cycles and the limited reproductive function of women is due primarily to the action of hormones produced by the endocrine glands, which are themselves controlled by the nervous system. Therefore, the failure of reproduction may lie at any of these locations in the body.

Review Questions

1. Describe the mechanism by which the hypothalamus controls the phenomenon of reproduction.

2. Describe how hermaphrodites may be produced.

3. Describe the role of the various hormones in the menstrual cycle as it prepares for pregnancy.

4. For the infertile man and woman, what laboratory tests may be performed to determine where an abnormality exists?

BIBLIOGRAPHY

Albert, A.: The mammalian testis. *In* Young, W.C. (ed.): Sex and Internal Secretions, Vol I, 3rd ed. Baltimore, Williams & Wilkins, 1961, p. 305.

Baker, H.W.G., Bremner, W.J., Burger, H.G., et al.: Testicular control of follicle-stimulating hormone secretion. Recent Prog. Horm. Res. *32*:429, 1976.

Blyth, B., and Duckett, J.W., Jr.: Gonadal differentiation: A review of the physiological process and influencing factors based on recent experimental evidence. J. Urol. *145*:689, 1991.

Franchimont, P., Chari, S., Hazee-Hagelstein, M.T., et al.: Evidence for existence of inhibin. *In* Troen, P., and Nankin, H.R. (eds.): The Testis in Normal and Infertile Men. New York, Raven Press, 1977, p. 253.

Ghirardini, G., Tridenti, G., Vadora, E., et al.: Human reproduction and a D.D.D. (determination, differentiation, development) pathogenetical classification of genital anomalies in phenotypic females. Acta Eur. Fertil. *21*:257, 1990.

Graves, J.A., and Short, R.V.: Y or X—which determines sex? [news]. Reprod. Fertil. Dev. *2*:729, 1990.

Hutson, J.M., Williams, M.P., Fallat, M.E., et al.: Testicular descent: New insights into its hormonal control. Oxford Rev. Reprod. Biol. *12*:1, 1990.

Irvine, D.S., and Aitken, R.J.: Seminal fluid analysis and sperm function testing. Endocrinol. Metab. Clin. North Am. *23*:725, 1994.

Jensen, T.K., Toppari, J., Keiding, N., et al.: Do environmental estrogens contribute to the decline in male reproductive health? Clin. Chem. *41*:1896, 1995.

Johnson, L.A.: Sex preselection by flow cytometric separation of X and chromosome-bearing sperm based on DNA difference: A review. Reprod. Fertil. Dev. *7*:893, 1995.

Jost, A., Vigier, B., Prepin, J., et al.: Studies on sex differentiation in mammals. Recent Prog. Horm. Res. *29*:1, 1973.

Lee, V.W.K., Keogh, E.J., Burger, H.G., et al.: Studies on the relationship between FSH and germ cells: Evidence for selective suppression of FSH by testicular extracts. J. Reprod. Fertil. Suppl. *24*:1, 1976.

Mastroianni, L., Jr.: Forty years of infertility management—exponential progress and demanding future. Nurse Pract. Forum *7*:87, 1996.

McNatty, K.P., Sawer, R.S., and McNeilly, A.S.: A possible role for prolactin in control of steroid secretion by the human Graafian follicle. Nature *250*:653, 1974.

Motta, P.M., Nottola, S.A., Familiari, G., et al.: Ultrastructure of human reproduction from folliculogenesis to early embryo development: A review. Ital. J. Anat. Embryol. *100* (4):9, 1995.

Orgebin-Crist, M.-C., Danzo, B.J., and Davies, J.: Endocrine control of the development and maintenance of sperm fertilizing ability in the epididymis. *In* Hamilton, D.W., and Greep, R.O. (eds.): Handbook of Physiology, Sect. 7: Endocrinology, Vol. 5: Male Reproductive System—Male. Baltimore, Williams & Wilkins, 1975, p. 319.

Pauerstein, C.J., Eddy, C.A., Croxatto, H.D., et al.: Temporal relationships of estrogen, progesterone, and luteinizing hormone levels to ovulation in women and infrahuman primates. Am. J. Obstet. Gynecol. *130*:876, 1978.

Ross, L.S., and Niederberger, C.S.: Male infertility: Diagnosis and treatment. Compr. Ther. *21*:276, 1995.

Scheele, F., and Schoemaker, J.: The role of follicle-stimulating hormone in the selection of follicles in human ovaries: A survey of the literature and a proposed model. Gynecol. Endocrinol. *10*:55, 1996.

Simpson, J.L.: Disorders of gonadal development in humans. Arch. Biol. Med. Exp. *22*:1, 1989.

Stansberry, J.: The infertile couple: An overview of pathophysiology and diagnostic evaluation for the primary care clinicians. Nurse Pract. Forum *7*:76, 1996.

Van Blerkom, J.: The influence of intrinsic and extrinsic factors on the developmental potential and chromosomal normality of the human oocyte. J. Soc. Gynecol. Invest. *3*:3, 1996.

Vekemans, M., Delvoyc, P., L'Hermite, M., et al.: Serum prolactin levels during the menstrual cycle. J. Clin. Endocrinol. Metab. *44*:989, 1977.

Yen, S.S.C., and Lein, A.: The apparent paradox of the negative and positive feedback control system on gonadotropin secretion. Am. J. Obstet. Gynecol. *126*:942, 1976.

Yen, S.S.C., Tsai, C.C., Naftolin, F., et al.: Pulsatile patterns of gonadotropin release in subjects with and without ovarian function. J. Clin. Endocrinol. Metab. *34*:671, 1972.

Yen, S.S.C., Vela, P., Rankin, J., et al.: Hormonal relationships during the menstrual cycle. JAMA *211*:1513, 1970.

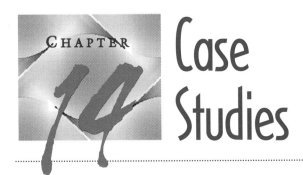

CHAPTER

14

Case Studies

Answers to the case studies can be found in Appendix B at the back of this book.

CASE STUDY 1

A 65-year-old white man is admitted to the hospital with myalgia, severe headache, and a stiff neck. Physical findings show that the patient is lethargic and febrile. The physician suspects meningitis with associated bacteremia and requests the following tests: CBC, blood culture, and lumbar puncture for CSF aspiration to include leukocyte count, protein and glucose levels, and bacterial culture.

The following laboratory results are obtained:

- CBC shows increased leukocyte count; other parameters within normal reference ranges
- Blood culture: growth
- CSF WBC: 1,200 cells/μl (reference range: adult, 0–5/μl)
    Protein: 150 mg/dl (reference range: 20–40 mg/dl)
    Glucose: 35 mg/dl (reference range: 45–60 mg/dl)
    Culture: growth

Questions

1. Define the following terms:
    myalgia   bacteremia
    meningitis   lethargy
    lumbar

293

2. Why was a lumbar puncture requested on this patient?

3. In which area of the laboratory would the following tests be performed?
   Blood and CSF culture
   CSF protein and glucose levels
   CBC and CSF cell count

4. Explain why the glucose level is decreased and the protein level is elevated.

CASE STUDY 2

A 12-year-old child presents to the emergency room with abdominal pain, fever, nausea, and vomiting. The child also reports a few diarrheal episodes. On physical examination, the child's abdomen is tender, particularly in the lower right quadrant.

The following laboratory results are obtained:

- Leukocyte count $12.0 \times 10^9/l$
- Cell differential: 85% neutrophils
                     10% bands
                     5% lymphocytes
- Urinalysis: normal

Questions

1. Based on the anatomic location of the pain, what organ could possibly be affected?

2. Why is the child febrile?

3. Give the significance of the leukocyte count and differential results.

4. What risks may be involved in this condition if it is not immediately treated?

CASE STUDY 3

A four-year-old girl underwent a physical examination after arriving in the United States with her parents. The doctor noted an abnormal gait. She measured 40 inches in height and 35 lbs. She had an enlarged head, a marked abdominal protuberance, and bowing of the legs. Apart from the distinct muscular weakness, she appeared to be in good health. The following is a partial list of the laboratory results.

Analyte	Value	Reference range
Calcium (S)	9.4 mg/dl	8.5–10.5
Phosphorus (S)	2.0 mg/dl	3.6–6.2
Alkaline phosphate (S)	1647 U/l	100–330
1,25 (OH) vitamin D_2 (S)	92.6 pg/ml	20–40
25 (OH) vitamin D	7.1 ng/ml	15–45
PTH (S)	123 pg/ml	<65

Questions

1. What are the important clues you picked up from this case?

2. What do you suspect the child is suffering from?

3. What is the source of the serum alkaline phosphatase?

4. What is the importance of the elevated levels of the 1,25-dihydrovitamin D in the blood?

5. Can her condition be treated or is it too late to treat?

CASE STUDY 4

A 45-year-old obese woman comes to the physician complaining of polydypsia, weight loss, and polyuria. Family history includes a father who had an acute myocardial infarction at age 60 and a diabetic grandmother. The physician requests a routine chemistry profile, a urinalysis, and a CBC. The CBC and chemistry results are all within normal reference ranges except for glucose, which is elevated. The urine shows 2+ glucose and trace protein.

Questions

1. Define the following terms:
   polydypsia
   polyuria

2. Based on the chemistry results, what condition do you suspect?

3. What is the underlying cause of this disease?

4. What follow-up tests might be performed to confirm the diagnosis?

5. List two complications that may develop if the disease is not treated.

6. Why is the urine glucose test positive?

CASE STUDY 5

A 25-year-old mother of two presents to the physician with complaints of diarrhea, back pain, nausea, and vomiting. On physical examination, she is febrile and slightly jaundiced. Further examination reveals hepatomegaly. She denies hematemesis. The physician requests laboratory tests to rule out hepatitis, pancreatitis, and food poisoning. Laboratory test results rule out pancreatitis and hepatitis. Stool examination shows leukocytes. The culture grows *Salmonella* species.

Questions

1. Define the following terms:
   hepatomegaly
   pancreatitis
   hematemesis
   hepatitis

2. Why did the physician suspect this group of conditions?

3. What laboratory test(s) would be used to rule out pancreatitis?

4. Name two laboratory tests that might have elevated results in hepatitis.

5. What is the significance of isolating *Salmonella* species from the stool? How does this relate to the presence of leukocytes in the stool?

CASE STUDY 6

A 23-year-old man complains of fever, dysuria, polyuria, and lower back pain. The physician suspects a urinary tract infection and orders a complete urinalysis (UA) and complete blood count (CBC). The CBC shows a normal hemoglobin level but an elevated leukocyte count. The UA results are positive for nitrite, protein, and leukocyte esterase. Microscopic examination of the urine shows numerous leukocytes and casts, and many bacteria.

Questions

1. Define the following terms:
   dysuria
   polyuria

2. Explain which of the clinical symptoms support the diagnosis of a urinary tract infection.

3. What is cystitis?

4. What urinalysis results confirm the diagnosis of urinary tract infection? Explain.

5. Explain why the leukocyte count is elevated. What specific leukocyte would be present in increased numbers in this patient?

CASE STUDY 7

A 10-year-old boy has been experiencing diarrhea for the last 3 days. He has severe abdominal cramping but no nausea or vomiting. He also has no fever. Antidiarrheal medication has not relieved any of the symptoms. He has not eaten anything for the last 2 days and has not increased his liquid intake. His family has traveled to Mexico within the last 2 weeks and stayed for 10 days. The doctor requests bacterial stool culture and an examination of the stool for ova and parasites (O&P). The stool culture grew no significant bacterial pathogens. The O&P demonstrated the presence of *Entamoeba histolytica*.

Questions

1. How is this organism transmitted?

2. What complication may arise with infection by this organism?

3. Name two bacterial pathogens and two other parasites that may cause diarrheal illnesses.

CASE STUDY 8

A 50-year-old obese white man is admitted to the cardiac intensive care unit with complaints of crushing chest pains that radiate into his left arm, mild nausea, and dyspnea. The patient states that the pain is similar to previous episodes of angina, only worse. He has a history of diabetes, elevated cholesterol, hypertension, and atherosclerosis. The patient is placed on a cardiac monitor.

The following test results are obtained:

- Blood pressure: 180/100 mm Hg
- Pulse: 100 beats/min
- CBC: within normal limits
- Chemistry profile: elevated cholesterol and cardiac enzymes
- ECG: shows changes consistent with acute myocardial infarction (AMI)

Questions

1. Define the following terms:
   dyspnea
   hypertension
   myocardial infarction
   angina
   atherosclerosis

2. Which value in the blood pressure is the systolic reading? Diastolic? Explain what each indicates.

3. List three cardiac enzymes that would be tested for in a suspected AMI.

4. Describe how this patient's elevated cholesterol levels contributed to his coronary disease.

CASE STUDY 9

A 4-year-old girl is examined by her pediatrician for a harsh cough and fever that has persisted for 2 days. Her mother states she thinks that the child has a cold because of the cough and congestion. The child's breathing is labored and she appears slightly hypoxic, with slight cyanosis of the nail beds.

The following test results are obtained:

- CBC: elevated leukocyte count with an increased number of bands and segmented neutrophils
- Blood gases: slight decrease in the partial pressure of oxygen and carbon dioxide
- Chest radiograph: abnormal infiltrate of the left lower lobe
- Sputum Gram's stain: gram-positive diplococci

She is diagnosed with pneumonia and admitted to the hospital for treatment.

Questions

1. Define the following terms:
   hypoxia
   pneumonia
   cyanosis

2. List two common bacterial agents of pneumonia.

3. What is the significance of the elevated leukocyte count and cell differential?

4. What is the purpose of a bacterial culture of the sputum?

CASE STUDY 10

A 25-year-old woman is seen in the emergency room. She complains of painful urination and also states that she feels as if she has to urinate all the time. A midstream "clean catch" urine specimen is collected for a routine urinalysis and culture.

The following urinalysis results are obtained:

- Physical exam:
    Color: yellow
    Clarity: cloudy
    Specific gravity: 1.015

■ Chemical exam:

pH: 6.0   Glucose: negative
Bilirubin: negative   Ketones: negative
Blood: 1+   Protein: trace
Urobilinogen: normal   Nitrite: positive
Leukocyte esterase: positive

■ Microscopic exam:

5–10 RBC/hpf   Moderate bacteria
20–30 WBC/hpf   Few squamous epithelial cells

Questions

1. Based on these results, what is the most likely diagnosis? Explain which values are significant in the diagnosis.

2. List four reasons that a urine specimen may have a cloudy or turbid appearance.

3. How are most infections of this type acquired? What is the most common organism identified upon urine culture?

4. What would you suspect if this patient also had leukocyte casts present?

CASE STUDY 11

A 30-year-old woman is admitted to the hospital complaining of decreased urinary output, weight gain, and puffy eyes in the morning. Upon examination, it is noted that she also has a mild edema around her ankles and abdomen. Routine blood work revealed hypoproteinemia and hyperlipidemia.

The following urinalysis results are obtained:

■ Physical exam:

Color: straw
Clarity: hazy
Specific gravity: 1.010

■ Chemical exam:

pH: 6.0   Glucose: negative
Protein: 4+   Bilirubin: negative
Ketones: negative   Blood: 1+
Urobilinogen: normal   Nitrite: negative
Leukocyte esterase: negative

■ Microscopic exam:

2–5 RBC/hpf   3–5 hyaline casts/lpf
Few squamous epithelial cells   0–2 waxy casts/lpf
Few oval fat bodies   2–5 fatty casts/lpf

Questions

1. Define the following terms:
   hypoproteinemia
   hyperlipidemia
   edema

2. Explain how casts are formed in the urinary tract.

3. What is the significance of the presence of fatty casts and waxy casts in the urine?

4. What is the most likely diagnosis for the patient based on the blood and urinalysis results?

CASE STUDY 12

A 38-year-old woman is admitted for diagnostic evaluation. She has a history of irregular menses, but currently has amenorrhea. Her chief complaints are easy fatigability and muscle weakness. Physical examination reveals an obese individual with lean arms and legs. The physician notes a nontender hump between her back and neck. Her face appears moon shaped.

The following laboratory results are obtained:

	Patient results	Reference range
Serum cortisol	716 nmol/l	138–635 nmol/l
Serum ACTH	1.0 pmol/l	2.2–18.7 pmol/l
24-hr urinary free cortisol	400 nmol/24 hr	27.6–276 nmol/24 hr

Questions

1. What medical term describes the serum cortisol result?

2. Based on the patient's history, physical examination, and laboratory findings, what is the presumptive diagnosis?

3. What additional laboratory procedure would be appropriate?

CASE STUDY 13

A patient presents with complaints of nausea, anorexia, malaise, and an upper right quadrant tenderness. She does not appear to be icteric. Her travel history includes a trip to Mexico in the last 3 weeks, where she lived with a local family. She drank their water and ate meals with them. The physician suspects hepatitis and ordered a chemistry profile, CBC, and hepatitis profile.

Questions

1. Define the following terms:

    icteric   anorexia

    hepatitis   malaise

2. Which of the hepatitis viruses does the physician suspect? Why?

3. Which of the chemistry profile results would you expect to be abnormal?

4. How would the physician confirm his initial diagnosis using the hepatitis profile results?

CASE STUDY 14

A 42-year-old man visits an infertility clinic after it is determined that a fertility problem may not lie with his wife. On examination, he is found to have a decreased beard and he has never developed underarm hair. He had a testicular problem as a child.

Questions

1. What test should the doctor order?

2. What results would you expect?

CASE STUDY 15

A 17-year-old boy is seen at a neighborhood health clinic. His chief complaints are a lack of energy, slight fever, and sore throat. The physician's examination reveals a well-nourished teenager who appears lethargic and has slight cervical lymphadenopathy.

The following laboratory results are obtained:

	Patient results	Reference range
Erythrocyte count	$5.12 \times 10^{12}/l$	$4.40–5.90 \times 10^{12}/l$
Hemoglobin	14.2 g/dl	13.3–17.7 g/dl
Hematocrit	43%	40–52%
Leukocyte count	$14.9 \times 10^9/l$	$3.9–10.6 \times 10^9/l$
Platelet count	$234 \times 10^9/l$	$150–440 \times 10^9/l$
Leukocyte differential		
Segmented neutrophil	35%	54–62%
Lymphocyte	56%	20–40%
Monocyte	8%	4–10%
Eosinophil	1%	1–3%

Comment: The majority of the lymphocytes are reactive lymphocytes.

Questions

1. What medical term describes the leukocyte count?

2. What are three possible conditions associated with an elevated leukocyte count?

3. Based on the patient's history, physical examination, and laboratory findings, what is the presumptive diagnosis?

4. What additional laboratory procedure would confirm the diagnosis?

CASE STUDY 16

A 28-year-old woman is seen for a routine prenatal examination. During her examination, she complains about being unusually tired. This is her second pregnancy in 2 years, and she does not recall that she required the same amount of rest during her first pregnancy. Her physician is concerned about this complaint and orders a complete blood cell (CBC) examination.

The following laboratory results are obtained:

	Patient results	Reference range
Erythrocyte count	$3.28 \times 10^{12}/l$	$3.80–5.20 \times 10^{12}/l$
Hemoglobin	7.5 g/dl	11.7–15.7 g/dl
Hematocrit	25%	35–47%
Leukocyte count	$7.6 \times 10^9/l$	$3.5–11.0 \times 10^9/l$
Platelet count	$378 \times 10^9/l$	$150–440 \times 10^9/l$
Leukocyte differential		
Segmented neutrophil	60%	54–62%
Lymphocyte	35%	20–40%
Monocyte	5%	4–10%

Erythrocyte morphology: The erythrocytes appear hypochromic and microcytic.

Questions

1. What medical term describes the patient's erythrocyte count?

2. What condition is associated with a decreased erythrocyte count, hemoglobin, and hematocrit?

3. Based on the patient's history and laboratory findings, what is the presumptive diagnosis?

4. If a blood sample is sent to the clinical chemistry laboratory for a serum iron procedure, what would you expect the patient's result to be (decreased, increased, or normal)?

CASE STUDY 17

A 40-year-old woman is admitted for diagnostic evaluation. Her chief complaints are heart palpitations, heat intolerance, and fatigue. The patient also states that her husband is concerned about her recent weight loss and her increased irritability. On physical examination, the physician notes exophthalamus (bulging eyes) and an enlarged thyroid gland (goiter).

The following laboratory results are obtained:

	Patient results	Reference range
T_3	4.13 nmol/l	1.54–3.08 nmol/l
T_4	200 nmol/l	65–155 nmol/l
TSH	0.14 mIU/l	0.32–5.0 mIU/l

Questions

1. What medical term describes the T_3 and T_4 results?

2. Based on the patient's history, physical examination, and laboratory findings, what is the presumptive diagnosis?

3. Which cells of the thyroid are responsible for the synthesis of T_3 and T_4?

4. What is the precursor substance for T_3 and T_4?

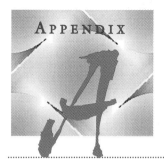
Answers to Review Questions

REVIEW QUESTIONS—CHAPTER 3

1. Specialized areas in microbiology include parasitology, virology, mycology, and mycobacteriology.

2. Glucose testing is performed in the clinical chemistry section.

3. Compatibility testing is used to determine if the unit of blood from a donor is compatible with blood of a patient who is about to receive a transfusion. The test involves mixing a small amount of the patient's serum with a small amount of the erythrocytes from the donor's unit.

4. Hematology is the area in the laboratory where complete blood cell counts, coagulation studies, and body fluid examinations are performed. These tests are important in the diagnosis of disease states such as anemia, leukemia, bleeding disorders, infections, and other malignancies.

REVIEW QUESTIONS—CHAPTER 4

1. Desired units are deciliters (10^{-1}), existing units are milliliters (10^{-3}). The calculation is $-3 - (-1) = -2$; $10^{-2} = 0.01$; $220 \times 0.01 = 2.2$ dl; *or*

$$\frac{220}{1{,}000} = \frac{x}{10}$$
$$1{,}000x = 2{,}200$$
$$x = 2.2$$

Therefore, 220 ml is equal to 2.2 dl.

2. Desired units are milligrams (10^{-3}), existing units are grams (10^{0}). The calculation is $0 - (-3) = 3$; $10^3 = 1{,}000$; $0.01 \times 1{,}000 = 10$ mg; *or*

$$\frac{0.01}{1} = \frac{x}{1,000}$$
$$1x = 10$$

Therefore, 0.01 g are equal to 10 mg.

3. Calculation:

$$75 - 32 = 43$$
$$43 \times 0.556 = 23.9$$

Therefore, 75° F is equal to 23.9° C.

4. A mole is the molecular weight of a substance, referred to as the gram molecular weight of that substance; it contains 6.02×10^{23} particles of the substance. A mole of a compound is equal to the total of the molecular weights of each substance and is referred to as the formula weight.

5. Calculation for a:

$$M = \frac{g/l}{MW}$$

$$M = \frac{60 \text{ g}/0.3 \text{ l}}{40 \text{ g}}$$
$$40 \text{ M} = 60 \text{ g}/0.3 \text{ l}$$
$$40 \text{ M} = 200$$
$$M = 5$$

Therefore, 60 g of NaOH in 300 ml water is a 5.0M (or mol/l) solution.

Calculation for b:

$$M = \frac{112 \text{ g}/0.7 \text{ l}}{233 \text{ g}}$$
$$233 \text{ M} = 112 \text{ g}/0.7 \text{ l}$$
$$233 \text{ M} = 160$$
$$M = 0.7$$

Therefore, 233 g of $BaSO_4$ in 700 ml buffer is a 0.7M solution.

6. Calculation for molarity:

$$M = \frac{50 \text{ g}/0.5 \text{ l}}{58 \text{ g}}$$

$$M = \frac{100}{58}$$
$$M = 1.7$$

Calculation for normality:

$$N = \frac{mol/l}{eq\ wt}$$

$$N = \frac{50\ g/0.5\ l}{eq\ wt}$$

$$equivalent\ weight = \frac{MW}{equivalents}$$

$$eq\ wt = \frac{58}{1} = 58$$

$$N = \frac{100}{58}$$

$$N = 1.7$$

Calculation for percent (w/v):

$$50\ g/500\ ml = 10\ g/100\ ml$$
$$percent\ w/v = 10\%$$

Therefore, for a solution of 50 g of NaCl in 500 ml of distilled water, the molarity is 1.7, the normality is 1.7, and the percent w/v is 10%.

7. Calculation:

$$\frac{3}{100} = \frac{6}{x}$$
$$3x = 600$$
$$x = 200$$

Therefore, 200 ml of a 3% solution can be made if 6 g of solute are available.

8. Calculation:

$$N = \frac{100\ g/0.45\ l}{eq\ wt}$$

$$equivalent\ weight = \frac{MW}{equivalents}$$

$$eq\ wt = \frac{98}{2} = 49$$

$$N = \frac{222.2}{49}$$

$$N = 4.5$$

Therefore, 100 g of H_2SO_4 in 450 ml of buffer is a 4.5N (or eq/l) solution.

9. (a) The formula for calculating the molarity of a substance in solution is

$$\frac{number\ of\ grams\ of\ solute}{liter\ of\ solution} \div the\ gram\ molecular\ weight$$

10. (a) The formula for calculating the equivalent weight of a compound is

$$\frac{\text{gram molecular weight}}{\text{\# of replaceable hydrogens or valence}}$$

11. Calculation:

$$0.1 + 5 + 4.9 = 10$$
$$0.1 \text{ in } 10 \text{ is equal to } 0.1:10$$
$$\frac{0.1}{10} = \frac{1}{x}$$
$$0.1x = 10$$
$$x = 100$$

Therefore, the dilution of 0.1 ml of serum in 5 ml of reagent and 4.9 ml of water is 1:100.

12. The Henderson-Hasselbalch equation is:

$$pH = pK + \log \frac{[HCO_3^-]}{[H_2CO_3]}$$

13. Calculation:

$$\frac{\text{Absorbance}_{unk}}{\text{Absorbance}_{std}} \times \text{Concentration}_{std} = \text{Concentration}_{unk}$$

$$\frac{0.03}{0.018} \times 4.0 = 6.7 \text{ g/dl}$$

Therefore, the protein concentration of a sample with an absorbance of 0.03, if the standard concentration is 4.0 g/dl and the absorbance of the standard is 0.018, is 6.7 g/dl.

14. Calculation:

$$\frac{s}{x} \times 100\% = CV$$

$$\frac{7.0}{89} \times 100\% = 7.9\%$$

Therefore, the coefficient of variation when one standard deviation (s) equals ± 7 mg/dl and the mean is 89 mg/dl is 7.9%.

15. (a) In a Gaussian distribution, the $\pm 2s$ range includes 95.5% of the values.

16. Calculation:

$$\frac{100 + 120 + 150 + 140 + 130}{5} = \bar{x}$$
$$128 = \bar{x}$$

Therefore, the mean of the values 100, 120, 150, 140, and 130 is 128.

17. (b) The formula for standard deviation is

$$\text{square root of } \frac{\text{(sum of squared differences)}}{n-1}$$

18. Calculation:

Glucose values (in mg/dl): 109, 102, 104, 97, 105, 98, 100, 96, 103, 97, 96, 97, 97, 104, 99, 105, 94, 95, 97, 100.

$$\text{Mean} = \frac{\text{sum of values}}{\text{number of values}}$$

$$\frac{1,995}{20} = 99.75$$

Mode is the value occurring with the greatest frequency, 97.
Median is the value that lies in the middle of the values when they are arranged in increasing magnitude, 98.5.

$$\text{Standard deviation} = \sqrt{\frac{\Sigma(x-x_i)^2}{n-1}} = \frac{317.7}{19} = 16.72 = 4.1$$

$$CV = \frac{s}{x} \times 100\%$$

$$= \frac{4.1}{99.75} \times 100\%$$

$$= 4.1\%$$

Therefore, for the values listed, the mean is 99.75, the mode is 97, the median is 98.5, the standard deviation is 4.1, and the coefficient of variation is 4.1%.

REVIEW QUESTIONS—CHAPTER 5

1. The musculoskeletal system provides three basic functions: movement, support and protection. The bones of the system have been variously modified to form joints across which muscles attach and allow movement. The bones in the spinal column provide points of attachment for anchoring the muscles of the body. Additionally, the bones are modified to form the skull, the rib cage, and the spinal column to provide protection for the delicate organs such as the brain, heart, and the spinal cord.

2. A joint is the junction formed when ligaments attach muscles across individual bones. The knee is the largest joint in the body.

3. The apparently inert bone is actually the major determinant of blood calcium levels.

4. The presence of elevated levels of CK and LD enzymes in the blood is indicative of damage to any number of tissues in the body and so their isoenzymes are measured to determine which specific tissues are damaged.

5. There are three main classes of muscles in the body: cardiac, skeletal (striated) and smooth. Their classification is based predominantly on their physical location in the body and appearance.

REVIEW QUESTIONS—CHAPTER 6

1. The three major types of blood vessels are:

   ■ The arteries that are responsible for carrying blood away from the heart.

   ■ The veins that are responsible for carrying blood from the tissues to the heart.

   ■ The capillaries that service the tissues. The capillaries allow the transfer of nutrients to the tissues and the removal of metabolic byproducts from the tissue.

2. The respiratory system is responsible for

   ■ The movement of air in and out of the lungs

   ■ Exchange of oxygen and carbon dioxide between the air in the lungs and the blood

   ■ Transport of oxygen and carbon dioxide by the blood

   ■ Exchange of oxygen and carbon dioxide between the blood and the tissues

   ■ Utilization of oxygen in cellular metabolism

3. Infectious conditions associated with the cardiopulmonary system include the following:

   ■ Rheumatic heart disease: a complication that results from a previous group A streptococcal infection

   ■ Bacterial endocarditis: bacteria colonizes the interior lining of the heart

   ■ Pneumonia: acute inflammation of the lungs that causes a fibrous exudate produced within the alveoli

The most common bacterial agent of pneumonia in adults is *Streptococcus pneumoniae*. Noninfectious conditions associated with the cardiopulmonary system include the following:

   ■ Myocardial infarction, or heart attack: when the cardiac muscle is deprived of blood for a period of time that leads to tissue death

   ■ Stroke: caused by decreased blood flow to a portion of the brain resulting in tissue death

   ■ Arteriosclerosis: hardening of the arteries when atherosclerotic plaques become calcified

REVIEW QUESTIONS—CHAPTER 7

1. (a) Urine flows through the nephron in the following order: Bowman's capsule, proximal convoluted tubule, loop of Henle, distal convoluted tubule, collecting duct.

2. (d) Reduction is not a function of the nephron.

3. (b) The structure that conducts urine from the bladder to the kidney is the ureter.

4. (c) Renin, which is produced by the juxtaglomerular apparatus, regulates blood pressure through its action on angiotensin.

5. (d) The primary constituent of urine is water.

6. (a) Bacteriuria is not characteristic of chronic renal failure.

7. (a) A strong ammonia odor in urine is caused by the breakdown of urea by bacteria.

8. (d) The creatinine clearance test is considered to be the most sensitive indicator of renal function.

REVIEW QUESTIONS—CHAPTER 8

1. Definitions:

diarrhea:	abnormal increase in stool liquidity and frequency, usually accompanied by abdominal discomfort and pain
febrile:	having increased body temperature; feverish
hepatomegaly:	enlargement of the liver
pancreatitis:	inflammation of the pancreas
nausea:	sensation that usually culminates in vomiting
jaundice:	yellowish discoloration of the skin, mucous membranes, and whites of eyes
hepatitis:	inflammation of the liver

2. The enzymes responsible for digesting these substances are

Starch:	(b) amylase
Lipids:	(c) bile
Proteins:	(a) trypsin

3. (c) Peristalsis is the involuntary wave-like contraction of the gastrointestinal tube that propels food through the digestive system.

4. (b) Absorption of nutrients during digestion occurs primarily in the small intestine.

5. (c) Inflammation of the gallbladder is referred to as cholecystitis.

REVIEW QUESTIONS—CHAPTER 9

1. (c) The conversion of glucose to glycogen is called glycogenesis.

2. (c) Bilirubin is a breakdown product of hemoglobin.

3. (c) Acute HBV.

4. (d) Urine bilirubin is increased; urine urobilinogen is decreased.

REVIEW QUESTIONS—CHAPTER 10

1. (c) Microglia play a major role in protecting the CNS from infection.

2. (d) Gray matter is composed of unmyelinated neurons.

3. (b) The reticular formation is not part of the diencephalon.

4. (c) Cerebrospinal fluid is formed primarily in the ventricles.

5. (d) The spinal cord is responsible for transmitting messages back and forth between various parts of the body and the brain.

6. (d) The correct order of the layers of the meninges from outside in is dura mater, arachnoid mater, pia mater.

7. (b) This laboratory picture is most consistent with a bacterial infection.

8. (a) These results are most likely due to a traumatic tap.

9. (b) Xanthochromia in a centrifuged sample of CSF is a good indication of subarachnoid hemorrhage.

10. (c) The tubes should be distributed as follows: tube 1—chemistry; tube 2—microbiology; tube 3—hematology.

REVIEW QUESTIONS—CHAPTER 11

1. (d) Hematopoiesis is not performed by the blood.

2. (a) The neutrophil is responsible for the phagocytosis of bacteria.

3. (c) The eosinophil is characterized by a segmented nucleus and the presence of large red-orange granules in the cytoplasm.

4. (b) The thymus is responsible for the differentiation and maturation of pre-T lymphocytes into immunocompetent T lymphocytes.

5. (a) Splenic "culling" refers to the spleen's ability to remove senescent erythrocytes by phagocytosis.

6. (c) Acute leukemia is associated with an increased leukocyte count and the presence of 30% or more blasts in the bone marrow.

7. (c) The factor assay is not considered a coagulation screening test.

REVIEW QUESTIONS–CHAPTER 12

1. (c) Cholesterol is the precursor substance for testosterone.

2. (a) Norepinephrine and epinephrine are released into the bloodstream by pinocytosis.

3. (d) Prolactin's mode of action is through cAMP, a second messenger.

4. (b) Growth hormone is synthesized and released by the pituitary.

5. (a) Graves' disease is associated with excess production of thyroid hormones.

6. (c) The dexamethasone suppression test is useful in the diagnosis of Cushing's syndrome.

REVIEW QUESTIONS–CHAPTER 13

1. The hypothalamus secretes GnRH, which stimulates the anterior pituitary gland to produce LH and FSH. In men, these hormones control the production of testosterone and sperm; in women, they stimulate the maturation of ovarian follicles.

2. Hermaphrodites, or persons with ambiguous genitalia, may be produced due to improper processing of chemical signals to the developing fetus within a time-limiting window. This is usually between weeks 8 and 12 of gestation.

3. Estradiol is involved with endometrial growth. After ovulation, progesterone becomes the dominant hormone that further prepares the endometrium for blastocyst implantation. Progesterone is the pregnancy-maintaining hormone.

4. The following laboratory tests may be performed to determine the location of an abnormality.

   ■ Hypothalamic function test. Administration of an estrogen antagonist should lead to a rise in pituitary gonadotropin levels. A negative response indicates defective hupothalamic function.

   ■ Pituitary function test. Administration of synthetic GnRH should produce a rise in FSH and LH in normal individuals. Failure to produce increased levels of these gonadotropins indicates a pituitary disorder.

   ■ Testicular function test. Injection of hCG should lead to increased tesosterone production. If there is no increase, then the testes may be defective.

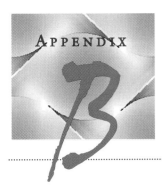

Answers to Case Studies

CASE STUDY 1 (refer to Chapter 10 for further information)

1. Definitions:
   myalgia: muscular pain
   meningitis: inflammation of the meninges
   lumbar: the part of the back between the thorax and the pelvis
   bacteremia: presence of bacteria in the bloodstream
   lethargy: drowsiness

2. Lumbar puncture is performed to obtain cerebrospinal fluid (CSF), a fluid that fills the ventricles and subarachnoid space that surround the brain. Based on the clinical symptoms presented by the patient, the physician requests laboratory testing of the CSF, which will provide indicators of infectious disease processes or any other anomalies. The CSF is collected in three to four different sterile tubes, which are taken to several different areas in the laboratory depending on the tests to be performed.

3. Blood and CSF cultures are performed in microbiology, glucose and protein levels are determined in the clinical chemistry area, and cell count is done in hematology.

4. Whenever the CSF glucose level is determined, a blood glucose level must also be determined. Under normal conditions, the CSF glucose level is about 65 to 70% of the blood glucose level (70 to 110 mg/dl). The decreased CSF glucose level in this case is most likely due to increased utilization by the leukocytes and the infectious agents present in the fluid. The increased protein level may be attributed to the damage to the blood-CSF barrier, resulting in an increased membrane permeability, increased numbers of leukocytes, and increased synthesis of immunoglobulins.

CASE STUDY 2 (refer to Chapter 8 for further information)

1. Based on the anatomic location of the pain, the appendix could be affected.

2. The child is febrile because of the inflammatory and infectious process taking place.

3. The leukocyte count and the differential results are indicators of an infectious process; the leukocyte count becomes elevated during an infection, and the cell differential shows which particular cell line is increased. Increase in neutrophils is usually indicative of a bacterial infection, while an increase in lymphocytes may be indicative of a viral agent. Bands (immature neutrophils) are increased because of the increased demand on the bone marrow.

4. If the condition is not properly and immediately resolved, risks such as rupture of the appendix with subsequent perforation and peritonitis may occur.

CASE STUDY 3 (refer to Chapter 5 for further information)

The important clues are:

1. Recent emigration to the United States, possibly from a developing country, an enlarged head, a marked abdominal protuberance, bowing of the legs and muscular weakness.

2. Rickets, as a result of nutritional vitamin D deficiency.

3. Alkaline phosphatase is released from the bone possibly due to a defective bone mineralization.

4. The child may be suffering from the failure to absorb vitamin D rather than a dietary deficiency.

5. Because this developed before the age of 4 years, this can be treated and the present symptoms are not permanent.

CASE STUDY 4 (refer to Chapters 7 and 10 for further information)

1. Definitions:
   polydypsia: increased thirst
   polyuria: frequency of urination

2. Based on the chemistry results, diabetes mellitus is the likely diagnosis.

3. Diabetes mellitus is a disorder in glucose or carbohydrate, protein, and fat metabolism

that may be due to either decreased pancreatic insulin production or dysfunctional insulin production.

4. A fasting glucose test and a glucose tolerance test can be performed to confirm the diagnosis.

5. Renal nephropathy and peripheral neuropathy of the sensory and motor nerves in the lower extremities may develop if the diabetes is not treated.

6. Glucose appears in the urine when the renal threshold is exceeded because of the elevated glucose level in the plasma.

CASE STUDY 5 (refer to Chapters 8 and 9 for further information)

1. Definitions:
   hepatomegaly: enlargement of the liver
   pancreatitis: inflammation of the pancreas
   hematemesis: vomiting of blood
   hepatitis: inflammation of the liver

2. The physician suspected hepatitis because jaundice and hepatomegaly are present. Jaundice, the yellowish discoloration of the skin and whites of the eyes, is usually associated with hepatitis. Pancreatitis and food poisoning have similar presenting symptoms, such diarrhea, nausea, and vomiting.

3. Serum amylase and serum lipase levels would be used to rule out pancreatitis. Serum amylase shows an elevation in acute pancreatitis within hours of onset. Lipase also becomes elevated and remains increased for up to 14 days.

4. Bilirubin and liver enzyme (serum transaminases and alkaline phosphatase) levels may be elevated in hepatitis.

5. *Salmonella typhi*, the bacterial agent that causes typhoid fever, may also infect the gallbladder and biliary tree. Finding this organism in the stool may explain the symptoms that the patient has presented. Salmonellosis is an infectious process that stimulates the increased production of leukocytes or neutrophils (versus intoxication, where there are no leukocytes present).

CASE STUDY 6 (refer to Chapter 7 for further information)

1. Definitions:
   dysuria: painful urination
   polyuria: increased urinary output or urination

2. Fever, dysuria, and low back pain are common symptoms of urinary tract infection (UTI).

3. Cystitis is an infection of the urinary bladder.

4. Positive nitrite and leukocyte esterase tests are used to screen for possible UTI. Positive *nitrite* indicates the presence of bacterial species that can reduce nitrate to nitrite. The nitrite is detected by the reagent in the strip. A negative result, however, does not always indicate the absence of UTI. Results must be correlated with the microscopic exam results, which show increased numbers of leukocytes, casts, and bacteria. *Leukocyte esterase* is present in certain types of leukocytes, which are increased in UTI.

5. The leukocyte count is elevated as an immune response to infection. Neutrophils, or polymorphonuclear leukocytes, will be increased.

CASE STUDY 7 (refer to Chapter 8 for further information)

1. *Entamoeba histolytica* is acquired by ingesting contaminated water or food.

2. Amebic dysentery, which may lead to the production of amebic ulcers and extraintestinal infection in the liver, may be a complication of *E. histolytica* infection.

3. *Salmonella, Shigella,* and *Escherichia coli* are among several bacterial pathogens that may cause diarrheal illness. *Giardia lamblia* and *Cryptosporidium* are other intestinal parasites that cause gastrointestinal diseases.

CASE STUDY 8 (refer to Chapter 6 for further information)

1. Definitions:
   dyspnea: shortness of breath or difficulty in breathing
   hypertension: high blood pressure
   myocardial infarction: heart attack
   angina: tightness or heaviness of the chest
   atherosclerosis: hardening of the arteries because of plaques or calcification

2. Systolic pressure measures the contraction phase of the heart and is the higher reading, while diastolic pressure is the pressure when the blood enters the relaxed chamber.

3. Cardiac enzymes used to detect the presence of a suspected AMI include creatine kinase (CK), lactate dehydrogenase (LDH), and aspartate transaminase (AST). Isoenzymes of CK and LDH are used as specific indicators of cardiac injury.

4. Elevated cholesterol levels for a long period of time lead to the deposition of lipid materials or plaques along the walls of blood vessels. The presence of plaques creates re-

stricted blood flow through the affected areas, which leads to the formation of thrombus or clots, further narrowing of the blood vessel, and eventually deprivation of blood flow to the heart, resulting in a heart attack, or myocardial infarct.

CASE STUDY 9 (refer to Chapter 6 for further information)

1. Definitions:
   hypoxia: insufficient oxygen available to the tissues
   pneumonia: inflammation of the lungs
   cyanosis: bluish discoloration of the skin and mucous membranes due to hypoxia

2. *Streptococcus pneumoniae* and *Haemophilus influenzae* are two common bacterial agents that cause pneumonia

3. An elevated leukocyte count with an increased number of neutrophils indicates the presence of bacterial infection.

4. Sputum is used to recover and then identify the bacterial agent that causes the pneumonia.

CASE STUDY 10 (refer to Chapters 5 and 6 for further information)

1. The most likely diagnosis is lower urinary tract infection (UTI) because of positive nitrite and leukocyte esterase, bacteria, and leukocytes present on microscopic examination of the urine, as well as painful urination and urinary urgency.

2. Erythrocytes, leukocytes, nitrite, leukocyte esterase, protein, and epithelial cells all may cause a cloudy appearance of the urine.

3. *Escherichia coli* is the most common organism identified in urine cultures. Infections are acquired when bacteria ascend from the urethra to the bladder.

4. If leukocyte casts were also present, this patient might have acute pyelonephritis.

CASE STUDY 11 (refer to Chapter 7 for further information)

1. Definitions:
   hypoproteinemia: decreased protein level in the blood
   hyperlipidemia: increased lipid (cholesterol and triglycerides) levels in the blood
   edema: swelling

2. Casts are formed in the distal convoluted tubule when conditions favor cast formation.

These conditions include an acidic pH environment, the presence of a special protein called Tamm-Horsfall, a high salt concentration, and a reduced urine flow.

3. Fatty and waxy casts are found in nephrotic syndrome and toxic renal poisoning. Fatty casts incorporate large fat molecules that have leaked through the damaged glomerulus.

4. The most likely diagnosis is nephrotic syndrome, caused by lesions that develop in the glomerular membrane. It may be indicated by hyperlipidemia, proteinuria, edema, and hypoproteinemia.

CASE STUDY 12 (refer to Chapter 12 for further information)

1. The medical term that describes an elevated serum cortisol level is hypercortisolism (*hyper-* = increased or elevated).

2. The presumptive diagnosis would be Cushing's syndrome. The laboratory findings are suggestive of an adrenal adenoma being the cause of the elevated cortisol production.

3. The dexamethasone suppression test would help confirm the diagnosis of Cushing's syndrome and its cause.

CASE STUDY 13 (refer to Chapter 9 for further information)

1. Definitions:
   icteric: jaundiced
   hepatitis: inflammation of the liver
   anorexia: loss of appetite
   malaise: feeling of not being well

2. The physician probably suspects hepatitis virus A, which is the most common enterically transmitted hepatitis virus in the United States. However, he may also suspect hepatitis virus E, which is endemic in developing countries such as Mexico and also can be transmitted via the fecal-oral route. Both viruses are acquired by drinking contaminated water and eating contaminated food.

3. In hepatitis, liver enzymes such as AST, ALT and bilirubin will be expected to be elevated.

4. Hepatitis profile results would show the following: anti-HAV/IgM—positive; anti-HCV, anti-HBc/IgM, and HBsAg negative.

CASE STUDY 14 (refer to Chapter 13 for further information)

1. The physician would request a hypothalamic function test, a testicular function test, and pituitary function studies because the problem may lie at any of the three levels governing male fertility: hypothalamus, pituitary, or testes.

2. A reduced testosterone level would be expected in this patient. If it is a testicular problem, an hCG test will not produce an increased testosterone level.

CASE STUDY 15 (refer to Chapter 11 for further information)

1. The medical term that describes an elevated leukocyte count is leukocytosis (*-osis* = increase).

2. An elevated leukocyte count is observed in bacterial infections, viral infections, inflammation, stress, vigorous exercise, and other conditions (see Table 11–3).

3. The presumptive diagnosis is infectious mononucleosis, a viral infection. The presence of lymphadenopathy, a mildly elevated leukocyte count, and reactive lymphocytes is highly suggestive of infectious mononucleosis.

4. A monospot test could be used to confirm a diagnosis of infectious mononucleosis. The monospot test would detect the presence of infectious mononucleosis heterophil antibodies.

CASE STUDY 16 (refer to Chapter 11 for further information)

1. The medical term that describes a decreased erythrocyte count is erythrocytopenia (*-penia* = reduction in number).

2. Anemia is characterized by a decreased erythrocyte count, hemoglobin, and hematocrit.

3. The presumptive diagnosis is iron-deficiency anemia. In iron-deficiency anemia, the erythrocytes appear hypochromic and microcytic. The patient would also present with a decreased erythrocyte count, hemoglobin, and hematocrit. The patient's iron-deficiency anemia is most likely the result of increased requirements associated with pregnancy.

4. The patient's serum iron level would be decreased. In iron-deficiency anemia, there is insufficient iron for hemoglobin production.

CASE STUDY 17 (refer to Chapter 12 for further information)

1. The medical term that describes elevated T_3 and T_4 levels is hyperthyroidism (*hyper-* = increased or elevated).

2. The presumptive diagnosis is Graves' disease. Graves' disease is a common form of hyperthyroidism and is characterized by elevated levels of T_3 and T_4 and a decreased TSH (thyroid-stimulating hormone).

3. The follicular epithelial cells are responsible for the synthesis of T_3 and T_4.

4. The amino acid tyrosine is the precursor substance for T_3 and T_4.

Index

Note: Page numbers in *italics* refer to illustrations; page numbers followed by *t* refer to tables.

Abdomen, quadrants of, 20, *23*
Abdominal cavity, 20, *22*
Abdominal pain, differential diagnosis of, case study of, 294
Abdominopelvic region(s), 20–21, *23*
Absorbance, of solutions, 63–65, *64*
Absorption, of nutrients, 153
Accessory digestive organ(s), 156–157
Achlorhydria, 159
Acid(s), properties of, 61
Acid-base balance, respiration and, 104–105
Acid-base relationship, 62
Acidic solution(s), 61
Acidosis, metabolic, 105
    respiratory, 104
Acromegaly, 257
ACTH (adrenocorticotropic hormone), and Cushing's syndrome, 261, 261t
    stimulation test for, 264
Activated partial thromboplastin time (APTT), 232
Acute lymphoblastic leukemia, 226
Acute myeloblastic leukemia, 226
Acute poststreptococcal glomerulonephritis, 124–125
Acute-phase reactant(s), 173
Addison's disease, 260–261
ADH (antidiuretic hormone), action of, 121, *122*
    and diabetes insipidus, 258
Adrenal gland, anatomy of, 254, *254*
    disorders of, 260–262, 261t
    hormones secreted by, 248t, 254–255
Adrenocorticotropic hormone (ACTH), and Cushing's syndrome, 261, 261t
    stimulation test for, 264
AFP (alpha-fetoprotein), 181
Albumin, production of, 172
Alcoholic liver disease, 178
Aldosterone, 248t, 255

Alimentary tract. See *Digestive system.*
Alkaline phosphatase, in bone, 79
    in liver disease, 181
Alkaline solution(s), 61
Alkalosis, metabolic, 105
    respiratory, 104
Allergic rhinitis, 106
Alpha$_1$-antitrypsin, deficiency of, 181
Alpha-fetoprotein (AFP), 181
Alveoli, anatomy of, *102*
American Medical Technologist (AMT), 15
American Society for Clinical Laboratory Science (ASCLS), 14–15
American Society of Clinical Pathologists (ASCP), 15
    Board of Registry of, 4–5, 13
Amine(s), aromatic. See *Aromatic amine(s).*
Aminoaciduria, 180
Aminotransferase, 180
Ammonia, in liver disease, 181
Ampulla of Vater, 170
AMT (American Medical Technologist), 15
Amylase, in pancreatitis, 162
Androgen(s), 278
Anemia, case study of, 302–303
    from cirrhosis, 178
    iron-deficiency, 223
    pernicious, 158
    sickle cell, 223–224
Aneurysm(s), 106
ANF (atrial natriuretic factor), 249t, 256
Angina pectoris, 105
Anisotropic band(s), 83
Anorchia, 279–280
Antibiotic susceptibility study(ies), 39–40
Antidiuretic hormone (ADH), 247t, 252
    action of, 121, *122*
    and diabetes insipidus, 258
Aorta, *92*, 93

Appendicitis, 159
    case study of, 294
Appendicular skeleton, 77
APTT (activated partial thromboplastin time),
    232
Arachnoid mater, 194, *195*
Aromatic amine(s), biosynthesis of, 238, *239*
    degradation of, 239
    secretion of, 239
Arteriolar nephrosclerosis, 126
Arteriole(s), *97*, 98
Artery(ies), *97*, 98
    cardiac, *92*, 93
ASCLS (American Society for Clinical Labora-
    tory Science), 14–15
Ascorbic acid, in urine, 132t, 134
ASCP (American Society of Clinical Patholo-
    gists), 15
    Board of Registry of, 4–5, 13
Asthma, 107
Astrocyte(s), 189
Atherosclerosis, 105
Atrial natriuretic factor (ANF), 249t, 256
Atrium (atria), 92–93, *93*
Autoanalyzer(s), for clinical chemistries, 41
Autoantibody(ies), in liver disease, 182
Axial skeleton, 75–76, *75–76*
Axon(s), 188

Bacterial endocarditis, 106
Bacterial flora, normal, 39
Bacteriuria, 136
Base(s), properties of, 61
Basophil(s), properties of, 215t, 217
Becker muscular dystrophy, 85
Beer's law, 63–65
Bile, 156
    production of, 167, 171–172
Biliary cirrhosis, 178
Bilirubin, in urine, 132t, 133, 134t–135t, 181
    metabolism of, 171, *172*
    tests for, 180
Bioassay(s), 263
Biologic safety cabinet(s), 40, *40*
Biopsy, bone marrow, 231
    renal, 139
Bladder, 113, *114*
Blast cell(s), in leukemia, 226
Bleeding, gastrointestinal, 158, 160
    subarachnoid, 199
Bleeding time, 231–232
Blood, See also *Hematopoietic system.*
    circulation of, through heart, 95
    compatibility testing of, 43–44
    composition of, 36, 99, 210, *211*

Blood (*Continued*)
    functions of, 210–212, *212–213*
    in stool, 160–161
    in urine, 132t, 133
    oxygenation of, 94
    pH of, maintenance of, 62
Blood cell(s), terminology for, 30
Blood chemistry, 37t, 108
Blood component(s), 44
Blood donor(s), processing of, 43
Blood gas(es), 62, 108
Blood pressure, 98–99
Blood smear, 230, 231t
Blood urea nitrogen (BUN), 138
Blood vessel(s), 96–99, *97*
    terminology for, 30
Blood-brain barrier, 196
Board of Registry, of American Society of Clini-
    cal Pathologists, 4–5, 13
Body cavities, 20, *22–23*
Body direction, terminology for, 20–24, *21–24*
Body fluids, clinical chemistries of, 41–42, 42t
Body planes, 20, *21*
Bone, anatomy of, 77, *78*
    cellular elements of, 79–80
    diseases of, 81–82
    physiology of, 74, 79
    tumors of, 82
Bone marrow, 212–216, *214*, 215t, *216*
    analysis of, 231
    biopsy of, 231
    stem cells in, 214–215, *216*
    types of, 212–213, *214*
Brain, anatomy of, 190–193, *191–193*
    terminology for, 33
Brain stem, anatomy of, 190, *191*
Brain tumor(s), tests for, 198t, 199
Breathing, physiology of, 103
Broad casts, 137
Bronchitis, 108
BUN (blood urea nitrogen), 138

Calcium, blood levels of, 80, *80*
Calculi, in bile duct or gallbladder, 179
    renal, 126–127
cAMP (cyclic adenosine monophosphate), ac-
    tion of, 242, *243*
Cancellous bone, 77, *78*
Candidiasis, oral, 157–158
Capillary(ies), *97*, 98
Carbohydrate(s), digestion of, 153
Carbon dioxide, and exchange of oxygen, *102*
    partial pressure of, 103
Cardiac cycle, 95–96, *96–97*
Cardiac enzyme(s), 108

Cardiac muscle, 82, 84
Cardiovascular disorder(s), tests for, 108–109
Cardiovascular system, anatomy of, 90–99,
    91–97
    disorders of, 105–108. See also specific disor-
        der, e.g., *Hypertension.*
        infectious, 106
        noninfectious, 105–106
    physiology of, 94–96, *95–97,* 98–99
        electrical events in, 95–96, *96–97*
        mechanical events in, 94, *95*
    terminology for, 30
Caries, dental, 158
Casts, in urine, 136
Categorical practitioner(s), 8
Cavity(ies), body, 20, *22–23*
CBC (complete blood count), 38–39
    with differential, 108
Cecum, anatomy of, 154
Cell count, Coulter principle in, *229*
    of cerebrospinal fluid, 201
Celsius temperature scale, 52
Cementum, 149, *149*
Central nervous system (CNS), anatomy of,
        188–190, *189*
    bleeding within, 199
    control of reproduction by, 271, 274, *275*
    diseases of, 196–199, 197t-198t. See also
        specific disease, e.g., *Meningitis.*
        diagnostic trends in, 199
    integrative function of, 188
Central tendency, measures of, 65–66
Cerebellum, anatomy of, *191,* 192
Cerebrospinal fluid (CSF), 195–196
    appearance of, 201
    cell count of, 201
    chemical analysis of, 202–203
    collection of, 200
    culture of, 202
        case study of, 293–294
    glucose in, 203
        case study of, 293–294
    gram stain of, 202
    leukocyte differential of, 202
    serologic examination of, 203
Cerebrovascular accident, 105–106
Cerebrum, anatomy of, *191,* 192–193, *193*
Certification examination(s), 13–14, 13t
Ceruloplasmin, 181
Cervical vertebra(e), 21, *24*
Chemistry(ies), blood, 37t, 108
    cerebrospinal fluid, 202–203
    clinical, 41–42, 42t
Chemistry laboratory(ies), in hospitals, 10
Chemoreceptor(s), and control of respiration,
    104

Cholecystitis, 159, 179
Cholelithiasis, 179
Cholestasis, 179
Cholecystokinin, 249t, 256
Cholinesterase, 189
Chronic lymphocytic leukemia, 227
Chronic myelogenous leukemia, 226
Chyme, 154
Circulatory shock, 106
Circulatory system. See also *Cardiovascular
        system; Heart.*
    anatomy of, 90–99, *91–97*
Cirrhosis, 178
CK (creatine kinase), 86
Clinical chemistry(ies), 41–42, 42t
Clinical laboratory science, history of, 4–5
Clinical laboratory scientist(s), 6–9
    certification examinations for, 13–14, 13t
    education of, history of, 4–6
    employment settings for, 10–12, 11t
    future opportunities for, 15–16
    professional organizations for, 14–15
    role of, 3, 6–7
    skills needed by, 12–13
CNS. See *Central nervous system (CNS).*
Coagulation cascade, 210–211, *213*
Coagulation factor(s), assays of, 232
    metabolism of, 173
Coagulation study(ies), 37t, 39
Coagulation test(s), 231–232
Coefficient of variation, 67
Colds, 107
Colitis, 159–160
Collagen, properties of, 79
Colon, 154, *155*
Common cold, 107
Common logarithm(s), 61–62
Compatibility testing, 43–44
Complete blood count (CBC), 38–39
    with differential, 108
Component therapy, 44
Computed tomography (CT), of urinary system,
        139
Concentration, expression of, 54–61
    as molarity, 54–56
    as normality, 56–58
    as osmolarity, 59–60
    as percent, 58–59
    as specific gravity, 60–61
Conduction system, cardiac, 95–96, *96–97*
Confidence limits, 66
Congestive heart failure, 106
Conjugated bilirubin, 133
Conn's syndrome, 261–262
Control chart, Levy-Jennings, 66, *67*

Convoluted tubules, anatomy of, 116
Corporate setting(s), for employment, 12
Corpus luteum, formation of, 285
Cortical bone, 77, *78*
Corticotropin-releasing hormone (CRH), 246t, 250
Cortisol, 248t, 255
Coulter principle, *229*
Cranial cavity, 20, *22*
Creatine kinase (CK), 86
Creatinine, serum, 137
Creatinine clearance, 138
Cretinism, 259, 259t
CRH (corticotropin-releasing hormone), 246t, 250
Crigler-Najjar syndrome, 175
Crohn's disease, 160
Cryptorchidism, 279
Crypts of Lieberkuhn, 153
CSF. See *Cerebrospinal fluid (CSF).*
Culture media, 39
Cushing's syndrome, 261, 261t
  case study of, 300
Cyclic adenosine monophosphate (cAMP), action of, 242, *243*
Cyst(s), hydatid, 183
Cystic fibrosis, 107
Cystitis, 125
Cystoscopy, 139
Cytogenetic technologist(s), role of, 9
Cytologic study(ies), of urinary system, 139
Cytometry, flow, 37t, 38
Cytotechnologist(s), role of, 7–8

Defecation, 154, 156
Density, specific gravity and, 60–61
Dental caries, 158
Dentin, 148–149, *149*
Dentition, 148–149, *149*
Dexamethasone suppression test, 264
Diabetes insipidus, 258
Diabetes mellitus, 262
  and renal function, 126
  case study of, 295
Diaphysis, of bone, 77, *78*
Diarrhea, 159
Diastole, 94
Diastolic pressure, 99
Diencephalon, 190, *191,* 192
Digestion, in large intestine, 154
  in mouth, 150
  in small intestine, 153
  in stomach, 151
  of carbohydrates, 153
  of lipids, 153
  of proteins, 153

Digestive system, anatomy of, 146–157, *147–155*
  disorders of, 157–160
  hormones secreted by, 249t, 256
  organs of, 147–156. See also specific organ, e.g., *Stomach.*
    accessory, 156–157
  terminology for, 31
  tests for, 160–162
Dilutions, serial, 53–54
  simple, 53
Dipstick test(s), 131–132, 132t
Direction, anatomic, terminology for, 20–24, *21–24*
Diverticulitis, 160
Dorsal cavity, of body, 20, *22*
Dorsal surface, of body, 20
Duchenne muscular dystrophy, 85
Duodenum, anatomy of, 153
Dura mater, 194, *195*
Dwarfism, 257–258
Dysentery, 159

Echinococcus granulosus, 183
Education, of clinical laboratory personnel, history of, 4–6
Electrical activity, in heart, 95–96, *96–97*
Electrocardiography, 96, *97*
Electrophoresis, 42
  protein, 180–181
Elimination, physiology of, 154, 156
ELISA (enzyme-linked immunosorbent assay), 264
Embryo, development of, 270–271, *272–273*
Emphysema, 107
Employment, settings for, 10–12, 11t
Enamel, 149, *149*
Encephalitis, 197–198, 198t
Endocarditis, bacterial, 106
Endocardium, 92
Endocrine gland(s), 243–256, *245–254,* 246t–249t. See also specific gland, e.g., *Adrenal gland.*
  disorders of, 257–263, 259t, 261t
  hormones secreted by, 238–242, *239–244.* See also *Hormone(s).*
Endometrium, 286, *287*
End-stage renal disease (ESRD), 127
Entamoeba histolytica infection, 183
  case study of, 296–297
Enzyme(s), cardiac, 108
  digestive, 153
  liver, assays for, 180–181
  pancreatic, 157
Enzyme-labeled immunoassay, 263–264

Enzyme-linked immunosorbent assay (ELISA), 264
Eosinophil(s), properties of, 217
Ependymal cell(s), 189
Epicardium, 91
Epididymis, 274, *276*
Epigastric region, of abdomen, 21, *23*
Epinephrine, 248t
   biosynthesis of, 238, *239*
   secretion of, 239
Epiphysis, of bone, 77, *78, 79*
Epithelial cell(s), in urine, 136
Equivalent weight, 56–58
Erythrocyte(s), in urine, 136
   properties of, 216
Erythrocyte casts, 137
Erythrocyte count, 228, *229,* 229t
Erythroid cell(s), in hematopoiesis, 215t
Erythropoietin, 249t, 256
Esophagus, anatomy of, 150
   disorders of, 157–158
ESRD (end-stage renal disease), 127
Estradiol, production of, 285
Estrogen, 248t, 255–256
   functions of, *275*
Extracellular matrix, 79

Factor VIII, and hemophilia, 227
Fahrenheit temperature scale, 52
Fasciola hepatica, 183
Fat, fecal, 162
Feedback loop, in hormone secretion, 242, *242*
Females, fertility in, tests for, 288–289
   reproductive system of, 281–288, *282–287.*
      See also *Reproductive system, female.*
Fertility tests, in females, 288–289
   in males, 280–281
Flow cytometry, 37t, 38
Fluid volume, regulation of, 121, *122*
Follicle(s), ovarian, development of, 283–285, *284*
Follicle-stimulating hormone (FSH), 285
   action of, 274, *275*
Follicular phase, of menstrual cycle, 286, *287*
Food, digestion of. See *Digestion.*
Food poisoning, from *Salmonella,* case study of, 295–296
4+1 educational program(s), 6
Frontal lobe, of brain, 192, *193*
Frontal plane, of body, 20, *21*
FSH (follicle-stimulating hormone), 285
   action of, 274, *275*
Fulminant hepatitis, 177

Gallbladder, anatomy of, 157, 170
   diseases of, 179
Gallbladder disease(s), 179
Gallstones, 179
Gamma-glutamyl transpeptidase, 180
Gas exchange, 103–104
Gastric analysis, 162
Gastrin, 249t, 256
   serum analysis of, 161–162
Gastritis, 158
Gastroesophageal sphincter, 150
Gastrointestinal system. See *Digestive system.*
Gender, determination of, 270–271, *272–273*
GFR (glomerular filtration rate), 119–120
GH-RH (growth hormone–releasing hormone), 246t, 250
Gigantism, 257
Glomerular filtration rate (GFR), 119–120
Glomeruli, 116
Glomerulonephritis, chronic, 125
   poststreptococcal, 124–125
Glucagon, 248t.254
Glucose, in cerebrospinal fluid, 203
   case study of, 293–294
   in urine, 132t, 133
   regulation of, 173
Glucose level(s), serum, 41
Glycogenesis, 173
GnRH. See *Gonadotropin-releasing hormone (GnRH).*
Gonadotropin-releasing hormone (GnRH), 246t, 251, 288–289
   action of, 274, *275*
Gonads. See also *Ovary(ies); Testes.*
   embryology of, 270–271, *272–273*
Gram equivalent weight, 56–58
Gram stain, of cerebrospinal fluid, 202
Granulosa cell(s), 283, *284*
Graves' disease, 258, 259t
   case study of, 303
Great vessel(s), 93–94
Growth factor(s), hematopoietic, 215t
Growth hormone, 247t, 251
Growth hormone–releasing hormone (GH-RH), 246t, 250

Hand, physiology of, 77
Hashimoto's thyroiditis, 258–259, 259t
hCG (human chorionic gonadotropin), 249t, 256
Heart, anatomy of, *91–93,* 91–94
   external, 91–92, *92–93*
   internal, 92–93, *93*

Heart (*Continued*)
  disorders of, 105–106
  electrical activity in, 95–96, *96–97*
  hormones and, 249t
  physiology of, 94–96, *95–97*
  terminology for, 30
Helicobacter pylori infection(s), 158
Hematemesis, 158
Hematocrit, 228
  reference values for, 229t
Hematology laboratory(ies), in hospitals, 10
Hematology test(s), 36–39, 37t, 228–231, *229,*
    229t-231t
  Coulter principle in, *229*
  reference values for, 229t
Hematopoietic system, 210–218, *211–216,*
    215t, 218t
  blood cells in, 216–218, 218t
  blood in, 210–212, *211–213.* See also *Blood.*
  bone marrow in, 212–216, *214,* 215t, *216.*
      See also *Bone marrow.*
  compartments of, 215–216, 215t, *216*
  disorders of, 223–227, 224t
    tests for, 227–232, *229,* 229t-231t
  growth factors in, 215t
Hematuria, 132t, 133
Hemoglobin, reference values for, 229t
  structure of, 210, *212*
  tests for, 228, 229t
Hemolytic disease of newborn, 175
Hemophilia, 227
Hemorrhage, gastrointestinal, 158, 160
  subarachnoid, 199
Hemostasis, 210–211
Henderson-Hasselbalch equation, 62
Hensen's zone(s), 83
Hepatitis, 160, 175–177, 176t
  case study of, 300–301
  tests for, 182–183, 182t
Hepatocarcinoma, 178–179
Histocompatibility testing, 44–45
Histotechnologist(s), role of, 7–8
HLAs (human leukocyte antigens), testing for,
    44–45
Homeostasis, definition of, 90
  endocrine system in, *238*
  skeletal, control of, 80, *80*
Hormone(s), 238–242, *239–244.* See also spe-
    cific hormone, e.g., *Follicle-stimulating
    hormone (FSH).*
  biosynthesis of, 238–239, *239–241*
  definition of, 238
  degradation of, 239, 241
  effects of, specific vs. global, 238
  mode of action of, 242, *243–244*

Hormone(s) (*Continued*)
  regulation of menstrual cycle by, 286, *287,*
    288
  secretion of, 239
    regulation of, 242, *242*
Hospital laboratory(ies), clinical disciplines in,
    9–10
hPL (human placental lactogen), 249t, 256
Human chorionic gonadotropin (hCG), 249t,
    256
Human leukocyte antigens (HLAs), testing for,
    44–45
Human placental lactogen (hPL), 249t, 256
Hyaline casts, 136–137
Hydatid cyst(s), 183
Hydrochloric acid, 151
Hyperaldosteronism, primary, 261–262
Hypercortisolism, 261, 261t
Hyperinsulinemia, 262–263
Hyperparathyroidism, 260
Hypertension, 105
  and arteriolar nephrosclerosis, 126
Hypochondriac region, of abdomen, 21, *23*
Hypocortisolism, 260
Hypogastric region, of abdomen, 21, *23*
Hypoparathyroidism, 260
Hypoproteinemia, 41
Hypothalamus, 190, 192, 244, 246t, 250
Hypothyroidism, 258–259, 259t

Immunity panel, for hepatitis, 183
Immunization, for hepatitis, 177
Immunoassay(s), 263–264
Immunoglobulin(s), functions of, 45
Immunohematology, 37t, 43–45
Immunology, 45–46
Incident light, 63
Infectious disease(s), cardiac, 106
  immunologic studies for, 45
  of central nervous system, 196–199, 197t-
    198t
  urinary, 125–126
Inferential statistics, 65–66
Infertility. See also *Fertility.*
  in males, case study of, 301
Influenza, 107
Inguinal region, of abdomen, 21, *23*
Inhibin, 248t, 255
Insulin, 254, 258t
Insulin-dependent diabetes mellitus, 262
Insulinoma, 262–263
Integrated educational program(s), 6
Intensity of transmitted light, 63
International Society for Clinical Laboratory
    Technology (ISCLT), 14

Interstitial fluid, 218–219
Intravenous pyelography (IVP), 138–139
Iron-deficiency anemia, 223
ISCLT (International Society for Clinical Laboratory Technology), 14
Isoenzyme(s), 86
Isotropic band(s), 83
IVP (intravenous pyelography), 138–139

Jaundice, 174–175
  neonatal, 175
Jejunum, 153

Kallman's syndrome, 280
Kelvin temperature scale, 52
Ketone(s), in urine, 132t, 133
Kidney(s). See also entries under *Renal.*
  anatomy of, 113, *113–115*, 115–116, 116t
  biopsy of, 139
  blood supply to, 117–118, *118–119*
  hormones secreted by, 249t
  radiographic studies of, 138–139
  terminology for, 32
Kidney stone(s), 126–127
Klinefelter's syndrome, 82
Kupffer cell(s), 167

Laboratory(ies), hospital, clinical disciplines in, 9–10
  professionals in, 6–9
  public health, 12
  reference, 11
  tests performed in, 37t
Laboratory personnel. See *Clinical laboratory scientist(s).*
Lactase, in cerebrospinal fluid, 203
Lactate dehydrogenase (LD), 86
Lambert-Beer's law, 228
Large intestine, 154–156, *155*
Laryngitis, 107–108
Larynx, anatomy of, 100, *101*
LD (lactate dehydrogenase), 86
Leukemia, 225–227
Leukocyte(s), function of, 211
  in urine, 136
  properties of, 217–218, 218t
  types of, 37
Leukocyte count, 228–230, 229t
  case study of, 301–302
Leukocyte differential, 202, 230, 231t
Leukocyte esterase, 134
Leukocytosis, 224–225, 224t
Levy-Jennings control chart, 66, *67*

LH (luteinizing hormone), action of, 274, *275*
  production of, 286
Light, measurement of, 63–64
Lipase, in pancreatic disease, 162
Lipid(s), digestion of, 153
  synthesis of, 174
Lipid profile(s), 108
Liver, anatomy of, 156–157, 166–170, *167–170*
  blood supply to, 167, *170*
  lobes of, 166, *169*
  physiology of, 171–174, *172*
    bile production and, 171–172
    bilirubin metabolism and, 171, *172*
    coagulation factor metabolism and, 173
    glucose regulation and, 173
    lipid synthesis and, 174
    protein metabolism and, 172
    vitamin storage and, 173
  terminology for, 31–32
Liver disease, 174–179, 176t
  parasitic, 183
  tests for, 179–183, 182t
Liver enzyme(s), assays for, 180–181
Liver function test(s), 179–181
Logarithm(s), types of, 61–62
Long bone(s), anatomy of, 77, *78*
Loop of Henle, anatomy of, 116
  tubular reabsorption in, 120
Lumbar puncture, 200
  case study of, 293–294
  traumatic, 199
Lumbar region, of abdomen, 21, *23*
Lumbar spine, anatomy of, 21, *24*
Lung(s). See also entries under *Pulmonary; Respiratory.*
  anatomy of, *102*, 103
  gas exchange in, 103–104
Luteinizing hormone (LH), action of, 274, *275*
  production of, 286
Lymph, properties of, 218–219, *220*
Lymph node(s), 219–221, *220*
Lymphatic system, 218–222, *219–222*
  lymph in, 218–219, *220*
  lymph nodes in, 219–221, *220*
  spleen in, 221–222, *222*
  thymus in, 221
Lymphoblastic leukemia, 226
Lymphocyte(s), function of, 211
  properties of, 217–218
Lymphocytic leukemia, 227
Lymphocytosis, 225
Lymphokine(s), activity of, 218t

Males, fertility in, case study of, 301
  tests for, 280–281
Mean, in statistics, 65–66

Measurement system(s), 50–52, 51t
Media, for cultures, 39
Median, in statistics, 65–66
Medical terminology, components of, 24–29, 25t, 28t-29t
  prefixes as, 25–26, 28t
  root terms as, 24, 25t
  suffixes as, 25–26, 29t
  construction of, 27, 30–33
  for body direction, 20–24, *21–24*
Medulla oblongata, 190
Megakaryocyte(s), in hematopoiesis, 215t
Melanocyte-stimulating hormone releasing factor (MSH-RF), 246t, 250
Melatonin, production of, 243–244
Menarche, 284
Meninges, 194, *195*
Meningitis, 197, 198t
  tests for, case study of, 293–294
Menstrual cycle, hormonal regulation of, 286, *287, 288*
mEq (milliequivalent), 56
Messenger RNA (mRNA), mechanism of action of, 242
Metabolic acidosis, 105
Metabolic alkalosis, 105
Metaphysis, of bone, 77, *78*
Metric system, 50, 51t
MI (myocardial infarction), case study of, 297
Microbial culture(s), 109
Microbiology, 37t, 39–41, *40*
Microbiology laboratory(ies), in hospitals, 10
Microglia, 190
Millequivalent (mEq), 56
Milliosmole (mOsm), 60
Mode, in statistics, 65–66
Molarity (M), of solution, 54–56
Monocyte(s), function of, 211
  properties of, 215t, 217
Mononucleosis, 225
mOsm (milliosmole), 60
Mouth, anatomy of, 147–150, *148–149*
  digestion in, 150
  disorders of, 157–158
MSH-RF (melanocyte-stimulating hormone releasing factor), 246t, 250
Müllerian ducts, 271, *272*
Multiple myeloma, 82
Multiple sclerosis, 198–199
Muscle(s), anatomy of, 82–85
  microscopic, 82–84, *83*
  cardiac, 82, 84
  contraction of, 84–85
  skeletal, 82, 84
   disorders of, 85

Muscle(s) (*Continued*)
  smooth, 82, 84
Muscular dystrophy, 85
Musculoskeletal system, anatomy of, 73–74
  disorders of, tests for, 85–86
  terminology for, 32
Mycobacteriology, 40
Mycology, 40, *40*
Myelitis, 198
Myeloblastic leukemia, 226
Myelogenous leukemia, 226
Myeloma, multiple, 82
Myocardial infarction (MI), case study of, 297
Myocardium, 91
Myofibril(s), 82, *83*
Myopathy, 85

National Certification Agency (NCA), for Medical Laboratory Personnel, 14
Natural logarithm(s), 61–62
NCA (National Certification Agency) for Medical Laboratory Personnel, 14
Neonatal jaundice, 175
Nephron, anatomy of, *115*, 115–116, 116t, *117*
  blood supply to, 117–118, *118–119*
  physiology of, 122, *123*
Nephrosclerosis, arteriolar, 126
Nephrotic syndrome, 125
Nervous system, control of respiration by, 104
  terminology for, 33
Neuron(s), structure of, 188, *189*
Neurosyphilis, 197, 198t
Neurotransmitter(s), 189
Neutrophil(s), in hematopoiesis, 215t, 217
Neutrophilia, 225
NMR (nuclear magnetic resonance), proton, for urinalysis, 140
Non–insulin-dependent diabetes mellitus, 262
Norepinephrine, 248t
  biosynthesis of, 238, *239*
  secretion of, 239
Normality, of solution, 56–58
Nose, anatomy of, 100, *101*
Nuclear magnetic resonance (NMR), proton, for urinalysis, 140
Nuclear medicine imaging, of urinary system, 139
Nutrient(s), absorption of, 153

Occipital lobe, 193, *193*
Oligodendrocyte(s), 189
Opisthorchis sinensis, 183
Oral cavity. See *Mouth.*
Orchitis, 280

Osmolarity, 59–60
Osmotic diarrhea, 159
Osteoblast(s), 79
Osteoclast(s), 80
Osteocyte(s), 79–80
Osteomalacia, 81
Osteoporosis, 81–82
Ovarian function test(s), 288–289
Ovary(ies), anatomy of, *282, 283*–285, *284*
    disorders of, 285
    hormones secreted by, 248t, 255–256
Oviduct(s), anatomy of, *282, 283*
Ovulation, 284–285
    disorders of, 288–289
Oxygen, and exchange of carbon dioxide, *102*
    partial pressure of, 103
    transport of, 210, *212*
Oxygenation, of blood, 94
Oxytocin, 247t, 252

P wave, 96, *97*
Packed cell volume, 210
Pancreas, anatomy of, 157, *245,* 253–254
    disorders of, 262–263
        tests for, 162
    hormones secreted by, 248t, 253–254
Pancreatitis, 160
Parasite(s), and liver disease, 183
    in stool, 161
Parasitology, 41
Parathyroid gland, disorders of, 260
    hormones secreted by, 247t, 253
Parathyroid hormone (PTH), and calcium, 80,
        80
Parietal lobe, 192, *193*
Parotitis, 158
Partial pressure, of respiratory gases, 103
Pectoral girdle, anatomy of, 77
Pelvic girdle, anatomy of, 77
Pepsinogen, 151
Percent concentration, of solutions, 58–59
Percent purity, of solvents, 60
Peripheral blood smear, 230, 231t
Peritonitis, 159
Peritubular capillary(ies), 118, *118*
Pernicious anemia, 158
pH, and acid-base balance, 104
    measurement of, 61
    of blood, maintenance of, 62
    of urine, 132, 132t
Pharynx, 100, *101*
Pheochromocytoma, 262
Phlebitis, 106
Phlebotomist, role of, 7
Photometry, 63–64

Pineal gland, 243–244, *245,* 246t
Pituitary gland, anatomy of, *250,* 250–251
    disorders of, 257–258
    hormones secreted by, 246t-247t, 251–252
Pituitary-hypothalamic-gonadal axis, 271, 274
Placenta, hormones secreted by, 249t, 256
Plane(s), of body, 20, *21*
Plasma, composition of, 99
Platelet(s), functions of, 218
Platelet count, 229t-230t, 230
Pneumonia, 108
    case study of, 298
Pneumothorax, 107
Poisoning, food, from *Salmonella*, case study of,
        295–296
Pons, 190
Postcoital test, 281
Posthepatic jaundice, 174
Postrenal acute renal failure, 127
Poststreptococcal glomerulonephritis, acute,
        124–125
Prefix(es), for units of measure, 51t
    in medical terminology, 25–26, 28t
Prehepatic jaundice, 174
Prenatal test(s), 44
Prerenal acute renal failure, 127
Professional organization(s), 14–15
Progenitor cell(s), 215
Progesterone, 248t, 256
    functions of, *275*
Progesterone withdrawal test, 288–289
Prolactin, 251
Protein(s), digestion of, 153
    functions of, 41, 42t
    in cerebrospinal fluid, 202
    in urine, 132t, 133
    metabolism of, 172
Protein electrophoresis, 180–181
Protein hormone(s), biosynthesis of, 238, *241*
Prothrombin time, 232
    in liver disease, 181–182
Proton nuclear magnetic resonance urinalysis,
        140
PTH (parathyroid hormone), and calcium, 80,
        80
Public health laboratory(ies), 12
Pulmonary. See also entries under *Lung(s)*.
Pulmonary circuit, 94
Pulmonary vein(s), 93–94
Pulse, 98
Pyelography, intravenous, 138–139
Pyelonephritis, 125–126
Pyorrhea, 158

QRS complex, 96, *97*
Quadrant(s), abdominal, 20, *23*

Radioimmunoassay(s), 263

Radionuclear imaging, of urinary system, 139

Range, in statistics, 65–66

Rapid transit pathway, 221

Rectum, anatomy of, 154

Red blood cell(s). See *Erythrocyte(s)*.

Reference laboratory(ies), 11

Renal. See also entries under *Kidney(s)*.

Renal arteriole(s), 117–118, *118*

Renal calculi, 126–127

Renal disease, 123–127, 124t

  case study of, 299–300

  diabetes mellitus and, 126

Renal failure, 127

Renal function tests, 127–138, 128t-135t. See
    also *Urinalysis*.

Renal plasma threshold, 120

Renal system, terminology for, 32

Renin, 249t, 256

Renin-angiotensin-aldosterone system,
    120–121, *121*

Reproductive system, central nervous system
    control of, 271, 274, *275*

  female, 281–288, *282–287*

    anatomy of, 281, *282*

    disorders of, ovarian, 285

    hormones regulating, *275*

      ovaries in, *282*, 283–285, *284*

      uterus in, *282*, 285–286

  male, 274–280, *276–277*, 279t

    disorders of, 279–280

    hormones regulating, *276*

    spermatogenesis in, 274, *277*, 278

  terminology for, 33

Respiration, and acid-base balance, 104–105

  control of, 104

  physiology of, 103

Respiratory acidosis, 104

Respiratory alkalosis, 104

Respiratory system, anatomy of, 100–103, *101–102*

  lower, *102*, 103

  upper, 100, *101*

  disorders of, 106–108

  physiology of, 103–105

  terminology for, 31

Reticular formation, 190

Rheumatic heart disease, 106

Rhinitis, allergic, 106

Rib(s), anatomy of, 77

Rickets, 81

  case study of, 294–295

Root term(s), 24, 25t

Sacral spine, 21, *24*

Safety cabinet(s), 40, *40*

Sagittal plane, of body, 20, *21*

Salivary glands, 150

Salmonella food poisoning, case study of,
    295–296

Sarcomere(s), 83–84

Scrotum, varicocele in, 280

Secretin, 249t, 256

Secretory diarrhea, 159

Secretory phase, of menstrual cycle, 286, *287*,
    288

Segmented neutrophil(s), 217

Semen, analysis of, 281

  composition of, 278, 279t

Serial dilutions, 53

Serology laboratory(ies), in hospitals, 10

Serum, dilution of, 53–54

  gastrin in, 161–162

  glucose levels in, 41

  osmolarity of, 60

  proteins in, 41

Serum amylase, in pancreatitis, 162

Serum creatinine, 137

Serum lipase, in pancreatic disease, 162

Sexual differentiation, 270–271, *272–273*

Shock, circulatory, 106

SI (Systeme Internationale) units, conversion
    from standard lab units to, 51–52

Sickle cell anemia, 223–224

Sinoatrial (SA) node, electrical activity in,
    95–96, *96*

Skeletal muscle, anatomy of, 82–84, *83*

  disorders of, 85

Skeletal system, anatomy of, 74–82, *75–80*

  appendicular, 77

  axial, 75–76, *75–76*

  homeostasis in, control of, 80, *80*

  visceral, 77

Skull, anatomy of, *76*

Slow transit pathway, of splenic blood, 222

Small intestine, 151–154, *152*

Smooth muscle, 82, 84

Solutes, 53

Solutions, 53–54

  absorbance of, 63–65, *64*

  acidic, 61

  alkaline, 61

  molarity of, 54–56

  normality of, 56–58

Solvents, 53

Somatostatin, 254

Specialist(s), 9

Specific gravity, 60–61

  of urine, 131

Sperm, motility of, 281

Spermatogenesis, 274, *277*, 278

Sphincter of Oddi, 156, 170
Spinal column, 21, *24*
    vertebrae in, 75–76, *75–76*
Spinal cord, 194
Spinal tap, 200
  traumatic, 199
Spleen, 221–222, *222*
SRτ gene signal, 271
Standard curve(s), for absorbance of solutions, *64,* 64–65
Standard deviation, 66–67, *67*
  formula for, 66
Statistics, 65–67, *67*
Stem cell(s), in hematopoiesis, 214–215, *216*
Steroid(s), and spermatogenesis, 278
  biosynthesis of, 239, *241*
  degradation of, 241
  mechanism of action of, 242, *244*
  secretion of, 239, 255
Stimulation test(s), 264
Stock solutions, 53
Stomach, anatomy of, 150–151, *151*
  disorders of, 158–159
Stomatitis, 158
Stool, analysis of, 160–161
    case study of, 296–297
    fat in, 162
Striated muscle, 82, 84
Stroke, 105–106
Subarachnoid space, 194, *195*
  bleeding within, 199
Suffix(es), in medical terminology, 25–26, 29t
Suppression test(s), 264
Synapse(s), 189
Systeme Internationale (SI) units, conversion from standard lab units to, 51–52
Systemic circuit, 94
Systole, 94
Systolic pressure, 99

T wave, 96, *97*
Teeth, anatomy of, 148–149, *149*
  decay in, 158
Temperature, measurement systems for, 52
Temporal lobe, 193, *193*
Testes, anatomy of, *276*
  disorders of, 279–280
  hormones secreted by, 248t, 255
Testosterone, 278
Thalamus, 190
Thoracic cavity, 20, *22*
Thoracic spine, 21, *24*
3+1 educational program(s), 6
Thrush, 157–158

Thymus, 221
  hormones secreted by, 247t, 253
Thyroid gland, disorders of, 258–259, 259t
Thyroid hormone(s), 247t, 252–253
  biosynthesis of, 238, *240*
  degradation of, 241
  secretion of, 239
Thyroid-releasing hormone (TRH), 246t, 250
Thyroid-stimulating hormone (TSH), 246t, 251
Tongue, anatomy of, 148, *148*
Tonsillitis, 107
Trachea, anatomy of, *102,* 103
Transmittance, of light, 63
Transverse plane, of body, 20, *21*
Traumatic spinal tap, 199
TRH (thyroid-releasing hormone), 246t, 250
TSH (thyroid-stimulating hormone), 246t, 251
Tuberculosis, 108
Tubular reabsorption, of urine, 120–121, *121–122*
Tubular secretion, of urine, 122
Turner's syndrome, 285
2+2 educational program(s), 6

Ulcer(s), gastric, 158
Ultrasonography, 139
Urea nitrogen, 138
Urethra, 113, *114*
Urinalysis, 42–43, 128–137, 128t–135t
  automated, 137
  components of, 129–130, 129t
  history of, 128–129, 128t
  macroscopic, chemical tests in, 131–135, 132t, 134t-135t
    physical inspection in, 130–131, 130t
  microscopic, 135–137
  proton nuclear magnetic resonance in, 140
Urinary system, anatomy of, 113–118, *113–119,* 116t
    gross, 113, *113–114*
    microscopic, 116–117, 116t, *117*
  blood supply to, 117–118, *118–119*
  cytologic studies of, 139
  kidneys in, 113, *113–115,* 115–116, 116t
  physiology of, 119–123, *121–122,* 123t
  radiographic studies of, 138–139
  tests for, 127–138, 128t–135t. See also *Urinalysis.*
Urinary tract infection(s), 125–126
  case study of, 296, 298–299
Urine, ascorbic acid in, 132t, 134
  bacteria in, 136
  bilirubin in, 132t, 133, 134t-135t, 181
  blood in, 132t, 133

Urine (*Continued*)
  casts in, 136
  color of, 130–131, 130t
  composition of, 123
  crystals in, 136
  epithelial cells in, 136
  erythrocytes in, 136
  formation of, 119–123, *121–122,* 123t
    glomerular ultrafiltration in, 119–120
  glucose in, 132t, 133
  ketones in, 132t, 133
  leukocytes in, 136
  pH of, 132, 132t
  protein in, 132t, 133
  specific gravity of, 60–61, 131
    tubular reabsorption of, 120–121, *121–122*
    tubular secretion of, 122
  volume of, 131
Urobilinogen, 132t, 133–134, 134t-135t
  in liver disease, 181
Uterus, anatomy of, *282,* 285–286

Vaccination, for hepatitis, 177
Variance, of data, 66
Variation, coefficient of, 67
Varicocele(s), 280
Varicose vein(s), 106

Vasa recta, 118, *118*
Vasopressin. See *Antidiuretic hormone (ADH).*
Vein(s), *97,* 98
  varicose, 106
Ventral surface, of body, 20
Ventricle(s), of brain, 193
  of heart, 92–93, *93*
Venule(s), *97,* 98
Vertebra(e), 21, *24,* 75–76, *75–76*
Virology, 40
Visceral skeleton, 77
Vitamin(s), storage of, 173
Vitamin C, in urine, 132t, 134
Vitamin D, and rickets, 81

Weight, equivalent, 56–58
Weight per volume (w/v), 58
White blood cell(s) (WBCs). See *Leukocyte(s).*
White muscle fiber(s), 84
Wisdom teeth, 149. See also *Teeth.*
Wolffian ducts, 271, *272*
Working solution(s), 53
w/v (weight per volume), 58

Zollinger-Ellison syndrome, 161
Zwischenscheibe line, 83